Advanced First Aid for
First Responder on Scene

Contents

Chapter 6

Chapter 7

Chapter 12

Chapter 15

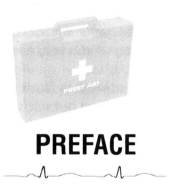

PREFACE

The level of pre-hospital emergency care that we have available to us at the end of the phone every day and night gives a great level of comfort to everyone in every community knowing that in the event of sickness or accident, help is only three numbers away. The three practitioner levels of pre-hospital care that we hear about and see only too often responding to various types of accidents, cardiac arrests, shootings, muggings, drug overdoses, and a 1,000 other incidents are the Emergency Medical Technicians, Paramedics, and Advanced Paramedics, each with their own level of expertise. These practitioners do most definitely save lives both because of their high standard of medical knowledge and the skills that go with it. However, we have three other levels of care that aren't as visible, but yet, they too make a difference and are the reason why, because of their interventions, many people are alive today. These are the occupational first aider (OFA), cardiac first responder (CFR), and emergency first responder (EFR). Any level of care, whether they can give vast varieties of drugs and carry out complicated procedures or just perform basic first aid, truly has its place when it comes to helping someone who has become ill or injured, and quite often, it's the first-aider or responder that is first on scene.

The aim of this book is to identify each of these non-practitioner levels of expertise and their particular skill set and present them in a way that is easily followed. It is worth remembering that the basics in pre-hospital care carry all the way from the basic first-aider right through to the advanced paramedic. Those of us you, will call for help and provide the basics until help arrives. If you can learn the basics and become skilful and efficient in those, you will be a great asset to your community. If I can just get that message across, then I have done my job well. If you can deal with life-threatening emergencies such as stopping a bleed, helping someone who is choking, recognising the signs of stroke and performing CPR effectively, and give comfort and a sympathetic ear to someone who needs it and know your limits, everything else is easy. That's what this book is all about.

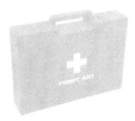

ACKNOWLEDGEMENTS

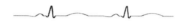

I thank the following most sincerely for all their assistance. Without their help, it would not have been possible to produce this manual or textbook.

The Pre-Hospital Emergency Care Council of Ireland (PHECC), for allowing me to use their Clinical Practice Guidelines (CPGs).

At their request, I must advise that while the guidelines provided for this book are current at the time of publication, you are advised to check the PHECC website occasionally on www.phecc.ie to view any updated versions. For more information, see chapter 15.

Medscape (http://emedicine.medscape.com/);

Thank you, Kathy, for allowing me access to your vast database on healthcare subjects as a reference source.

The following is a list of Universal Resource Locations (URLs) for the subjects adapted from Medscape:

http://emedicine.medscape.com/article/166320-treatment—Heatstroke Treatment and Management. http://emedicine.medscape.com/article/772753-overview—Drowning. http://emedicine.medscape.com/article/770296-overview—Emergency management of Frostbite. http://emedicine.medscape.com/article/287555-overview—Nicotine addiction.

The National Heart, Lung and Blood Institute; National Institutes of Health;

US Department of Health and Human Services (http://nhlbi.nih.gov):

Thank you so much for giving me permission to use your website as a source of reference and to reprint in whole or in part, any relevant materials.

The following is a list of Universal Resource Locations (URLs) for the subjects adapted from your website:

http://www.nhlbi.nih.gov/health/health-topics/topics/oxt/—Oxygen therapy (Part 2).

http://www.nhlbi.nih.gov/health/health-topics/topics/hlw/system.html—The Respiratory System.

http://www.nhlbi.nih.gov/health/health-topics/topics/stroke/types.html—Types of stroke.

http://www.nhlbi.nih.gov/health/health-topics/topics/arm/—Aneurysm.

http://www.nhlbi.nih.gov/health/health-topics/topics/copd/—C.O.P.D.

http://www.nhlbi.nih.gov/health/health-topics/topics/brnchi/—What is Bronchitis.

http://www.nhlbi.nih.gov/health/health-topics/topics/rf/causes.html—Respiratory failure.

http://www.nhlbi.nih.gov/health/health-topics/topics/vv/atrisk.html—Varicose veins.

Xlibris:

I thank Mary and Rachel who are part of the Xlibris publishing team for all their advice and encouragement over the past twelve months. Whenever I had questions, they were always there to guide me in the right direction.

Photo acknowledgements

I thank my two sons Paul and Ivan, for their assistance both as models and in the editing and production of the vast amount of illustration photographs used in this project. I also thank Kingdom Crash Repairs, Tralee (Ireland), for allowing me access to their premises and giving permission to take photographs required for this project.

All photographs and graphs used in this manual were produced by me and must not be used in any form without my permission.

Illustration acknowledgements

All Animated photographs and illustrations used in this project are by kind permission of The National Heart, Lung and Blood Institute; National Institutes of Health; US Department of Health and Human Services (http://nhlbi.nih.gov).

I also acknowledge a local graphic design company Collins/Shannon Design and Print, Tralee (Ireland), for their help in designing the graph on stages of childbirth.

Personal acknowledgement

Finally I would like to thank Fiona, John and Brigid who helped and encouraged me to become an instructor. Their friendship and expertise in their individual medical fields have influenced me greatly over the years and the inspiration for this book grew both out of this relationship and the personal satisfaction I get out of giving a course. It's always a bonus working with people who like me are passionate about their work. Also thanks to my wife Mary for her support and patience during this project.

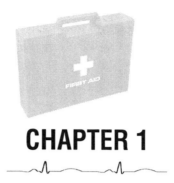

CHAPTER 1

1.1. Becoming an Advanced First-Aider

People do first-aid courses for many reasons. Some will do it as the first stepping stone to greater things. For example, you might be involved in sport or other community projects where accidents could, and often do, happen, and you feel you would be the right person and that you have what it takes to assist someone who is injured. You may also want to join voluntary organisations such as the Civil Defence, the Order of Malta, Red Cross, the Coast Guard, or get involved in a Community First Responder programme. You may have an interest in joining the ambulance service as a future career, and a first-aid course can give you a flavour of what it's all about though in a more simplistic and understandable manner.

People mainly take first-aid courses in order to be able to help a family member or a neighbour in their own community. On the other hand, they may be interested in becoming a first-aider in their place of work. While a paramedic and emergency medical technician (EMT) are at a much greater level than first-aiders or first responders, a good first-aider is a valuable asset in any community and is often the person who can make the difference when the emergency services are delayed or when you live in a place where the nearest ambulance is an hour away, which in not uncommon nowadays.

It's a great feeling to be able to help someone with the knowledge that you know exactly what you are doing. Not only will you learn how to help that person, you will also learn how to reassure them. You may not know it, but the confidence you show in stressful circumstances radiates to your patient and helps to reduce their stress level until the professionals arrive.

Anyone who has the ability to administer first aid regardless of their level holds a privileged position both in their local community and in their place of work. The level of trust that is placed on you is not like that of any other job. People who are sick or injured, be they old or young, or rich or poor, are being treated every day for various injuries by both voluntary and professional people in the emergency services, and more often than not, they are people you are meeting for the first time. The very fact that people will allow a responder, who may be a total stranger, to physically examine them or their children, regardless of age or gender, without question speaks volumes.

All this is about the mutual respect that has been built up over many years between the sick and injured and those who come to their aid, and it's up to everyone who takes up the challenge and follows in the footsteps of previous first-aiders, responders, and paramedics to ensure that this mutual trust and respect continues.

The first two lines of Rudyard Kipling's famous poem 'IF' describes in an odd way how you should carry out your duties as a first-aider.

If you can keep your head when all about you are losing theirs and blaming it on you, if you can trust yourself when all men doubt you, but make allowance for their doubting.

It summarises three essential points. In a stressful situation, you must be the person in control when everyone else is losing the plot. As a trained first-aider, you must put your trust in your training and decide what's best for your patient, even if others doubt you. You also have to make allowances for others with a lesser understanding and reassure them that you are a competent first-aider.

Primum non Nocere is a Latin phrase meaning 'first, do no harm'. It is one of the principal precepts of medical ethics that all medical students are taught in medical school and is a fundamental principle for emergency medical services (EMS) around the world. Regardless of the level of care you choose, whether it is basic or advanced, make this motto yours and reflect on it from time to time.

There are three questions that people get asked in every first aid class by their instructor. The instructor asks these questions in order to confirm that the learner has grasped the concept and has a reasonable understanding of what first aid is all about. When you sit a first-aid exam, apart from the practical section, you'll have to attend a written exam which is usually twenty short answer or multiple choice questions. These three questions will without a doubt be part of the exam, and the answers should enable you to have a full understanding of what you are about to take on as an advanced first-aider or responder.

Q. What is First Aid?

A. First aid is the provision of initial care for an illness or injury. It is usually performed by a non-expert person to a sick or injured person until definitive medical treatment can be given. It generally consists of a series of simple and in some cases, potentially life-saving techniques that an individual can be trained to perform with minimal equipment.

Q. What are the aims of a first-aider?

A. It is

1. To preserve life, and
2. To prevent the patient's condition from getting worse and to promote recovery.

Q. What are the responsibilities of the first-aider?

A. It is

1. To assess the situation/get help,
2. To protect the casualty and others from danger,
3. To assess the casualty,
4. To identify the casualty's injury/illness,
5. To provide treatment and understand the concept of triage,
6. To arrange transport,
7. To remain with the casualty until help arrives,
8. To pass on information regarding casualty,
9. To prevent cross infection.

1.2 Legal Aspects

1.2.1. Understanding the Legal Aspects Associated with First Aid.

Q. Can I be sued for helping someone?

A. Good Samaritan Act

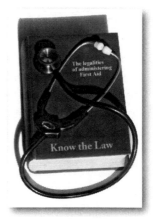

In the USA, there is what is known as the Good Samaritan Act. It's there to protect caregivers from prosecution as long as they are acting in a voluntary manner without any expectation of reward or financial gain. This Act has now come into play in Ireland under the Civil Law (Miscellaneous Provisions) Act 2011. You can download this information by logging on to http://www. irishstatutebook.ie/pdf/2011/en.act.2011.0023.pdf. However, if you do provide first aid, you will still be held accountable for your actions. If you give treatment to someone who is sick or injured, you have assumed a duty of care. This duty of care requires that you assess and treat the casualty but only in accordance with the rules and guidelines that your level of first aid allows. Confine yourself to your guidelines, and you will have no legal liability.

The difference between a first-aider volunteering their help and someone working with the emergency services is clearly defined and there are no grey areas. The professional is trained and expected to know what they are doing and is legally accountable for their actions. All professionals such as EMTs, paramedics, nurses, and doctors always work within their individual scope of practice and clearly understand their limits.

Consent

Before you do anything, introduce yourself. Tell the patient you are a first-aider and tell them you would like to help. You must have the consent of the conscious, alert casualty before you treat them. It can be expressed by either a nod of the head or verbally (expressed consent). When the casualty is unresponsive, mentally incompetent, or a child whose parents or guardian is not available and whose condition is life-threatening, you may assume that you have consent. This is known as implied consent. What this means is that you assume for all the right reasons, that the parent(s) or nest of kin would want you to assist and treat that casualty. However, if a person is alert, they have the right to refuse treatment, and you must respect their decision. You may advise them of the consequences associated with their refusal, but if they still say no, then you must not touch them. Any form of physical touch without consent could be interpreted as common assault.

Confidentiality

Sometimes a patient may tell you things they want passed on to family etc. if they think they are dying. This is confidential and must not be repeated to anyone other than the person or persons it's meant for. The same applies when sharing information about their injuries. This is also confidential and must only be shared with the appropriate people such as when handing over to the ambulance crew or other medical personnel. Disclosure of this information to another party must have the full permission of the casualty.

1.3. Equipment

What equipment do I need in order to give effective first aid?

First aid is about improvising when an emergency arises. Doing what you can with what you have available to you at that moment summarises it. The purists will say in order to deliver first aid, you must have X, Y, and Z, but you can stop a bleed with your bare hands if you know where to apply pressure. A magazine or a newspaper can become a splint. You can cool a burn with water. In a cardiac arrest, by giving a breath, you can supply oxygen to a person's lungs, and with a pair of hands, by doing compressions, you can circulate oxygenated blood throughout the body keeping the brain and other vital organs alive. However, a good first aid kit will make life easy and depending on your needs, it's not expensive to put one together.

Putting a first-aid kit together

All workplaces, leisure centres, homes, and cars should have a first-aid kit. The kits for the workplace and leisure centres, however, must conform to legal requirements, and in some cases, these kits may be tailored to suit what is required, such as adding additional equipment for a specific use. The first-aid kit should be clearly marked and easily accessible for the trained first-aider. For the home or the car, a complete basic first-aid kit can be bought or you can assemble a kit yourself.

If you decide to assemble your own kit, use a clean waterproof container. Mark it clearly and store it in a dry place. Check your kit regularly and replace items as soon as possible after your kit has been used. If for any reason you carry ointments, creams, aspirin, paracetamol, etc., in your kit, always make sure that they are in date and the packaging is intact. The important thing is not to go overboard when putting a kit together. Some people get completely carried away and end up with a bag that a surgeon on the battlefront would envy.

Apart from the weight and cost of putting such a kit together, the owner will never use half the contents. Be practical, and if you are unsure, get some advice. Any first-aider, EMT, or paramedic will be glad to advise you. As a guideline, I have given a list of contents that will help you. A small flashlight or pen torch that can fit in your kit can be worth having as an add-on. For your car, a high visibility vest is a good purchase and should be kept within easy reach. The ideal place is under your seat. A current, pocket-size first-aid book is also worth having as a reference.

First-Aid Boxes

Recommended Contents for First-Aid Boxes or Kits

Materials	Quantity 1-10 Persons	Quantity 11-25 Persons
Assorted adhesive plasters	20	40
Triangular bandages	2	4
Sterile eye pads	2	4
Safety pins	6	12
Medium sterile wound dressings	6	12
Large sterile wound dressings	4	6
Extra large sterile wound dressings	2	4
Non-alcoholic cleaning wipes	10	20
Crepe roller bandage	1	2
Pair of disposable latex gloves	5	10
Sterile eye wash (500 ml)	1	2
Tweezers	1	1
Pocket mask or disposable face shield	1	1
Paramedic shears or good quality scissors (blunt point)	1	1
Ice pack	2	2
Adhesive tape	1	1
Elasticised roller bandage	1	2
Small burn dressing	1	1
Large burn dressing	1	1
Gauze pads (small pack)	1	1
Safety glasses	1	1

Other Items You Might Consider

Flash light or pen torch	1	1
High visibility vest	1	1
Space blanket	1	2
Thermometer	1	1
Small notepad and pen	1	1
Current pocket-size first-aid book	1	1

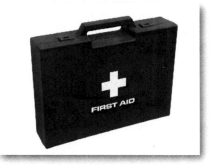

Note: This list is only a guideline based on the minimum amount of supplies required for an average first-aid box. You can use this as a building block when putting your own first-aid kit together.

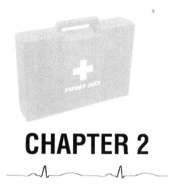

CHAPTER 2

2.1. Scene Safety

In order to understand what scene safety is all about, ask yourself the following questions:

Q. Would I run out into the middle of a busy street to help someone who has fallen off their bike?

Q. A car has just crashed at a bend on a busy road; would I stop my car as near as possible, dash over and try to assist him?

Q. As you walk past a building site, a man falls from very unstable scaffolding. Some of the scaffold bars have already fallen and more are just hanging there. Should you go to assist him in case the whole thing collapses?

Q. You are at home and hear a shout. When you go to look, you see your sister or roommate lying on the ground. There's water on the bathroom floor, and she's holding an old hairdryer she's had for years and there appears to be a crackling sound where her hand is in contact with the water. Will you rush to see if she's OK?

A. If these scenarios were real and you answered yes to any of the questions, you would probably be the next casualty or worse.

Scene safety is all about taking a step back and having a good long look at the situation. Even when you've checked, check again! Only when you are completely sure that there is no danger and the scene is safe should you then move to treat the casualty. It's called looking after number one! If you never remember anything else about safety, remember that the first-aider is the most important person at the scene of an accident. If you get injured, you are useless to the casualty. It's a time to be selfish and put your own safety first.

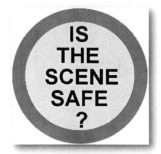

2.1.1. Understanding Scene Safety

Approaching the scene

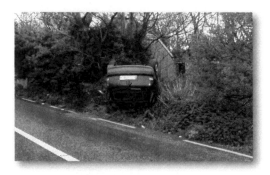

When approaching any accident scene as a first-aider, no matter what the circumstances, you must try to act in a professional manner. It may not be an easy or pleasant situation, but if you are the only person there that can potentially be a lifesaver, you should try to do the best you can. If the incident is very serious where, for example, there may be a fatality involved, unless you're prepared for such an event, it can be extremely traumatic. Even seasoned responders sometimes have problems dealing with death. The dead person may resemble a family member or friend maybe because of their size, shape, the colour of their hair, the scent of perfume or aftershave, or the clothes they are wearing. If you feel the situation is too much for you to handle and it's freaking you out, wait for the emergency services. If the person is dead, there is nothing you can do, apart from keeping others away and making sure the scene is safe. Doing that alone could be more important than you think.

You may be dealing with a crime scene, and by keeping people away, you are preserving the crime scene for forensic examination. It's important not to touch anything, although that's easier said than done because your impulse is to help that person and you won't know how the casualty is until you examine them. If you have to move something, try to remember where it was beforehand. Events where severe trauma or death is present are not the average person's every day event. In fact, in a lot of cases, attending a funeral may be the only time a person will ever witness death.

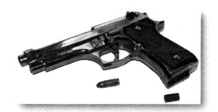

Approaching a road traffic collision or RTC as it is known is another minefield. You could write a book on the amount of things that can happen at one of these. Things can be calm one minute, and as you approach, the car may burst into flames, or there may be people there before you trying to get someone out, not knowing the consequences of their actions. A car could have ended up on its side with the person still trapped inside. Any movement from either rescuer or casualty could cause the car to fall over on top of the rescuer or cause more serious injuries to the casualty. The common one is when the person rushes to help and oil from the vehicle has spilled on to the road surface. The rescuer can slip and get hurt or break a limb, or other traffic can skid and lose control and possibly injure or kill someone. The same applies where ice is concerned. Dealing with an accident on an icy surface is extremely hazardous. Trying to stay standing is difficult enough let alone deal with what's going on around you. Accidents at night are an even bigger nightmare because the darkness alone brings even more danger. You can be seriously injured or even killed in a flash. Any scenario you can think of, you can multiply the danger by at least two when it's dark.

Using Your Four Senses

When approaching an incident, use your four senses.

- Look: Is the scene safe? Can you see anything out of the ordinary? Look up, down, left, and right. Do you see smoke, dangerous obstacles, hazardous material, or unstable objects?
- Listen: What can you hear? Approaching traffic? The hiss of gas? The sound of water or the crackle of flame? Are you able to interpret and understand the sounds?
- Smell: What can you smell? Gas, petrol, smoke, chemicals, or other fumes?
- Feel: What can you feel? Heat, cold, vibration, or any movement?
- Are there immediate life threats to the patient or to you?
- Approach the scene cautiously, and remember, if you don't control the scene, the scene will control you.
- If bystanders are not part of the solution, then they may become part of the problem; *Isolate them*, and make sure they are safe also.
- If bystanders volunteer their help, don't put them in harm's way.
- Time is an essential factor for the survival of a trauma patient.
- Is the environment safe and secure enough to proceed in order to the give adequate assistance?

Rule Number One, your safety comes first! Do not attempt to enter a dangerous environment unless it is safe to do so.

2.2. On Scene

When you get to the casualty or casualties, have another look around just to be really sure that you are safe. You may now notice dangers you hadn't already seen. When you have satisfied yourself that the area is safe to work in, check out the casualty. It may sound as if it takes forever from the time you first arrived at an incident to when you finally get to assess your casualty, but in reality, sizing up the situation and creating a safe working environment happens within a few minutes.

2.3. Body Substance Isolation

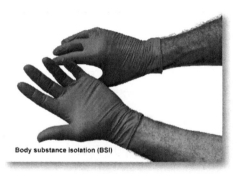

Body substance isolation (BSI)

Protecting Yourself

Before you make any physical contact with your casualty, you should take standard precautions as in using what we call body substance isolation or BSI for short. This means wearing surgical gloves at the very least. The reason for BSI is to isolate yourself as much as possible from infection transferred through direct contact with blood, open wounds or open sores.

Pathogens

A pathogen is a disease-causing microorganism. Diseases caused by pathogens can vary from the common cold to meningitis, from food poisoning right up to hepatitis and HIV. Healthcare professionals are faced with the real possibility of infection on a daily basis because of the volume of incidents they deal with. A scratch from a drug addict's needle can end your career quite rapidly to put it mildly! One of the most common ways a pathogen spreads is through personal contact from body fluids such as blood, urine, tears, saliva, faeces, and so on. BSI will reduce the chances of being infected. Professional responders, depending on the nature of an incident, would be expected to wear gloves, glasses, face masks, and a helmet.

BSI works both ways. It's something you should take seriously and practice it from the very start. It comes naturally in time, and you don't want to infect your patient either! Anywhere the skin is broken creates a doorway for infection to pass through. Infected blood and other bodily fluids can also inter your system through acne, sunburn, or broken blisters. You or your casualty may have cuts or scratches which could transfer infection, so you see why gloves are important. Likewise, glasses are important as infection can be introduced through the mucous membranes of the eye (conjunctiva) by blood splashes, sneezing, coughing, touching the eyes with contaminated fingers, or other objects or by someone spitting in your face. The eyes are susceptible to infection because they are not sterile. They rely on lysozyme (an enzyme found in the tears) to destroy bacteria. Bacteria line the surface of the eyelids (all the way down into the shaft of the eyelashes), which makes the conjunctiva predisposed to germs.

Surgical face masks are also used to protect you from airborne infections caused by inhalation or ingestion of pathogens through coughing, sneezing, spitting, etc. Even the water we drink can host pathogens. That's why we are sometimes asked to boil our tap water if there has been a problem with the water treatment processes. Hence, in reality, pathogens are never too far away from us, so don't play the hero. Protect yourself.

Three main points to remember:

1. Universal precautions: Necessary procedures used to control infection based on the assumption that blood is potentially infectious.

2. BSI: Concept that all bodily fluids are treated as potentially infectious.

3. Pathogen: A pathogen or infectious agent is a biological agent that causes disease or illness to its host.

Four-way spread of infection

1. Direct contact: Touching an infected person or coming into direct contact with sores, blood, or other bodily fluids.

2. Indirect contact: Coming into contact with articles of clothing, paper, or liquids that have been contaminated by blood, urine, faeces, or vomit.

3. Airborne infection: Germs are easily spread by droplets expelled through the nose and mouth through sneezing or coughing.

4. Carriers of infection and disease: Infection and disease can be carried over long distances by humans, animals, and insects.

Prevention of Cross Infection

Whenever possible, wash your hands with soap and water before and after treating your casualty. Be sure to wash both front and back of your hands, both thumbs, and all your fingers individually. Clean under your nails thoroughly. If you don't wear gloves while treating an injury, dirt and blood, even faeces, may bed in under your fingernails allowing the possibility of contaminating everything you touch. Remember, you may be faced with treating more than one casualty, so hygiene is paramount. If you are dealing with a casualty outdoors, use bottled water to wash with. Carry a hand sanitizer in your kit and use it. If you have cuts or grazes, be sure to cover them with waterproof dressings. If gloves aren't available and it's possible for the casualty themselves to apply a dressing to his or her wound, hand it to them and let them do it. Avoid touching the wound or the dressing where it has made contact with the wound. If you get blood splashes on your skin, wash it off right away. While treating the casualty, try not to cough, breathe, or sneeze over the wound, and likewise, be aware of the casualty sneezing and coughing in your direction. Surgical face masks are a great way of avoiding this, but again, it's not every day you see these in the average first-aid kit. First-aiders who wear glasses have an advantage over those that don't when treating casualties. Glasses help to protect the eyes from blood spatters and other fluids entering the eyes, and some first-aid kits, depending on their owner, may not carry safety glasses.

Although the risk of infection is very low, when giving rescue breaths, if possible, use a pocket mask or face shield as there is a risk that the casualty may vomit as a result of giving breaths with too much force. This is known as gastric inflation, and we will deal with this in great detail in a later chapter.

When wearing gloves and treating more than one casualty, it is important to remember, new gloves, new casualty. You must not wear the same gloves while treating multiple casualties. This is a classic example of cross contamination.

When disposing of waste, be sure to do so in a safe manner. If there is an ambulance on scene, they will as part of procedure take care of it for you. Be sure when removing gloves that you don't make contact with the outside part of the glove. This will be dealt with later in another chapter. Be sure all contaminated dressings, wipes, soiled objects, etc., are bagged. These should be incinerated. Ideally, they should be in a special yellow bag marked biohazard. Any sharp objects such as needles should be put in a clearly marked sharps box to avoid accidents and safely disposed of.

2.4. Common Infectious Diseases

The three most common infectious diseases that a first-aider or responder can be exposed to are human immunodeficiency virus (HIV), hepatitis B virus (HBV), and tuberculosis (TB). Although healthcare professionals and front line emergency services such as Fire and Rescue and Ambulance services are more likely to be exposed to these dangers, the risk is also there for the responder. While most first-aiders will on average deal only with family members or perhaps a neighbour, others are involved in voluntary organisations such as the Red Cross, Civil Defence, etc. These and other organisations from time to time are involved in giving first-aid cover for various events like concerts, festivals, and sports events. The more you're involved, the greater the risk of contact, so the greater the need for BSI.

I feel strongly about being informed of the risks involved when giving help to someone who is injured. Knowing that there are risks in the first place is half the battle, the rest is up to you. You won't put your hand into a fire because it's obvious that you will get burned, but it's far less obvious when you are giving first aid to someone whether or not they carry infection that can eventually kill you. In the next section 'Understanding these viruses', I try to give as much information as possible without getting too deep or technical. It's not pleasant reading, and the purpose is not to turn you off, but to give a heads up on what are to the first-aider the invisible dangers that emergency services all over the world strive to protect themselves from every day.

The biggest threat is the needle stick. Gloves will not stop a needle, so if a needle punctures the skin, you may be at risk of infection. If this happens, you should encourage the puncture site to bleed as quickly as possible by bruising, if necessary, while holding the wound under running warm water for two to three minutes. If you are not in a position where warm water is available, use cold water or as a last resort bottled water and ask someone to pour it slowly over the infected area while you encourage bleeding. The reason for using warm water is that it keeps the pores of the skin open allowing the blood to flow easier. Use whatever is available and do it quickly. Dispose of the needle safely. Do not attempt to suck the affected area for obvious reasons. Cover the wound with a clean dressing and get yourself to a hospital as soon as possible. An infected needle could present you with HIV, hepatitis C, or hepatitis B. The statistics for contamination are quiet staggering: 1 in 300 for HIV, 1 in 30 for Hep C, and 1 in 3 for Hep B. From these statistics, it's obvious that hepatitis B is the most dangerous and most common of the three blood-borne viruses, and any contact with blood should be avoided.

Understanding These Viruses

Hepatitis B, C, and A

For the first-aider or anyone that may come in contact with blood, it is important to know about blood-borne viruses. First, let's take a look at the hepatitis B virus (HBV). This is a very common virus. Worldwide, over 350 million people are infected with this virus. Although HBV is estimated to be 50-100 times more infectious than HIV, it cannot be spread through sneezing, coughing, hugging, or coming in contact with the faeces of someone who is infected. It is more commonly passed on through the exchange of bodily fluids with an infected person through exposure to blood during unprotected penetrative sex, through a blood transfusion in a country where blood is not screened for blood-borne viruses or what's known as blood on blood, whereby blood is transferred from one person to another through open wounds. This can happen quite easily in situations where responders are dealing with accidents. Cuts and scratches from sharp objects such as glass or metal may go unnoticed allowing cross contamination to occur. Sharing contaminated needles or by using non-sterilised equipment for tattooing, acupuncture, or body piercing are also ways to be infected. Even the very innocent can be infected whereby an infected mother can pass HBV on to her baby during delivery.

Hepatitis B can be either acute or chronic. Acute hepatitis B is the period of illness that occurs during the first four to sixteen weeks after acquiring the virus. Only 30%-50% of adults develop significant symptoms during acute infection. Rarely, acute hepatitis damages the liver so badly it can no longer function. Most people with acute infection will fully recover with no lasting health problems. Chronic hepatitis B, however, is more serious. Patients with chronic hepatitis B are at risk of severe liver disease such as cirrhosis (severe scarring of the liver). In patients with advanced cirrhosis, the liver begins to fail. The patient can also develop liver cancer. Unfortunately, 15% to 25% of patients with chronic hepatitis will eventually die from liver disease. Signs and symptoms of hepatitis B occur usually between eight and twenty-one weeks after exposure and can range from mild to severe.

Signs and symptoms of hepatitis A, B, and C include the following:

- Tiredness
- Yellow skin or yellowing of the whites of the eyes (jaundice)
- A short, mild, flu-like illness
- Loss of appetite
- Nausea, vomiting, and diarrhoea
- Stomach pain
- Weight loss
- Darker yellow urine and pale faeces
- Itchy skin

Now let's look at Hepatitis C

Hepatitis C virus (HCV), like other forms of hepatitis, causes inflammation of the liver. HCV is transferred primarily through blood and is more persistent than hepatitis A or B. HCV can be spread by sharing infected needles, the use of non-sterilised tattooing, acupuncture, or body-piercing equipment, and exposure to blood during unprotected sex with an infected person. Blood may be present because of genital sores, cuts, or menstruation. A mother infecting her baby during childbirth is rare, although the risk is much greater if the mother is also infected with HIV. Blood transfusion in developing countries where blood is not screened for HCV is a large contributor to infection. Snorting cocaine doesn't seem a likely way to become infected, but users usually use a rolled up banknote which can become contaminated with blood from the nose.

Hepatitis C cannot be passed on by hugging, sneezing, coughing, sharing food or water, sharing cutlery, or casual contact. The signs and symptoms are the same as that of hepatitis B. Most adults infected with the HBV fully recover and develop lifelong immunity. Between 2% and 10% of individuals infected as adults will become chronic carriers, meaning they will be infectious to others and can develop chronic liver damage. Infected children, especially newborn babies, are much more likely to become chronic carriers. A person living with the hepatitis B infection for a number of years may develop chronic hepatitis, liver cirrhosis, or liver cancer.

Our final look at hepatitis takes us to hepatitis A virus (HAV). We could have gone the alphabetical route, but I have put these three viruses in order of severity. Hepatitis A is the most common of all three mentioned. Infection with HAV leads to inflammation of the liver, but complications are rarely serious. It can affect all age groups. Once a person is exposed to the virus, it takes between two and six weeks to produce symptoms which are the same symptoms as hepatitis B and C. It is important to reiterate that early diagnosis is paramount. If you believe that you are showing any of the signs and symptoms, get yourself checked out.

HAV is found in the faeces of someone infected with the virus. It only takes a tiny amount of faeces getting inside another person's mouth to cause hepatitis A infection. Careful hand washing can minimise the risk of the virus being passed on. Hepatitis A is common in many parts of the world where sanitation and sewage infrastructure is poor. Often people become infected with HAV by eating or drinking contaminated food or water. Hepatitis A is also classed as a sexually transmitted disease. The HAV infection usually clears in up to eight to ten weeks, but may occasionally recur or persist longer in some people. Once a person has been infected and their body has fought off the virus, they are permanently immune. Occasionally, symptoms may be severe and require monitoring. Complications are rare and permanent liver damage is unlikely, but in very rare cases, infection can be fatal, particularly among the elderly.

HIV/AIDS

HIV infects cells of the immune system and destroys or impairs their function. Infection results in the progressive deterioration of the immune system, breaking down the body's ability to fend off infections and diseases. AIDS (Acquired immune deficiency syndrome) refers to the most advanced stages of HIV infection, defined by the occurrence of any of more than twenty opportunistic infections or related cancers. HIV can be transmitted through unprotected sexual intercourse (vaginal or anal) or oral sex with an infected person, transfusions of contaminated blood, and the sharing of contaminated needles, syringes, or other sharp instruments. Sharing a toothbrush also carries danger because of bleeding gums. It can also be transmitted between a mother and her baby during pregnancy, childbirth and breastfeeding. HIV/AIDS is the world's leading infectious killer claiming to date more than 27 million lives. An estimated 2 million people die every year from HIV/AIDS. Some people experience signs and symptoms of HIV as soon as they become infected, while others do not. When they occur, early signs and symptoms are often mistaken for the flu or a mild viral infection. Initial signs and symptoms of HIV include fever, headache, tiredness, nausea, diarrhoea, and enlarged lymph nodes in the neck, armpits, or groin.

The following signs and symptoms may be warning signs of late-stage HIV infection: rapid weight loss, dry cough, recurring fever or profuse night sweats, profound and unexplained fatigue, swollen lymph glands in the armpits, groin, or neck, diarrhoea lasting more than a week, white spots or unusual blemishes on the tongue, in the mouth, or in the throat, pneumonia, red, brown, pink, or purplish blotches on or under the skin or inside the mouth, nose, or eyelids, memory loss, depression, and other neurological disorders.

As you can see, the signs and symptoms of HIV infection are similar to those for many different viral infections. The only way to know for sure if you are infected with HIV is to be tested. Many people infected with HIV do not have any signs and symptoms at all for many years.

Tuberculosis

Tuberculosis, sometimes referred to as TB, is a disease caused by an organism called *Mycobacterium tuberculosis*. TB kills someone every twenty seconds. That's over 4,500 people every day, according to the estimates from the World Health Organization. TB is second only to HIV as the leading infectious killer of adults worldwide. At any given moment, more than 13 million people around the world are suffering from an active infection.

TB usually attacks the lungs, but it can spread to the joints, bladder, spine, brain, and other parts of the body. It is spread through the air when people who have the disease cough, sneeze, or spit. Most infections in humans result in an asymptomatic latent infection, and about one in ten latent infections eventually progresses to active disease, which, if left untreated, kills more than 50% of its victims.

The classic symptoms are a chronic cough that lasts three weeks or longer with blood-tinged sputum, fever, chills, night sweats, fatigue, loss of appetite, and weight loss. If TB affects the joints, it may cause a pain similar to that of arthritis. If TB affects the bladder, it may hurt when urinating, and there may be blood in the urine. TB of the spine can cause back pain and leg paralysis. TB of the brain can cause headaches, nausea, and brain damage (if left untreated).

Tetanus (Lockjaw)

Although tetanus is bacterial and not viral, I feel it's important to mention it because we all at some stage get cuts or scratches. When you treat a casualty for open wounds, it is important that you understand the implications of tetanus and that you always advise that person to have the wound looked at by a doctor. It's standard practice if you end up in the emergency room to be given a tetanus injection if you are being treated for any form of open wound. The doctor will always ask you if you have had a recent vaccination for tetanus, and if you can't remember when, you will get one before you leave. All healthcare professionals keep up to date with their vaccinations because of the dangers involved. If you get cut from anything rusty or dirty, let it be barbed wire, a tin can, a broken bottle, a nail, or a thorn, there could be at risk of tetanus, and it's best practice to have it checked out and cleaned properly, especially if the wound has been in contact with soil. Tetanus is an infection of the nervous system from the potentially deadly bacteria *Clostridium tetani (C. tetani)*. Spores of the bacteria live in the soil and are found around the world. The bacterium is also found in animal faeces. In the spore form, *C. tetani* may remain inactive in the soil, but it can remain infectious for more than forty years. Infection begins when the spores enter the body through an injury or wound and release bacteria that spread and make a poison called tetanospasmin. This poison blocks nerve signals from the spinal cord to the muscles, causing severe muscle spasms. The spasms can be so powerful that they tear the muscles or cause fractures of the spine. The time between infection and the first sign of symptoms is typically seven to twenty-one days. Sometimes, the spasms affect muscles that help with breathing, which can lead to breathing problems. Prolonged muscular action causes sudden, powerful, and painful contractions of muscle groups. Tetanus often begins with mild spasms in the jaw muscles (lockjaw). The spasms can also affect the chest, neck, back, and abdominal muscles. Other symptoms include drooling, excessive sweating, fever, hand or foot spasms, irritability, swallowing difficulty, uncontrolled urination, or defecation. Tetanus is completely preventable by vaccination, and in my view, everyone should look into it. Anyone can come in contact with the bacteria without being aware of it. For example, you get a flat tyre. As you are changing the wheel, the wheel brace slips and you bang your hand off the wheel or the body of the car resulting in a cut. More than likely, a lot of the dirt on the car is from soil.

If you are actively involved in first aid, it is your responsibility to look after yourself. Make sure you are protected and all your vaccinations are current.

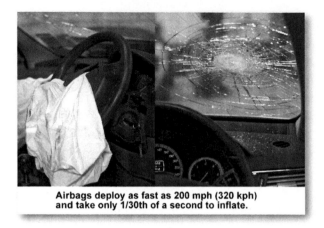

Airbags deploy as fast as 200 mph (320 kph) and take only 1/30th of a second to inflate.

2.5. What Should I Be Aware of on Scene?

Depending on the type and nature of the incident, there are obvious things to look out for. It's a bit like the soldier in battle using his heightened awareness of everything going on around him in order to survive, though not quite that dramatic. These are a few examples of hidden dangers to the less-experienced rescuer. Take for example; you arrive at a traffic accident. It's a single car verses pole. There's substantial damage to the front of the car and the pole carrying overhead power lines isn't too healthy looking either. In fact, it's tilted slightly, and there's a visible crack at the point of impact. You have secured the scene with the help of other bystanders, and you are in the process of approaching the single male occupant of the car who is clutching the steering wheel and is in obvious distress. Remember to the best of your knowledge the scene is safe. The bystanders who offered help are doing a great job with traffic control and keeping others away from danger so you can do your job. You make a judgement call on the pole and recon it's stable, so you turn your attention to the casualty to assess him before calling the emergency services.

There are no more surprises, so you manage to open the door to reassure the patient that everything is under control. He's bleeding slightly over his left eye and you lean in to examine it. You are now looking at him face to face when suddenly a hidden surprise literally pops out at you from behind at 200 mph in the form of the airbag, pushing your head forward into the casualty's face! This is something you won't think of unless you are involved in either Fire and Rescue or Ambulance service, and a lot of first-aid books don't mention it. This is a hidden killer, or at the very least, it will leave both you and your casualty with serious facial injuries such as broken teeth, cheek bones, jaw bone, nose, or even a fractured skull. It can happen on occasions that the airbag may not deploy at the time of impact and it may take very little movement of the vehicle to trigger it. Airbags normally deploy from between ten and twenty-five milliseconds after impact at a speed of around 200 mph (322 kph). The **powdery substance** released from the airbag is regular corn starch or talcum powder, which is used by the airbag manufacturers to keep the bags pliable and lubricated while they're in storage. This can be disorientating for a few seconds adding to the confusion. If you get between the casualty and the airbag as it deploys, you are in trouble. This is where experience counts, but now that you're aware of it, it may keep you out of trouble. If you have to assess someone in this situation, position yourself in front of the vehicle if it is safe to do so and access them visually through the windscreen. Pay attention to debris that may cause injury to you such as jagged metal or glass. Keep in mind also that the car could go on fire so always be sure you have a clear escape route. The fire service carries a device that covers the steering wheel allowing the airbag to deploy safely without it injuring the rescuer, so consider waiting for them to arrive.

Then there's the unconscious man. People can fall into this trap also from lack of experience. After a few minutes of assessing him, you discover that to the best of your knowledge his only problem was that he had a few drinks too many, fell or laid down, and fell asleep. You ask around if anyone knows him, but no one has a clue, so you check his pockets for identification. While going through his jacket pockets, you feel a sudden sensation as if you have just been stung by a bee. As you remove your hand, you notice a drop of blood on one of your fingers, and there's a small puncture wound. On further examination, you find that you've just been stuck by an uncapped needle! Is this person a drug addict or a diabetic or whatever? Has he got HIV/hepatitis? Are you infected or not? Be careful; never put your hands in someone's pockets or pat them down. leave the searching to the professionals.

2.6. Dangers in the Home

Dangers in the home are just as plentiful and varied, and what makes us more vulnerable is that we take too much for granted. How often do we check electrical appliances such as the hair drier, the iron, the kettle, and the radio? These are things we use every day, and they are only a small percentage of the electrical equipment in the average home. Frayed wiring, faulty sockets, or cracked appliances that allow water or steam to penetrate and make contact with the wiring are a great recipe for 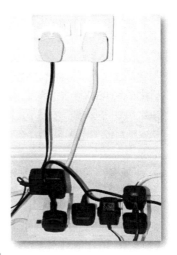 disaster. Other things that can be a danger and cause slips trips and falls are wet floors, children's toys, trailing appliance flex, or extension leads. Even the cat and the dog can be a danger! Always remember that a lot of our elder citizens spend a great deal of time on their own, and it's not uncommon for someone to fall and spend long hours on a cold floor with broken limbs waiting for someone to call, and in some cases, die waiting.

The DIY enthusiast is a regular visitor to our accident and emergency centres. Bank holiday weekends are notorious for carnage in the home. The desk jockey who spends all his time in an office setting suddenly becomes the weekend warrior with a toolbox and after watching a few DIY programs becomes the expert. The brand new power tools are not a problem, and after all, how hard can it be to rip down a few sheets of plywood with the skill saw, or cut those big overhanging branches in the garden with the new chainsaw? Nothing worse than looking for a finger or toe in the long grass! Power tools in the wrong hands are lethal, and the injuries can be horrific. Hand tools can be just as dangerous. Wood chisels, handsaws, knives, etc., can all cause serious injuries, and if you cut at the right place, you can bleed to death. Falls from ladders are also common occurrences. Overreaching with no one to hold the ladder can result in a helpless fall. This type of accident can result in the casualty being paralyzed or even killed. Breaking a limb is getting off light! Some people are naturally awkward, and without sounding nasty, they should let it to the professionals because in a lot of cases, DIY takes on the new meaning of 'destroy it yourself' rather than 'do it yourself'.

2.7. SBAR

This is worth discussing at this point. This simplistic approach to a situation may help you with scene safety, patient assessment, and reporting an incident, although we will deal with all this in the professional sense later on. This is an alternative method for gathering and reporting information to the appropriate agency and if it works for you then by all means use it. It's a technique that was adapted by the military and is now used for prompt and appropriate communication in some healthcare organisations. The US Navy developed the SBAR communication model which included a brief description of the situation at hand, pertinent background, an assessment of the problem, and a plan for resolution. So how are submarine and healthcare operations alike? Both exist in 'harms' way'. Both require timely action to avert disaster. Both operate 24/7. Both experience lots of turnover and cultural diversity. Both deal with fear, fatigue, interruptions, and distractions. Both sometimes have at the root of their situations unclear, in-concise, or inaccurate information.

The adoption of SBAR as a tool for the medical field was a touch of genius and simplifies what can be a very stressful situation by breaking it down to four primary parts. Why someone didn't think of it years ago is amazing as SBAR can be applied to everything and anything, be it industrial, educational as well as medical.

Four primary parts of SBAR:

S— Situation: Identify yourself and where you are calling from. Identify the patient by name, date of birth, age, sex, and reason for report. Describe the situation, reason for phone call, or current status of the patient (if urgent say so.)

B— Background: Give the patient's presenting complaint. Give the patient's relevant past medical history. Give a brief background summary.

A— Assessment: Vital signs include heart rate, respiratory rate, blood pressure, temperature, oxygen saturation, pain scale, and level of consciousness (LOC). List if any vital signs are outside of parameters; what is your clinical impression? How severe is the patient's injury or medical problem? Have your additional concerns worth mentioning.

R— Recommendation: Explanation of what you require, and how urgent the problem is. When and what action needs to be taken. Clarify what action you expect to be taken.

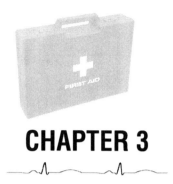

CHAPTER 3

3.1. Anatomy and Physiology

In order to do something, you need to know how to do it, why you do it, when to do it, and also what happens when you do it. Also, and very importantly, you need to know when not to do something! In this section, we will deal with the body in a way that is understood clearly without getting too technical. Knowing how all the parts are supposed to work can help you understand what to expect when treating a casualty. Treat this section more like an overview rather than an in-depth and complicated section. It's there as a reference to come back to and nothing else.

3.2. Topographic Anatomy

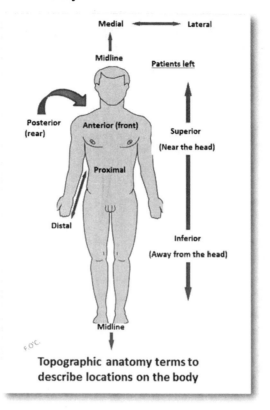

Topographic anatomy terms to
describe locations on the body

This section will briefly familiarise you with the topographic anatomy which is used to describe the location of injuries or area of pain on the body. Although it is important to be familiar with the terms, it isn't expected that anyone who isn't using these terms on a daily basis will remember them later on. If you can't remember, just describe in your own words where the injury or pain is when giving your information to EMS.

All medical personnel describe their findings based on the standard anatomic position. How this works is, you visualise the person standing in front of you, facing you with their arms by their side and their palms facing you. You always describe the injury or pain in relation to the patient's left or right side and not yours as you look at them. You will come across this in a number of situations such as, for example, when you look at illustrations in any medical book of the skeleton, or other organs such as the heart. These illustrations will be based on the person facing you unless specified otherwise. Topography gets its name from the Greek words 'topos' meaning place and 'graphia' which means writing. It refers to writing about local history but mainly concerned with local detail in general.

Topography is all about local detail and is easy enough to understand once it's explained. Take for example, Midline. This is an imaginary line drawn from the middle of the forehead all the way to the floor. This imaginary line divides the body into two parts, left and right. The word anterior simply means the front of the body, whereas posterior means the rear.

When you are referring to any injury or pain close to the centre of the body, it is referred to as medial, whereas anything away from the centre is referred to as lateral. As an example of this, the nose would be considered medial, whereas the eyes are considered lateral to the nose.

Next, we shall deal with superior and inferior. This is in relation to distance from the head. When an injury occurs in the patella (kneecap), it is classed as an inferior injury as it's closer to the feet than the head. The femur (thigh bone) would be considered superior to the patella as it is above the injured site. A shoulder or chest injury would be considered a superior injury as it is near the head and anywhere below that injury site is classed as inferior.

Finally, we shall deal with proximal and distal which is used mainly in relation to limbs. Consider this in a simplistic way. Take for example, where your arm is connected to the body at the shoulder joint. This is the proximal part as it is nearest to the torso. Your wrist would be distal to the shoulder. Exactly the same applies to the legs. If you had a fracture to a bone in the lower leg, it would be called a distal leg fracture, whereas if you fractured the top of your femur, it would be known as a proximal leg fracture. In relation to the knee, the foot is distal to the knee. Remember, the farthest away point is as the word suggests is distal.

3.3. The Respiratory System

The act of breathing is called respiration. The breathing mechanism is made up of three phases which are breathing in, breathing out, and a pause. The respiratory system is controlled by four sets of muscles. These are the diaphragm, the intercostal muscles (located between your ribs), the abdominal muscles, and the accessory muscles. The function of the respiratory system is to move air into and out of the body in order to bring in oxygen and expel carbon dioxide. It consists of the nose, the mouth, and the trachea, the bronchi, two lungs, and associated muscles.

Air, first enters your body through your nose or mouth, which wets and warms the air. (Cold dry air can irritate your lungs.) The air then travels through your voice box and down your windpipe (trachea). The windpipe splits into two bronchial tubes that enter your lungs. A thin flap of tissue called the epiglottis covers your windpipe when you swallow. This prevents food and drink from entering the air passages that lead to your lungs. Except for the mouth and some parts of the nose, all of the airways have special hairs called cilia that are coated with sticky mucus. The cilia trap germs and other foreign particles that enter your airways when you breathe in air. These fine hairs then sweep the particles up to the nose or mouth. From there, they're swallowed, coughed, or sneezed out of the body. Nose, hairs, and mouth saliva also trap particles and germs.

Lungs and blood vessels

Your lungs and linked blood vessels deliver oxygen to your body and remove carbon dioxide from your body. Your lungs lie on either side of your breastbone and fill the inside of your chest cavity. Your left lung is slightly smaller than your right lung to allow room for your heart. Within the lungs, your bronchi branch into thousands of smaller, thinner tubes called bronchioles. These tubes end in bunches of tiny round air sacs called alveoli. Each of these air sacs is covered in a mesh of tiny blood vessels called capillaries. The capillaries connect to a network of arteries and veins that move blood through your body. The pulmonary artery and its branches deliver blood rich in carbon dioxide (and lacking in oxygen) to the capillaries that surround the air sacs. Inside the air sacs, carbon dioxide moves from the blood into the air. At the same time, oxygen moves from the air into the blood in the capillaries. The oxygen-rich blood then travels to the heart through the pulmonary vein and its branches. The heart pumps the oxygen-rich blood out to the body. The lungs are divided into five main sections called lobes. Some people need to have a diseased lung lobe removed. However, they can still breathe well using the rest of their lung lobes. The diaphragm is a dome-shaped muscle, which separates the chest from the abdominal cavity. It is the major muscle and the one that begins the inhalation process. During inhalation, the diaphragm contracts and moves downwards, pushing out the abdomen and creating suction which draws in the air and expands the lungs.

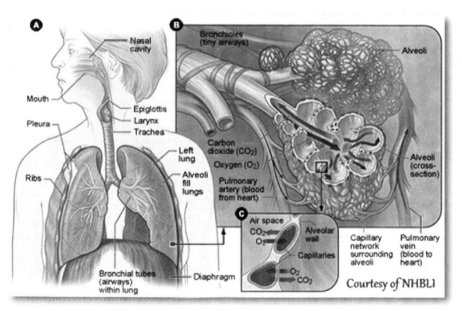

Figure A shows the location of the respiratory structures in the body. Figure B is an enlarged view of the airways, alveoli (air sacs), and capillaries (tiny blood vessels). Figure C is a close-up view of gas exchange between the capillaries and alveoli. CO2 is carbon dioxide, and O2 is oxygen.

What happens when you breathe?

Breathing In (Inhalation): When you breathe in, or inhale, your diaphragm contracts (tightens) and moves downward. This increases the space in your chest cavity, into which your lungs expand. The intercostal muscles between your ribs also help enlarge the chest cavity. They contract to pull your ribcage both upward and outward when you inhale.

As your lungs expand, air is sucked in through your nose or mouth. The air travels down your windpipe and into your lungs. After passing through your bronchial tubes, the air finally reaches and enters the alveoli (air sacs). Through the very thin walls of the alveoli, oxygen from the air passes to the surrounding capillaries (blood vessels). A red blood cell protein called haemoglobin helps move oxygen from the air sacs to the blood. At the same time, carbon dioxide moves from the capillaries into the air sacs. The gas has travelled in the bloodstream from the right side of the heart through the pulmonary artery. Oxygen-rich blood from the lungs is carried through a network of capillaries to the pulmonary vein. This vein delivers the oxygen-rich blood to the left side of the heart. The left side of the heart pumps the blood to the rest of the body. There, the oxygen in the blood moves from blood vessels into surrounding tissues.

Breathing Out (Exhalation): When you breathe out, or exhale, your diaphragm relaxes and moves upward into the chest cavity. The intercostal muscles between the ribs also relax to reduce the space in the chest cavity. As the space in the chest cavity gets smaller, air rich in carbon dioxide is forced out of your lungs and windpipe, and then out of your nose or mouth. Breathing out requires no effort from your body unless you have a lung disease or are doing physical activity. When you're physically active, your abdominal muscles contract and push your diaphragm against your lungs even more than usual. This rapidly pushes air out of your lungs.

What controls your breathing?

A respiratory control centre at the base of your brain controls your breathing. This centre sends ongoing signals down your spine and to the muscles involved in breathing. These signals ensure your breathing muscles contract (tighten) and relax regularly. This allows your breathing to happen automatically, without you being aware of it. To a limited degree, you can change your breathing rate, such as by breathing faster or holding your breath. Your emotions also can change your breathing. For example, being scared or angry can affect your breathing pattern. Your breathing will change depending on how active you are and the condition of the air around you. For example, you need to breathe more often when you do physical activity. In contrast, your body needs to restrict how much air you breathe if the air contains irritants or toxins. To adjust your breathing to changing needs, your body has many sensors in your brain, blood vessels, muscles, and lungs. Sensors in the brain and in two major blood vessels (the carotid artery and the aorta) detect carbon dioxide or oxygen levels in your blood and change your breathing rate as needed. Sensors in the airways detect lung irritants. The sensors can trigger sneezing or coughing. In people who have asthma, the sensors may cause the muscles around the airways in the lungs to contract. This makes the airways smaller. Sensors in the alveoli (air sacs) can detect fluid build-up in the lung tissues. These sensors are thought to trigger rapid, shallow breathing. Sensors in your joints and muscles detect movement of your arms or legs. These sensors may play a role in increasing your breathing rate when you're physically active.

3.4. The Cardiovascular System

The easiest way to remember this complicated subject is to think of it in simplistic terms. Think of it like this; the cardiovascular system is made up of three things: liquid, a vessel, and a pump. The liquid being blood, the vessel being the blood vessels, and the pump being the heart. How easy is that!

Functions of the Cardiovascular System

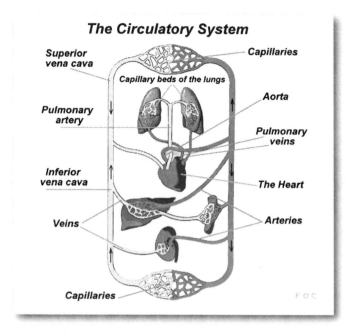

The cardiovascular system provides the transport system of the body. Using blood as the transport medium, the heart continually propels oxygen, nutrients, and many other substances into the interconnecting blood vessels that move past the body cells. The blood also carries waste products that are removed by the kidneys and carbon dioxide that is expelled by the lungs. Blood also helps control body temperature and maintains electrolyte balance. The cardiovascular system contains about 5 litres (8 pints) of blood which your heart continuously recirculates. Each day, your heart beats about 100,000 times and pumps about 23,000 litres (5,000 gallons) of blood.

3.5. The Heart

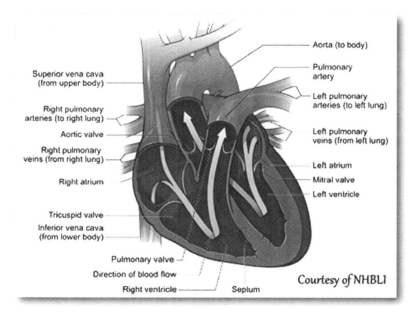

Superior vena cava (from upper body)

Right pulmonary arteries (to right lung)

Aortic valve

Right pulmonary veins (from right lung)

Right atrium

Tricuspid valve

Inferior vena cava (from lower body)

Pulmonary valve

Direction of blood flow

Right ventricle

Aorta (to body)

Pulmonary artery

Left pulmonary arteries (to left lung)

Left pulmonary veins (from left lung)

Left atrium

Mitral valve

Left ventricle

Septum

Courtesy of NHBLI

The heart is a two-sided double pump which weighs less than a pound (0.45 kg). It is also a muscle. It is slightly bigger than a fist and is located between the lungs in the thoracic cavity. It beats 40 million times per year (between 60 and 100 beats per minute). It is positioned partially to the left of the sternum. The heart is divided into four chambers called atria and ventricles. Blood enters the heart through the atria and leaves through the ventricles. The right and left sides of the heart are divided by the septum (a dividing wall).

With each contraction, or heartbeat, the heart pumps blood forward from the left side of the heart through the aorta (the main artery leaving the heart) and into the arteries. The arteries divide off into smaller and smaller branches to supply a microscopic network of capillaries, taking the blood to every part of your body. The blood then travels back to the heart from the capillaries into the veins. The branches of the veins join to form larger veins, which deliver the blood back to the right side of your heart. As the heart relaxes in between each heartbeat or contraction, blood from the veins fills the right side of the heart, and blood from the lungs fills the left side of your heart. The two sides of the heart are separate, but they work together. The right side of the heart receives dark, de-oxygenated blood which has circulated around your body. It pumps this to your lungs, where it picks up a fresh supply of oxygen and becomes bright red again.

The heart wall is made up of special muscle called myocardium. Like every other living tissue, the myocardium itself needs a continuous supply of fresh blood. This supply of blood comes from the coronary arteries which start from the main artery (the aorta) as it leaves the left ventricle. The coronary arteries spread across the outside of the myocardium, feeding it with a supply of blood.

Heart's Electrical System

Your heart has an electrical system which is a bit like the electrical wiring in your home. The heart's electrical system creates the signals that tell your heart when to beat, and your heartbeat is what pumps blood throughout your body. The heart's electrical system is also known as the *cardiac conduction system.*

Your heart's electrical system has three important parts:

1. S-A node (sinoatrial node)—known as the heart's natural pacemaker. The S-A node has special cells that create the electricity that makes your heart beat.

2. A-V node (atrioventricular node)—the A-V node is the bridge between the atria and ventricles. Electrical signals pass from the atria down to the ventricles through the A-V node.

3. His-Purkinje system—the His-Purkinje system carries the electrical signals throughout the ventricles to make them contract. The parts of the His-Purkinje system include His Bundle (the start of the system), Right bundle branch, Left bundle branch, and the Purkinje fibers (the end of the system).

Electrical signals and blood flow

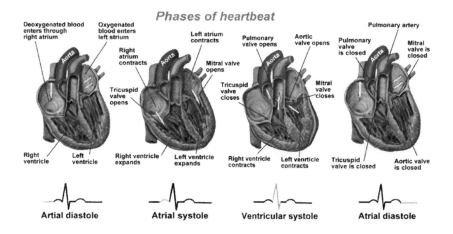

Phases of heartbeat

Deoxygenated blood enters through right atrium — Oxygenated blood enters left strium — Left atrium contracts — Pulmonary valve opens — Aortic valve opens — Pulmonary valve is closed — Pulmonary artery — Mitral valve is closed

Right atrium contracts — Mitral valve opens — Tricuspid valve closes — Mitral valve closes — Tricuspid valve opens

Right ventricle — Left ventricle — Right ventricle expands — Left ventricle expands — Right ventricle contracts — Left venrticle contracts — Tricuspid valve is closed — Aortic valve is closed

Artial diastole   Atrial systole   Ventricular systole   Atrial diastole

The S-A node normally produces 60-100 electrical signals per minute—this is your heart rate or pulse. With each pulse, signals from the S-A node follow a natural electrical pathway through your heart walls. The movement of the electrical signals causes your heart's chambers to contract and relax. In a healthy heart, the chambers contract and relax in a coordinated way, or in *rhythm*. When your heart beats in rhythm at a normal rate, it is called *sinus rhythm*. When working well, your conduction system automatically responds to your body's changing need for oxygen. When you run for example or do any vigorous exercise, you need more oxygen; therefore, your heart beats at a faster heart rate.

When you are sitting or sleeping, you need less oxygen; therefore, your heart beats at a slower rate. Your conduction system senses your need for oxygen and responds with the proper heart rate. A problem in your heart's electrical system can disrupt your heart's normal rhythm. Any kind of abnormal rhythm or heart rate is called an arrhythmia. It is normal and healthy for your heartbeat to speed up or slow down during the day as your activity level changes. But it is not normal for your heart to beat out of rhythm. When your heart beats out of rhythm, it may not deliver enough blood to your body.

Heart Disease

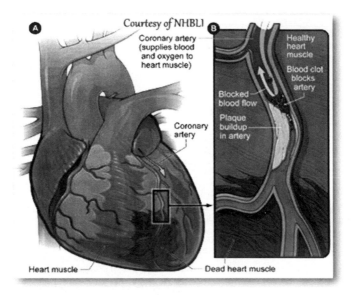

Any disease of the heart (cardio) and blood vessels (vascular) is called *cardiovascular disease.* When fatty material, or plaque, builds up in the walls of your heart's arteries, you have what is known as illustration shows 'A', a heart with dead heart muscle caused by a heart attack, and 'B' shows a cross-section of a coronary artery with a plaque build-up and a blood clot. A heart attack occurs if the flow of oxygen-rich blood to a section of heart muscle suddenly becomes blocked. If blood flow isn't restored quickly, the section of heart muscle begins to die. Cardiomyopathy affects the heart muscle itself. 'Cardio' means heart and 'myopathy' means muscle disease. People with cardiomyopathy often go on to develop more serious heart conditions. The heart muscle is like a rubber band, and as that rubber band stretches over time, it eventually loses its elasticity. Likewise, as the heart muscle stretches and the heart gets larger, the muscle loses some of its ability to pump or contract. Over time, as heart failure develops, the heart becomes less able to pump blood to the body as strongly as it did before.

3.6. The Musculoskeletal System

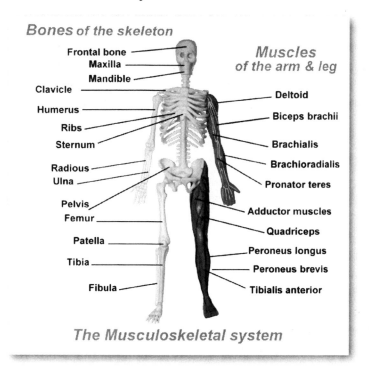

Bones *of the skeleton*

Frontal bone
Maxilla
Mandible
Clavicle
Humerus
Ribs
Sternum
Radious
Ulna
Pelvis
Femur
Patella
Tibia
Fibula

Muscles
of the arm & leg

Deltoid
Biceps brachii
Brachialis
Brachioradialis
Pronator teres
Adductor muscles
Quadriceps
Peroneus longus
Peroneus brevis
Tibialis anterior

The Musculoskeletal system

The musculoskeletal system is a system of muscles, tendons, ligaments and bones, joints, and associated tissues that move the body and maintain its form.

3.6.1. Muscles

There are three types of muscles: skeletal, smooth, and cardiac (heart). Two of these—skeletal and smooth—are part of the musculoskeletal system.

Skeletal

Skeletal muscles are controlled by the brain and are considered voluntary muscles because they operate with a person's awareness. These muscles are bundles of contractile fibers that are organised in a regular pattern. Skeletal muscles, which are responsible for posture and movement, are attached to bones and arranged in opposing groups around joints. For example, muscles that bend the elbow (biceps) are countered by muscles that straighten it (triceps). These countering movements are balanced in order to make movements smooth, which helps prevent damage to the musculoskeletal system. The size and strength of skeletal muscles are maintained or increased by regular exercise.

Smooth

Smooth muscles control certain bodily functions that are not readily under a person's control. Smooth muscle surrounds many arteries and contract to adjust blood flow. It surrounds the intestines and contracts to move food and faeces along the digestive tract. Smooth muscle also is controlled by the brain but not voluntarily. The triggers for contracting and relaxing smooth muscles are controlled by the body's needs, so smooth muscles are considered involuntary muscle because they operate without a person's awareness.

Cardiac

Cardiac muscle forms the heart and is not part of the musculoskeletal system. Like skeletal muscle, cardiac muscle has a regular pattern of fibres that also appear as stripes under a microscope. However, cardiac muscle contracts and relaxes rhythmically without a person's awareness.

3.6.2. Bone

The adult body has 206 bones. Bones serve as rigid structures to the body and create shields to protect delicate internal organs. They provide housing for the bone marrow, where the blood cells are formed. Bones also maintain the body's reservoir of calcium. Bones have two shapes: flat (such as the plates of the skull and the vertebrae) and tubular (such as the thighbones and arm bones, which are called long bones). All bones have essentially the same structure.

The skull

The skull rests on the upper end of the vertebral column. It is divided into two parts: the cranium and the face.

The cranium

The cranium is formed by a number of flat and irregular bones that provide protection for the brain. The bones that form the cranium are the frontal bone which is the forehead. It also forms the orbital cavities (*eye sockets*). Two parietal bones form the sides and roof of the skull. Two temporal bones are found on each side of the head and form fibrous immovable joints with the parietal, occipital, sphenoid, and zygomatic bones. The occipital bone forms the back of the head and part of the skull base. The sphenoid bone occupies the middle portion of the base of the skull which links the cranial and facial bones and cross-braces the skull. The ethmoid bone is at the front part of the base of the skull and forms the orbital cavity, the nasal septum, and lateral walls of the nasal cavity.

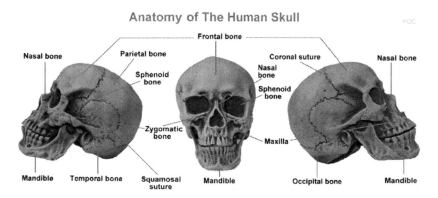

Anatomy of The Human Skull

The face

The skeleton of the face is made up of two zygomatic (*cheek*) bones that form the prominences of the cheeks and part of the floor and lateral walls of the orbital cavities. The maxilla forms the upper jaw, the front part of the roof of the mouth, the lateral walls of the nasal cavity, and part of the base of the orbital cavities. It also houses the upper teeth. On each side of the maxilla, there is a large air sinus (*the maxillary sinus)* lined with ciliated mucous membrane with openings into the nasal cavity. There are two nasal bones that form the sides and upper surfaces of the nasal bridge. Two lacrimal bones situated at the back and sides to the nasal bones form part of the medial walls of the orbital cavity. Both lacrimal bones facilitate a duct that carries tears from the eye to the nasal cavity. The vomer is a thin flat bone extending upwards from the middle of the hard pallet to form most of the lower part of the nasal septum. The palatine bones are two L-shaped bones that form the back of the hard palate and side walls of the nasal cavity. The upper extremities form part of the orbital cavities. The two conchae are scroll-shaped. They form the side wall of the nasal cavity, and together, they increase the surface area of the nasal cavity allowing inspired air to be warmed and humidified more effectively. The mandible is the lower jaw which holds the teeth and is the only movable bone of the skull.

3.6.3. Joints

Joints are the junction between two or more bones. Some joints do not normally move, such as those located between the plates of the skull. Other joints allow a large and complex range of motion. The configuration of a joint determines the degree and direction of possible motion. For example, the shoulder joints, which have a ball-and-socket design, allow inward and outward rotation as well as forward, backward, and sideways motion of the arms. Hinge joints of the knees, fingers, and toes allow only bending (flexion) and straightening (extension). The components of joints provide stability and reduce the risk of damage from constant use. In a joint, the ends of the bones are covered with cartilage—a smooth, tough, resilient, and protective tissue composed of collagen, water, and proteoglycans that reduce friction as joints move.

Bursa

Bursae are small fluid-filled sacs that can lie under a tendon, cushioning the tendon and protecting it from injury. Bursae also provide extra cushioning to adjacent structures that otherwise might rub against each other, causing wear and tear—for example, between a bone and a ligament or a bony prominence and overlying skin (such as in the elbow, kneecap, or shoulder area).

Tendons

Tendons are tough bands of connective tissue made up mostly of a rigid protein called collagen. Tendons firmly attach each end of a muscle to a bone. They are often located within sheaths, which are lubricated to allow the tendons to move without friction.

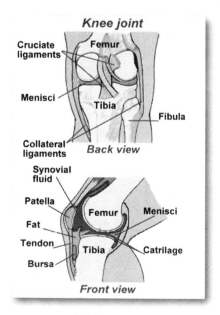

Ligaments

Ligaments are tough fibrous cords composed of connective tissue that contains both collagen and elastic fibres. The elastic fibres allow the ligaments to stretch to some extent. Ligaments surround joints and bind them together. They help strengthen and stabilise joints, permitting movement only in certain directions. Ligaments also connect one bone to another (such as inside the knee).

3.7. The Spinal column

The spine or backbone (also called the vertebral column or spinal column) is composed of a series of bones called vertebrae stacked one upon another. The spine runs from the base of the skull to the pelvis. It serves as a pillar to support the body's weight and to protect the spinal cord. There are four regions of the spine: Cervical (neck), thoracic (chest/trunk), lumbar (low back), and sacral (pelvic). There are three natural curves in the spine that give it an 'S' shape when viewed from the side. These curves help the spine withstand great amounts of stress by providing a more even distribution of body weight.

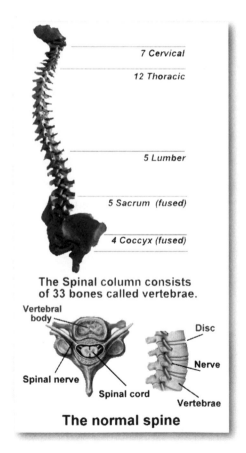

7 Cervical

12 Thoracic

5 Lumber

5 Sacrum (fused)

4 Coccyx (fused)

The Spinal column consists of 33 bones called vertebrae.

Vertebral body

Disc

Nerve

Spinal nerve

Spinal cord

Vertebrae

The normal spine

Cervical spine

The cervical spine is made up of seven cervical vertebrae. These are the smallest vertebrae. The main function of the cervical spine is to support the weight of the head which is approximately 10-12 lb. The first cervical vertebra, the atlas, is the bone on which the skull rests on. The cervical spine has the greatest range of motion.

Thoracic spine

The main function of thoracic spine is to protect the organs of the chest, especially the heart and lungs. There are twelve thoracic vertebrae with one rib attached on each side, to create a thoracic cage, which protects the internal organs of the chest.

The lumbar spine

The **lumbar spine** has five lumbar vertebrae, which are the largest vertebrae. These vertebrae are also aligned in a reverse 'C' like the cervical spine, creating a normal lumbar lordosis. The five lumbar vertebral bodies are the weight-bearing portion of the spine and are the largest in diameter compared to the thoracic and cervical vertebral bodies.

The sacrum

The **sacrum** is somewhat triangular in appearance. It is made up of five naturally fused vertebrae. The sacrum connects the spine to the pelvis and the lower half of the skeleton.

The coccyx

The coccyx (sometimes referred to as the tailbone) situated at the end of the sacrum consists of four terminal vertebrae fused to form a small triangular bone.

Intervertebral discs

Intervertebral discs (inter means 'between' or 'within') are flat, round cushioning pads that sit between the vertebrae and act as shock absorbers. Each intervertebral disc is made of very strong tissue, with a soft, gel-like centre called the nucleus pulposus surrounded by a tough outer layer called the annulus. When a disc breaks or herniates (bulges), some of the soft nucleus pulposus seeps out through a tear in the annulus. This can result in pain when the nucleus pulposus puts pressure on nerves.

The spinal cord

The spinal cord, the column of nerve fibres responsible for sending and receiving messages from the brain, runs through the spinal canal. It is through the spinal cord and its branching nerves that the brain influences the rest of the body, controlling movement and organ function. As the spinal cord runs through the spinal canal, it branches off into thirty-one pairs of nerve roots, which then branch out into nerves that travel to the rest of the body. The nerve roots leave the spinal cord through openings called neural foramen, which are found between the vertebrae on both sides of the spine. The nerves of the cervical spine control the upper chest and arms. The nerves of the thoracic spine control the chest and abdomen, and the nerves of the lumbar spine control the legs, bowel, and bladder.

3.8. The Nervous System

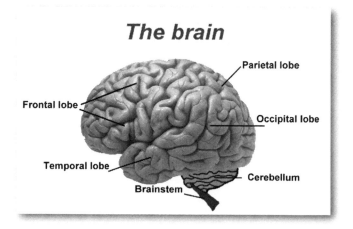

The brain

Parietal lobe

Frontal lobe

Occipital lobe

Temporal lobe

Cerebellum

Brainstem

The nervous system is what governs the functions of the body. It consists of the brain, the spinal cord, and all the individual nerves that extend throughout the body. The brain is where everything happens. Damage any part of it and it will prevent some part of the body from working. Your brain controls everything you do both in a voluntary (what you do consciously) and involuntary (automatic) capacity. Without getting too deep in human physiology, it is still important to understand what the brain regulates.

The brain stem

The brain stem is approximately the thickness of a pencil and controls the involuntary muscles such as breathing, heart rate, swallowing, and reflexes to seeing and hearing (startle response); controls sweating, blood pressure, digestion, and temperature (autonomic nervous system); and affects level of alertness, ability to sleep, and sense of balance (vestibular function).

The cerebrum

The cerebrum is the thinking part of the brain, and it controls your voluntary muscles—the ones that move when you want them to. Your memory lives in the cerebrum—both short-term and long-term memory. When you're thinking hard, you're using your cerebrum. The cerebrum has two halves, with one on either side of the head. The right half of the cerebrum controls the left side of your body, and the left half controls the right side. The cerebrum makes up 85% of the brain's weight.

The frontal lobe

The frontal lobe is responsible for concentration, emotional control, temperament, and goal-directed behaviour. Other functions include motor projection and association, coordination of messages from other lobes, and complex problem solving. It controls our speaking language, how we initiate activity in response to our environment, and judgments we make about what occurs in our daily activities.

Parietal lobe

The parietal lobe controls location for visual attention and touch perception and goal-directed voluntary movements and manipulation of objects. Another function is the integration of different senses that allows for understanding a single concept.

Occipital lobe

The occipital lobe receives and processes visual information.

Temporal lobe

The temporal lobe governs our hearing ability, memory acquisition, categorisation of objects, and some visual perceptions. It is also responsible for the function of our emotion and motivation and some language comprehension.

The cerebellum

The cerebellum is responsible for coordination of voluntary movement, balance and equilibrium, and some memory for reflex motor acts.

3.9. The Digestive System

The digestive system breaks down the food we eat, extracting nutrients and assimilating them for use throughout the body. Proper digestive-system function is essential for maintaining good health and energy levels. The body requires nutrients from all three-food categories (proteins, carbohydrates, and fats) to survive.

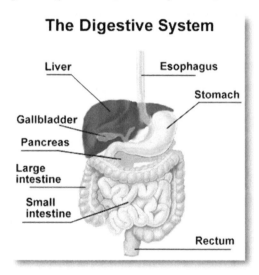

3.9.1. Activities of the Digestive System

This can be divided into five main headings.

Ingestion

This means taking in food into the alimentary tract by eating or drinking. Propulsion: This mixes and moves the contents along the alimentary tract.

Digestion

This comes about by the mechanical breakdown of food by mastication (chewing) and chemical digestion of food into small molecules by enzymes present in secretions produced by glands and other associated organs of the digestive system.

Absorption

This is when digested food substances pass through the walls of some organs of the alimentary canal into the blood and lymph capillaries for circulation and use by body cells.

Elimination

This is when food substances are eaten but are unable to be digested and absorbed is excreted from the alimentary canal as faeces by the process of defecation.

Alimentary tract

This is also known as the gastrointestinal (GI) tract and sometimes referred to as the digestive tract. It is approximately 35 feet long. It starts at the mouth and continues through the pharynx (throat), oesophagus (food tube), stomach, small and large intestine, rectum, and anal canal.

Accessory organs

Besides the digestive tract, the digestive system also includes the liver, the pancreas, and the gallbladder. One of the functions of the liver is to produce bile. Bile is stored in the gallbladder and released into the small intestine to help digest fats. The pancreas also has several digestive functions, but it is best known for the production of a hormone called insulin. Insulin is released directly into the bloodstream and helps with the body's usage of sugar. A disruption in the production of insulin causes diabetes.

3.10. The Skin

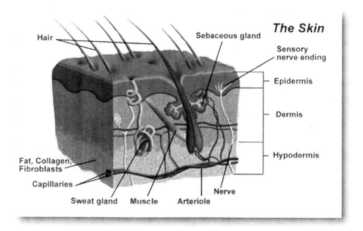

The skin completely covers the body. It protects the underlying structures from injury, bacteria, and viruses as long as it's not damaged. It is the largest organ in the body containing glands, hair, and nails. Our skin also regulates the internal temperature of our body. If the body gets too hot, the small blood vessels close to the skin dilate allowing more body heat to the surface where heat can be transferred to the air. Sweating is another source of cooling as it becomes released through the pores and evaporates. If we get cold, the blood vessels near the skin surface contract, transferring more body heat to the core of the body. The skin receives information from the environment such as degrees of cold and heat by special sensors. This information is then transmitted through the nerves and spinal cord to the brain where it interprets these sensations.

3.10.1. Three Layers

There are three main layers: the epidermis, dermis, and subcutaneous tissue.

The Epidermis

The epidermis (from the Greek Epi meaning on top, and derma meaning the skin) is the skin's outer structure which has a protective function. There are no blood vessels or nerve endings on the surface of the epidermis, but its deeper layers are moistened with fluid from the dermis which provides oxygen and nutrients. The epidermis varies in thickness and is at its thickest on the palms of the hands and the soles of the feet.

The Dermis

The dermis is the innermost section of the skin. The dermis contains blood and lymph vessels, nerves, sweat and oil glands, hair follicles, and arrector pili muscles. Arrector pili are tiny, smooth muscles attached to hair follicles, which cause the hair to stand upright when activated. The dermis nourishes and supplies blood to the epidermis.

Hypodermis

The hypodermis, also known as subcutaneous tissue, is the third of the three layers of skin. The subcutaneous layer contains fat and connective tissue that houses larger blood vessels and nerves. This layer is important in the regulation of temperature of the skin itself and the body. The size of this layer varies throughout the body and from person to person. It also thins with age.

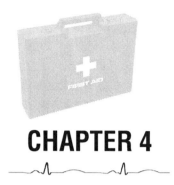

CHAPTER 4

4.1. Assessing the Casualty

Once you have made sure the scene is safe, you are now in a position to do your patient assessment. It is important to be able to perform a systematic patient assessment in order to determine the nature of their injuries or illness and to determine whether the complaint is serious and life-threatening or not.

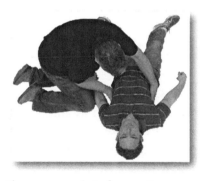

When performing your assessment, gather as much information as possible so that the casualty will get the level of care required. It's a good idea to practice this systematic approach to increase speed and accuracy of the process, but good judgement is also required. Although described in sequence, some of the steps may be taken simultaneously. The aim of good primary care is to prevent early trauma mortality. Early trauma deaths occur because of failure of oxygenation of vital organs or uncontrolled bleeding.

To assist you in your performance of patient assessment and treatment, you will find the more commonly used CPG algorithms associated with OFA, CFR, and EFR in the final section of this book under Clinical Practice Guidelines. These will give you step-by-step sequential assistance on how to access and treat a patient. CPGs are an invaluable resource and should be referred to for guidance. They are the practitioner's bible, and you will find a copy of these guidelines in every ambulance in the country.

Approaching the scene can tell you a lot. For example, if the casualty is lying on the ground at the bottom of a ladder, you might suspect fractures, a head injury, or a spinal injury. Is the casualty conscious or not, or will it turn out to be only a bruise or a sprain, depending on how far up the ladder they were before the fall? Nevertheless, because of what you see, all these things must be flagged as possibilities. You can apply this way of thinking to any scenario.

How the patient looks to you is very important. Do they look anxious? Are they what we call guarding a particular part of the body such as holding their hand or hands to protect their ribs or abdomen, or supporting a limb? Are they pale or sweaty? Are they having trouble breathing? Do they appear to be shivering? Can you see any obvious deformities or blood? When you take their hand, is it cold? Is there a smell from their breath? Sometimes we ignore the obvious. If they are able to speak, ask them what happened. It may be a medical problem that is ongoing. They may require assistance with their medication. For example, they may be diabetic or have a heart condition, or they may simply have had one drink too many. A lot of this information can be gained within seconds by just observing and perhaps talking to a witness or bystander as you carry out your scene size up.

Because we never stop reminding ourselves about scene safety, the first thing we must do before assessing the patient is to secure or make safe whatever hazard that might be potentially dangerous to both you and the patient. Good observation to establish what we call the mechanism of injury (MOI) is the key to a positive outcome. Remember, the aim of this initial evaluation or assessment is to stabilise the patient, identify life-threatening conditions in order of risk, and initiate supportive treatment. Consider also what other resources apart from the ambulance service are required such as Fire and Rescue or the police. Do you need to turn off electricity or gas? Is there a dog involved?

Remember, a dog will assume you are harming its master and may attack. If a dog is a threat, wait for help.

Good communication with your patient is also very important. Talking in a calm and controlled voice and explaining your actions can be very reassuring. It's worth remembering that even if the patient is unconscious, they may still hear you, so speak to them as if they were conscious and be careful what you say. Tell your patient the truth. If they ask a question about their condition, answer as best you can and don't make guesses. If you can't answer, say so. Don't fake it.

Standing over a patient regardless of age and talking down to them can be very intimidating. Bring yourself down to their level and try to make eye contact. If it gives them comfort to talk about football, the weather, or whatever, it can calm your patient and you gain their trust in return.

4.2. Primary Survey

The purpose of a primary survey is to locate and treat all life-threatening injuries. In order to do this, there must be a structured sequence to help you remember all the steps that make up this primary survey. For this, we use the first four letters of the alphabet. Indeed throughout this entire book, you will find that certain sections of the alphabet are used quite a lot. We also use various acronyms to help us remember sequential examinations. This method is standard in all levels of healthcare.

AVPU Scale		
A	Alert	Patient is fully alert and responsive.
V	Responsive to voice.	Patient unable to respond spontaneously but responds to voice.
P	Responsive to pain.	Patient is not alert and only responds to pain stimulus.
U	Unresponsive.	Patient unconscious and unresponsive, it's time to call 999 / 112.
When the patient is V, P or U on the AVPU scale, they must be transported to a hospital.		

Remember that Body Substance Isolation (BSI) is always important.

(A) Airway. Is the airway open and clear? In the case of trauma, you should consider the possibility of cervical spine (C-Spine) injury.

(B) Breathing. Is breathing present? Is it impaired? Is it fast or slow, or absent?

If you are a Cardiac First Responder-Advanced (CFR-A) or Emergency First Responder (EFR), you should consider Oxygen (O2) if breathing is inadequate.

(C) Circulation. Does the patient have a pulse? Is it fast or slow, strong or weak? Are they bleeding?

(D) Disability. Are they responsive? What is that response level (Use the AVPU Scale). The ABCD sequence has one simple rule. If 'A' isn't working, there's no point moving on to B until you fix 'A' first. Likewise with 'B', if your patient isn't breathing, you need to find out the reason. It's common sense. If the airway is blocked, you need to clear it; otherwise, they can't breathe. If the airway is clear and he's still not breathing, you need to start CPR and so on (Ref: CPG's Primary Survey—Adult).

Putting it together

When approaching an accident or an incident, remember, scene safety, gloves on. If the casualty appears conscious, introduce yourself as you approach. This will give you an indication of their level of consciousness (LOC). Try to approach from the front making eye contact so that the casualty won't be startled and have to turn their head to see you. If there is a suspected spinal injury, you don't want to aggravate it. If they are talking to you, you know that they at least have a patent airway and they are breathing. Just how well they're breathing is what you have to eventually determine. If the patient appears to be unconscious, try to determine their level of response (if any), keeping in mind that this may be a trauma situation. If you tap them and shout in their ear, the patient may be startled and move the head. This is not a good idea as you want to keep their head and neck in the position you found it in.

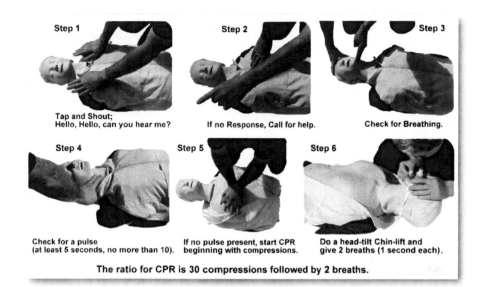

Step 1
Tap and Shout;
Hello, Hello, can you hear me?

Step 2
If no Response, Call for help.

Step 3
Check for Breathing.

Step 4
Check for a pulse
(at least 5 seconds, no more than 10).

Step 5
If no pulse present, start CPR
beginning with compressions.

Step 6
Do a head-tilt Chin-lift and
give 2 breaths (1 second each).

The ratio for CPR is 30 compressions followed by 2 breaths.

To assess this patient, if they are lying on the ground, you need to kneel down by their side. Check the ground for sharp objects or body fluids before kneeling as you don't want to injure yourself or be contaminated. Hold the patients head in position and then shout (not too loud) near their ear, 'Are you OK?' If the patient is in a sitting position, come down to their level so you are looking directly at them. Hold the head in the position it was in with both hands and then shout, 'Are you OK?' Realistically, an unresponsive casualty needs to be lying flat if possible on the ground in order to properly assess them and maintain a patent (open) airway. Just remember, if you must lay a casualty on the ground, be gentle, especially if you're dealing with a trauma patient as the head and neck should be protected from any unnecessary movement until a cervical collar is fitted. Fitting a cervical collar is a skillset only carried out at practitioner level and should never be attempted by a first aider or responder. Cervical Spine immobilisation will be done as a precaution by the emergency services on arrival as it is standard practice when dealing with a trauma patient. If there is no response to your verbal stimulus and you are still on your own, you need to call for help. Where two responders are dealing with this situation, one would hold the head, and the other would tap the patient's shoulders and shout, 'Are you OK?' Again, if there is no response, call for help (999/112). If your patient is conscious, and there are no C-Spine issues, you should allow them to adopt whatever position is most comfortable for them. However, if they are in shock, lay them down and raise their legs unless there is an injury. Once help is on the way, you can now continue your primary survey. It is better to assume that all trauma patients have spinal issues and should be handled with this in mind. Better sure than sorry!

Start with the airway (A). Is it clear? If yes, is he breathing (B)? If he is, how well is he breathing? Is it fast or slow? Is it deep or shallow? Can you see chest rise? Make notes to compare later! Now were on to (C) circulation. Is there a pulse? It's not a sure bet that you will be able to locate a pulse even if there is one but if you can find it, great!. In an out of hospital setting, healthcare professionals sometimes find it difficult to do this and they are trained.

If we have established that the patient is breathing, then it's a sure bet that they have a pulse of some sort. Circulation is all about blood, and it's supposed to travel around inside the body through blood vessels. However, if the patient is bleeding and it's severe, you need to stop it using direct or indirect pressure. Blood loss is the main preventable cause of death after trauma. Does their skin colour look OK? Now we're on to (D) disability (known also as mental status). This is where we use the AVPU scale.

The AVPU scale is used to determine the response level of the patient and to establish if they are they aware of their situation and surroundings. Are they responsive (A)? Did they respond to verbal stimulus (V)? Did they respond only to pain stimulus (P)? Or are they unresponsive (U)? Again, make a note. It's also important to note the time you started treatment, and also note the time if the patient got better or worse. If your patient is unconscious, there are several common reasons that may have caused the event. If a family member or friend was with them at the time of the collapse, they may know of any medical conditions, saving you valuable time in making your diagnosis. Or perhaps the event was witnessed by a passer-by. They would still be able to give you valuable information, for example, they may have seen the victim fall from a height, or they may have seen them grasping their chest before they collapsed indicating that they may have had a heart attack. Alternatively, if the event was un-witnessed, you could use the FISHSHAPED acronym to guide you through your process of elimination.

FISHSHAPED stands for fainting, intoxication, stroke, sepsis (infection), heart attack, shock, heat imbalance, anaphylaxis, poisoning, epilepsy, and diabetes.

4.3. Secondary Survey

This is the more detailed part of your assessment made up of two separate components comprising of a physical examination and obtaining a patient history (see CPG's Secondary Survey Trauma or Medical, whichever applies). A responder or first-aider working with the voluntary services doing this regularly will be able to carry out both components simultaneously. It does take practice to be able to focus on examining the patient while gathering their history at the same time, so for simplicity, we will take the two components separately. If you are dealing with a trauma patient, remember gloves on (BSI). Following on from your primary survey, if there were any minor or obvious injuries uncovered, now would be the time to treat them. If you have a partner, one of you should treat while the other continues the survey, recording the vital signs as they go.

The next part is to record the patient's history. This is the gathering of the patient's present symptoms, the event, and their medical history in a structured format. This is known as the SAMPLE history. The SAMPLE acronym is standard in healthcare. EMS may ask you as a matter of form for a sample history when they arrive. It's a brilliant memory aid to help you gather information. The key to getting a history is based on good relationship, asking questions in a sympathetic, non-judgemental, and logical manner. Listen to what the patient tells you, interrupt appropriately, make a note of what you see, hear, smell, and touch, and try to correctly interpret the information you have gathered.

SAMPLE history

S—Signs and symptoms

Signs are what you see. Symptoms are what the patient tells you. Don't put words into the patient's mouth; let them describe their symptoms in their own words.

A—Allergies

Is the patient allergic to any particular medication, food, or bee stings? Are they wearing a medical alert bracelet or pendant?

M—Medications

Is the patient on prescribed medication? Are they taking any non-prescription medicines? Are they taking herbal remedies? Some herbal remedies can have a medical quality and may have an effect on a particular treatment. Have they taken medication and when? The patient or witness may deny if drugs or excess alcohol was taken for legal reasons. This has implications for diagnosis.

P—Pertinent medical history

Does the patient have an existing medical history? For example, does the patient have a heart condition, diabetes, breathing problems, hypertension, and vertigo? Do they suffer from epilepsy? If so, are any of those symptoms related to the patient's current complaint?

L—Last oral intake

When was the last time the patient had anything to eat or drink? What did they eat and how much? What did they drink? Did they drink alcohol, how much?

E—Event

What was the patient doing that led to the injury or illness? The sequence of events that led to the event will give you a clue to what caused the problem. If the patient was found in an unconscious state, did they faint, trip, and bang their head? Did they complain of chest pain or headache? Were they drinking alcohol? If the patient was a diabetic, have they taken their insulin? Have they eaten lately? Where they exercising too vigorously? All this information is important.

When trying to decipher the patient's symptoms, it is not uncommon to discover that the patient may have more than one. What you must try to ascertain is what symptom led to their present complaint. If, for example, the patient banged their toe off a solid object, tripped, and as a result, fell and grazed the palms of their hands while getting to the phone to call for help because they had chest pain and felt light-headed, which one would be the bigger problem? Did the patient tell you or anyone else about the chest pain, or were they distracted by the other events? Perhaps the focus would be more on the pain in the toe and the grazed hands than on the chest pain because you can see the grazes and a little blood, and the toe is throbbing. These secondary injuries are called distraction injuries for obvious reasons. This is why you must ask all the right questions and not let the obvious distract you. Take them back to the start and get to the original or chief complaint. A few cuts and bruises won't kill them, but that chest pain needs attention.

Each problem must be discussed in detail with the patient and documented. Let the patient tell the story in his or her own words. Don't let them ramble off the subject. If they do, bring them back tactfully and keep them focused. When they have told you as much as they can, it's now your turn. Based on what you have heard, you can now home in on certain things they said and get them to elaborate more to help you make a diagnosis. Write everything down. You can put your information in chronological order later if there is more than one injury or medical complaint. The main thing is to sieve through all the information to get to the root of the problem, which is the chief complaint.

Physical examination

As part of your secondary survey, depending on whether your patient is conscious, semiconscious, or unresponsive, there are two approaches to this examination. You may be lucky with a responsive patient that while in the process of acquiring their SAMPLE history, they tell you something or you see something that leads you to discover that the complaint is not life-threatening and you don't need to investigate further. You should still call EMS if you have any doubts as it is sometimes possible to misinterpret your findings. It's no reflection on your skills; all you are doing is getting a second opinion from a higher level. It's always better to be sure than sorry!

However, in the case of an unresponsive patient, you may have some investigating to do. Exposing a patient is only done when necessary such as in the case of trauma or to carry out CPR. If such an incident happens in a public place, try to be tactful and only expose what you need to expose to treat the patient. Remember, we live in the age of technology where even a child has a mobile phone with a camera, so you don't want to see your actions played out on the internet. Having said that, it's all down to the nature of the incident and the severity of the injuries as to how much clothing has to go. You can only do your best but remember, modesty can kill too, so if it's necessary to expose the patient to find and treat the injury, do it! It's great when help arrives to support you, as dealing with a casualty can be stressful 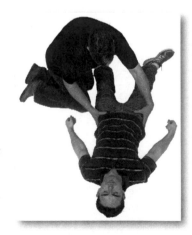 if it's not something you do every day. By sticking to a tried and tested standard sequence for examination (CPGs) as described in this book, you'll remember most of it, if not all when the time comes. The key is practice!

In the unconscious patient, if nothing is immediately apparent, continue on to the next step in the sequence known as the head-to-toe survey. This is a full hands-on examination and is very thorough, used on both responsive and unresponsive patients. If you're examining a conscious patient, look for a reaction to your actions. Ask the patient what they feel as you work your way down. Sometimes the unconscious patient may moan or grimace. Always assume the trauma patient has a spinal injury, so before you start, be sure to immobilise the head. A second first-aider or responder can keep the head from moving by holding it between the palms of their hands until EMS arrives. This is a very responsible job, so be comfortable before you start. It's best to lay down flat on your stomach so that your elbows are supported on the ground. Crouching down or kneeling isn't appropriate as you may be knocked off balance. Assuming you are satisfied that the patient has a clear airway and breathing adequately, carry on to the next step. For the head-to-toe survey, we use another acronym known as DCAP-BTLS. Everywhere you lay your hand from head to toe, you will be looking for DCAP-BTLS.

DCAP-BTLS

D—Deformities

A deformity is anything that structurally changes the normal shape of the body. The simplest example is a broken bone. This deformity can be very noticeable in some cases such as a bulge under the skin (closed fracture) or the bone may puncture the skin and stick out (open fracture). Dislocations and soft tissue swelling are also classed as deformities. Other less noticeable but palpable deformities are bone fragments. This happens when bone shatters as a result of blunt force trauma. When you palpate (feel) the area, you will feel the bone fragments grating off each other. This is known as crepitus.

C—Contusions

A contusion is a bruise. This is an injury without a break in the skin sometimes caused by blunt force, causing the capillaries or other blood vessels to leak or rupture. This is noticeable as a swelling due to leakage of plasma into the affected area. This will be tender and painful to the touch and may be followed by blood leakage from damaged vessels. When you see an area of skin that is black or blue, this is your classic sign of a contusion or bruise. When blood collects under the skin, it is known as a hematoma.

A—Abrasions

An abrasion is basically a scrape to the skin's surface. How often as a child did you trip and fall and skin your knee or elbow or the palm of your hand while trying to break your fall? This is an abrasion. Although painful, abrasions don't bleed that much. They tend to weep or ooze more than flow, so there is no significant blood loss. The thing to remember with about abrasions is that the skin is broken and open to infection, so it should be cleaned and dressed as soon as possible.

P—Punctures

Punctures can be deceptive, and although they are caused by sharp objects penetrating the skin, the depth of the puncture and the direction of the object determine the seriousness of the injury. This kind of injury involving nails is common in building sites. Splinters are also common as are thorns if you are a gardener. An injection is a puncture! Even a bee sting punctures the skin, so a puncture wound can be caused by a variety of objects. If an object is deeply bedded, it's best to secure it in place and seek medical assistance.

B—Burns

A burn can be caused by chemical, thermal, or electrical injury. There are three categories which are rated according to the depth of the burn. These are superficial (first degree) whereby the outer part of the skin (epidermis) is only burnt to a point that the skin is reddened. A perfect example of this is sunburn. Partial thickness burn (second degree) involves the outer part of the skin and the layer underneath (dermis). This is characterised by blistering which may or may not have redness. Finally, there is full thickness (third degree). This is very serious as the damage in most cases is irreversible. This type of burn has burnt through all the layers and may look black or charred, brown or dark red. It can even look translucent. In certain cases, veins and bone can be exposed. It is highly likely if they are conscious, the patient will feel no pain due to the nerves being burnt. This particular type of burn or indeed any burn where the skin has broken is very susceptible to infection.

T—Tenderness

Tenderness is the pain provoked by touching (palpation) the injured area. When you are feeling or palpating for underlying injuries, be mindful that when you find the injured area, you will aggravate it immensely, so be as gentle as possible.

L—Lacerations

Lacerations are generally caused by blunt or jagged objects such as barbed wire, saws, jagged metal, etc. A laceration tears the skin leaving the wound with jagged or irregular edges, whereas compared with an injury caused by a sharp object, the cut will be clean and easier to close and do less damage to surrounding areas. Because of the nature of a laceration, it tends to do more damage both to the injury locally and the surrounding area depending on the depth.

S—Swelling

Swelling is an abnormal enlargement of a body part or organ. This is caused by increased volume of fluid in blood vessels. Swelling can be quiet obvious during palpation because the indentations of your fingers will leave an imprint on the skin for a short time after palpation.

Putting DCAP-BTLS into action

Known officially as the 90-second head-to-toe examination, this is sometimes referred to as the 90-second quick feel! It doesn't matter what you call it once you can remember it. The DCAP-BTLS examination sequence seems like a lot to get through in ninety seconds, but in reality, that's all it takes.

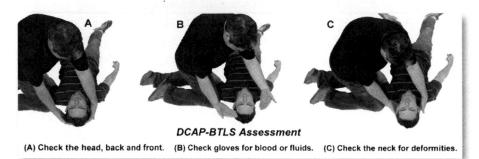

DCAP-BTLS Assessment

(A) Check the head, back and front.   (B) Check gloves for blood or fluids.   (C) Check the neck for deformities.

Starting with the head: Check for DCAP-BTLS. Look for visible signs such as blood on the scalp. Without moving the head, try to get your fingers underneath so that you can feel for any deformities or fluid. Check our gloves. Check the mouth for blood, vomit, or other fluids. Check the teeth. Are they intact? Is there any swelling or debris that may compromise the airway? Check behind the ears for bruising (battle signs). Check around the eyes for bruising (Raccoon eyes). This type of bruising could indicate a skull fracture. Look in the ears and nose for a yellow-tinged blood. You may notice a straw-coloured fluid (cerebral spinal fluid or CSF) weeping from the ears although it is more likely as with the nose to be mixed with blood. This is another sign of a skull fracture. If you suspect CSF to be present but are unsure due to the presence of blood, dip the end of a roller bandage in the blood and hold it up to the light. If CSF is present, a rainbow like pattern will be present on the bandage. Look in the eyes. Do they appear to be puffed or red-looking? Is there any blood or pus? Do the whites of the eyes look yellow (jaundiced)?

Moving on to the neck: Is there a medical alert pendent? Check for DCAP-BTLS. Pay particular attention to the neck and throat. Distended neck veins can be an indication of heart failure. Patients with right ventricular failure have jugular venous distension (JVD). JVD is also a sign of cardiac tapenade. This is the compression of the heart that occurs when blood or fluid builds up in the space between the heart muscle (myocardium) and the outer covering sac of the heart known as the pericardium. JVD can also be an indicator of a punctured lung (tension pneumothorax). A much later indicator of a punctured lung would be what is known as tracheal deviation. The trachea is the tube that carries air from the throat to the lungs commonly referred to as the windpipe. The most common cause of tracheal deviation is a pneumothorax, which is a collection of air inside the chest, between the chest cavity and the lung caused by either existing lung disease or as the result of a chest injury. Another common cause of tracheal deviation is a collapsed lung. When a lung has collapsed, the trachea or windpipe will shift toward the affected side. When you look at the windpipe, it should be in a straight line. If it is deviated or out of line, this is a late sign and the patient at this stage is seriously ill and time is not on their side.

Next, we move to the torso. Here, we examine the chest and abdomen. Again we apply DCAP-BTLS. Palpate the chest wall looking for deformities by fanning out your fingers as you work your way down the sternum (breastbone) and ribcage. Don't be afraid to apply a certain amount of pressure during palpation as sometimes depending on the size and weight of the patient, it can be difficult to diagnose a rib fracture. Be sure to get your hands as far under the patient as possible without moving them to check their back. Look at your gloves as there may be blood, indicating a wound which could be life-threatening. Treat as you find as quickly as possible and move on. Check for bilateral chest rise both visually and by palpation. Always compare one side of the chest with the other. This will help you notice any differences that may exist. Place your thumbs so that they touch together on the sternum as the patient exhales. As the patient inhales, your thumbs should move apart equally giving you an indication that both sides are symmetrical and also you should get a good indication of their depth of breathing. As you move on to the abdomen, apply DCAP-BTLS. What you're looking for here are indications that suggest organ damage or internal bleeding. You will be palpating for tenderness, rigidity, or distension.

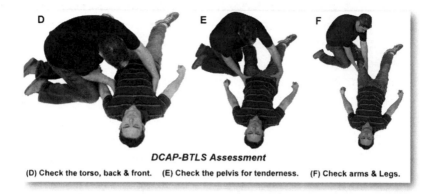

DCAP-BTLS Assessment

(D) Check the torso, back & front.   (E) Check the pelvis for tenderness.   (F) Check arms & Legs.

Now, we move down to the pelvis: Apply DCAP-BTLS. When examining the pelvis, the first-aider needs to be careful. Any unnecessary movement can cause significant blood loss. First, study at the Mechanism of injury (MOI) and the position of the patient to help you form part of your general impression. If the patient is conscious, ask them if they feel pain in the pelvic area or with their consent, *lightly* (and I stress the word lightly) feel for tenderness. If the patient is unconscious, and you are suspicious due to the MOI, then treat as a fracture. These are the new guidelines for pelvic assessment. Under no circumstances should you check for give or movement by pushing downwards or inwards. It's far better to assume there is a fracture and be told afterwards you were wrong. There's no shame in being wrong for all the right reasons! If the pelvis is completely broken, it is known as an open book fracture. The feet will be rotated and will have an open book like posture. For more detailed information, see section on pelvic fractures.

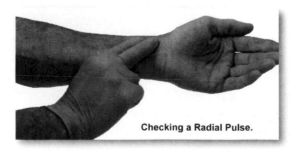

Checking a Radial Pulse.

Next, we examine the legs and hands. Once again using DCAP-BTLS, work your way from the groin down each leg,

checking front and back, again, check your gloves. Expose the feet and check for circulation, sensation, and movement (CSMs). Check for circulation first by checking the colour. It should be pink which is normal and not pale or cyanosed. Check for a pulse, palpable at the prominent arch of the top of the foot. Squeeze the toenail. When you squeeze the toenail, the nail bed should go white, and when you release the pressure, the colour should return within three seconds.

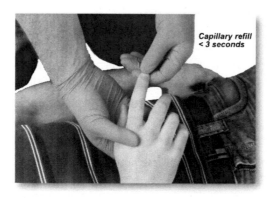

Capillary refill
< 3 seconds

This is known as capillary refill. It is worth noting; if the patient is hypothermic, capillary refill will be either very slow or non-existent. This will be dealt with in detail when we look at shock. If the patient is conscious, you can check for sensation by touching the area below the injury and compare the sensation with the same area on the other limb. Check movement by asking the patient to move their toes. Next, we move up to the shoulders checking the collar bones, again if unsure, comparing both sides. Check both arms and hands front and back. Is the patient wearing a medical alert bracelet? Check CSMs. Check a radial pulse on both wrists. Check capillary refill on the fingernails. Check sensation

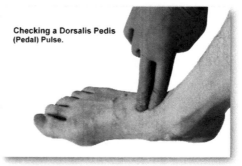

Checking a Dorsalis Pedis (Pedal) Pulse.

and movement. Note anything out of the ordinary. All this takes in or around ninety seconds to complete.

Providing ongoing assessment

The assessment is designed to determine the initial condition of your patient. However, things can change when you least expect them to. Your patient may appear stable one minute and become unstable the next. Therefore, it is important to keep a careful eye on them for any changes. These changes may be subtle or rapid depending on the circumstances. Normally, you should monitor your patient's vital signs every fifteen minutes. This includes airway, breathing, and pulse for quality and rate. Also check skin tone and temperature. Temperature is checked by un-gloving the back of your hand and placing it on the patient's forehead. If your patient is unstable, you should check their vitals every five minutes. If the condition of your patient changes, repeat your physical examination from scratch, checking all your interventions for effectiveness, and compare notes. If your patient is conscious, talk to them and tell them what you are doing. Keep reassuring them.

4.4. Paediatric Assessment Triangle

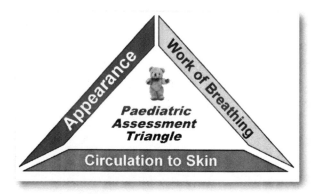

Paediatric assessment is somewhat different in its approach. An infant, for example, can't tell you how it feels, so you must rely on doorway observations. By doorway observations, I mean that you will conduct the bulk of your assessment as you enter the room. At a glance, you should assess the infant or child's environment for any signs of what may have caused the injury or what might have attributed to their illness.

There are a few important differences in the anatomy and physiology of an infant or child compared to that of an adult that you should consider when dealing with paediatrics. For example, when opening an adult's airway, we lift the chin and tilt the head well back. If we do this to an infant or small child, we could kink the trachea (airway) as it is still soft and not fully developed; therefore, when opening the airway, the head and neck should be kept in the neutral position or just marginally beyond it to what we refer to as the sniffing position. The tongue in relation to the airway is also large and is more than capable of blocking the airway in an unconscious child. New-born infants are considered obligate nasal breathers and are dependent on a patent (open/ clear)) nasal airway for ventilation for the first few months of life. New-borns will only breathe through their mouth when crying. If the responder has to administer oxygen, it should be humidified as it will help to loosen any secretions and clear the nasal passage. In fact, only humidified oxygen should be administered to children below eight years of age to prevent the mouth and airway from drying out, especially if they are suffering an attack of croup, asthma, or other respiratory conditions. An infant's head is larger also and should be protected from bobbing around. Apart from its weight, an infant's skull is not yet fully formed as one unit. It is in fact in five sections separated by soft membranes known as fontanels (also spelt fontanelle) or soft spots which enable the skull to flex allowing the head to pass through the birth canal during birth. The five cranial bones not yet fused together are the two frontal bones, two parietal bones, and one occipital bone. Even suctioning of an infant is carried out through the nasal passage, whereas in older children and adults, we suction through the mouth. So now you understand why we must look differently and handle more carefully when dealing with infants and children. To guide you in your assessment, we use what is known as the paediatric assessment triangle.

The paediatric assessment triangle or PAT for short is an important tool when dealing with young children and infants and can be completed in less than a minute. In that short space of time, you should be able to form a general impression. The assessment is based on three key points which are *appearance*, *work of breathing*, and *circulation* to skin. Because there is no hard and fast rule about which part of the assessment comes first, you can tailor it to suit yourself.

Appearance

Assessing appearance is generally done from a short distance (doorway observation). Remember that you are a stranger as far as the child is concerned, and they may react negatively toward you. They may get more upset if you have to physically examine them, but take that into account as this would be normal behaviour for some children. They may even go all shy on you and want to hide their face and that's normal too. Have a parent or someone they are familiar with hold the child on their lap, and gradually, with their help, you may gain the child's confidence. Spare a thought for the parent as they may be upset also and a bit of reassurance should be directed in their direction as well.

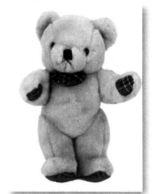

Use the child's favourite toy, call their name, or shine your pen torch in their direction to assess alertness. Your main concerns are ABC. If the child is screaming or crying out loud and jumping around, then things are good as this tells you that they have a patent airway, their breathing is adequate, and because they are moving about, their circulation is good and they have no immediate life-threatening problems. The fact that the child is jumping around also tells you that they do not have appendicitis or meningitis or other severe infections. If they did, they would be much quieter and lying still or would be far more upset.

Other things to look for are that the extremities move spontaneously with good muscle tone and that they can maintain good eye contact with objects such as your pen torch or a toy or their parent, or if they can be calmed easily. All these are good signs. You don't want a limp or floppy child that is drowsy, has no energy, or shows no interest in people or surroundings. When making your observations, casually check for any bruises or marks that seem out of place that might indicate mistreatment. Does the child appear to be well looked after from a nutritional point of view.

Child abuse is something we never want to come across, but it does go on. Sometimes you can see the fear on their face, especially when a parent says something that triggers a thought in the child's mind that a slap is inevitable. If you have genuine concerns, make mental notes of both the behaviour of the parent as well as the child and voice your concerns to the ambulance crew discreetly. They will note your concerns and deal with it through the appropriate channels.

Work at breathing

Ask the parent to remove the child's top. Again as this is part of your primary survey, checking their breathing can be a doorway observation. Once you know the age of the child, you should be able to get a reasonably accurate breathing rate just by watching the rise and fall of the chest (for breathing and pulse rates, see CPGs on Primary Survey—Paediatric). Make a note and compare it to later checks. Check for adequate and equal rise and fall of the chest. Listen to their breathing. Can you hear wheezing, gasping, hoarseness, or stridor? Stridor is a harsh raspy sound made during inspiration and is indicative of an upper airway obstruction. Acute stridor in children may indicate conditions such as epiglottitis, croup, tracheitis, anaphylaxis, or a partial foreign body airway obstruction (FBAO). This is a medical emergency. If the airway is severally compromised, this raspy sound can also be heard when the child tries to exhale. When you have a combination of stridor and what we call retractions, you need to be concerned. Retractions are when the child struggles to breathe in; the spaces between the ribs (intercostal muscles) are drawn in making the ribs stand out and look more pronounced. When you see this, the child is making a significant effort to breathe. If the child is standing and tripoding, they are also making a great effort to breathe. Tripoding is described as when someone is standing but leaning forward with their hands wresting on a table or other object of that height for support. A person with difficulty breathing can also be seen in the sitting position leaning forward wresting their hands on their knees. Tripoding optimizes the mechanics of respiration by taking advantage of the accessory muscles of the neck and upper chest to get more air into the lungs. Nasal flaring is also a sign of difficulty breathing especially in infants. When dealing with children in this type of situation, allow them to be in their own position of comfort. They may prefer to sit upright. When dealing with infants and young children, at the slightest hint of respiratory distress, call for help (999/112). If you are trained in oxygen administration, give the child 100% oxygen (15 Litres per minute) using a nebuliser mask and monitor their vital signs.

Circulation to skin

Look for a mottled-type pattern of red or reddish blue and porcelain blotches on the trunk as this may be an indicator of poor perfusion. This observation is based on the assumption that the room temperature is normal. However, if the room is cold, these patterns may occur naturally, especially on the hands and legs. Cyanosis of the peripheries is a normal occurrence in infants under twelve weeks in a cold environment. This is good to know so that you won't misinterpret what you see. If you find that the child's lips are cyanosed (blue), you will have to act quickly and oxygenate the child as this is a medical emergency and EMS must be notified. Young children may not tolerate an oxygen mask or may indeed be frightened of it. The hissing and bubbling sound of the oxygen flowing through the nebuliser mask may also unnerve them. If this is the case, just put the mask near their face and turn the regulator down slightly and they will still draw enough oxygen into their system to help them. It may even be necessary to remove the mask itself from the delivery hose and just let the oxygen flow as close to the mouth and nose as possible remembering not to point it directly into the face.

4.5. Handing over the Patient

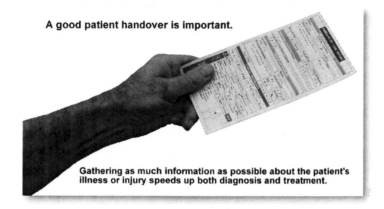

A good patient handover is important.

Gathering as much information as possible about the patient's illness or injury speeds up both diagnosis and treatment.

When the time comes to hand over your patient, it is important that you have collected as much information as possible. Remember that time can be of the essence in some cases, and as you may have been the only person dealing with the patient, your information and interventions are all that the emergency services may have to rely on. That's why it's so important to make notes as soon as you can. Your notes don't have to be word perfect once you can get the message across but always make an effort to note times if you assisted with medications.

The best way to put your report together is to remember the sequence of your patient assessment. For instance, when you approach your patient, you will obviously know if they are male or female! Then find out their age (if they are unconscious, guess). Then you have the history. Then there's the chief complaint. Give a description of their LOC and their vital signs (ABC's). Describe what you found during your physical examination. Using your SAMPLE format, find out whether they have any medical conditions. What were the interventions? Is the patient better or worse since you started treatment?

4.6. The Recovery Position

The recovery position, also known as the safe airway position, is designed to prevent suffocation due to obstruction of the airway during a period of unconscious. Putting someone in the recovery position correctly will ensure their airway remains clear and open while they remain in an unconscious state. Once an unconscious patient is put in this position, it ensures that any vomit or fluid will drain from the mouth and prevent them from choking. Every year, an unacceptable number of people die as a result of suffocation from non-fatal illnesses or injuries that render them unconscious.

There are many reasons as to why these illnesses or injuries caused the victim to lose consciousness, but they all have a common denominator, the victim, in the majority of cases, was discovered lying on their back (the supine position). Take for example a simple faint (syncope) where a person feels light-headed and drops to the floor. They may have banged their head on the way on the corner of a coffee table or other such hard surfaces, or perhaps they struck the sidewalk hard enough to prolong the unconscious period for several minutes. If that person landed on their back and remained there for several minutes, they obviously wouldn't be able to maintain an open airway and would suffocate as a result of flaccid tongue, whereby the muscles in the tongue relax allowing it to slump back in the throat blocking off the airway. You could also consider the person having succumbed to too much alcohol that falls into a deep sleep and vomits without waking up. If that person were on their back at this time, they wouldn't be able to clear their airway and would in all probability choke in their own vomit.

Children are also vulnerable. If, for example, there is a clash of heads while playing sports and one gets knocked unconscious. It has happened in the past whereby parents or staff who have had little or no first aid are looking at the child on the ground, wondering what to do. As the child starts to turn blue around the lips and earlobes, someone decides to call the local doctor, but the doctor isn't available, so eventually they phone for an ambulance. When they arrive, the child is long past being helped. So you see how important it is to be able to deal with this type of situation. It isn't called the safe airway position, or indeed the recovery position for nothing! So is there a right way or wrong way to carry out the recovery position?

The International Liaison Committee on Resuscitation (ILCOR) was formed in 1992 to provide a forum for liaison between principal resuscitation organisations worldwide. They provide a mechanism for collecting, reviewing, and sharing international scientific data on resuscitation. In relation to the recovery position, ILCOR does not recommend one specific recovery position, but it advises on six key principles to be followed:

1. The victim should be in as near a true lateral position (on their side) as possible with the head positioned to allow free drainage of fluid.
2. The position should be stable.
3. Any pressure of the chest that impairs breathing should be avoided.
4. It should be possible to turn the victim onto the side and return to the back easily and safely, having particular regard to the possibility of cervical spine injury.
5. Good observation of, and access to the airway, should be possible.
6. The position itself should not give rise to any injury to the victim.

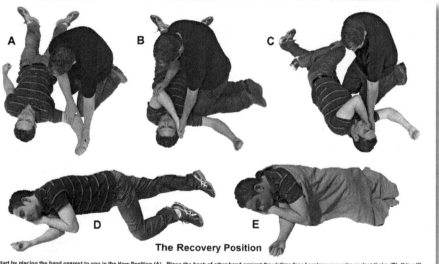

The Recovery Position

Start by placing the hand nearest to you in the How Position (A). Place the back of other hand against the victims face keeping your palm against theirs (B), this will allow you you control the head when you roll the patient. Bring the leg furthest from you upwards and tuck the toe in under the near leg as shown (C) and roll the victim by pulling the knee towards you. Raise the leg to stabalise the patient, then open the airway by tilting the head forward (D). Cover with a blanket to prevent heat loss (E).

The basic steps to put a patient into the recovery position are straight forward. First, ensure that there is nothing in their pockets such as keys, phone, or anything that might injure them when rolled onto that particular side. If you must remove something from a patient's pocket, try to have it witnessed by someone as you could be accused at a later stage of theft should the item be misplaced. If the patient is being transported by EMS, hand the items to them and they will see to it that they are kept safely. If they are wearing glasses, they should also be removed as they may mark the person's face. Kneeling at the patient's side, place the hand nearest to you palm side up in line with their head. This is often referred to as the how position, named after all those cowboy and Indian films where the Indian rides up, raises his hand and says, 'How' as a form of greeting. Next, by putting your hand under the knee, bring the leg farthest from you upwards to a comfortable angle where you are able to tuck the toes of that leg under the knee of the leg nearest to you. Once you have done this, take the palm of the patient's other hand into your palm and place it so that the back of their hand is against their cheek nearest to you. If there are any rings such as an engagement ring or any type of ring with a raised mounting on it, turn the mounted side into their palm to avoid marking the patient's face. While keeping the back of the patient's hand against their cheek, use your other hand to grab the knee that you lifted and pull it toward you until it touches the ground while ensuring your other hand remains in position palm to palm under the patient's head. What you are doing really is rolling the patient toward you with one hand and preventing injury to the head with the other. Once the patient is rolled, tilt the head back to open the airway and allow it to rest on the back of the hand that was against the cheek as if it was a pillow. Tucking both hands under the head palm to palm will raise the head a little higher but that's up to you. The main thing is to

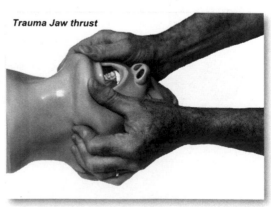

Trauma Jaw thrust

insure that the unconscious patient has an open airway when you're finished. Finally, bring the leg that was tucked under the knee upwards in the direction of the chest at around 45° to 50° from the body and bring the foot outwards for stability.

Be careful when putting an elderly person in this position, especially the latter part, as you could hurt or even cause a fracture due to brittle bone disease. When bringing the leg upwards, stop when you find any kind of resistance or if the patient shows signs of pain. Cover the patient with a blanket and monitor them. It is also advisable to move the patient on to their other side after twenty minutes to avoid sores occurring. One more note, if you suspect a spinal injury, do not under any circumstances move a patient or put them into the recovery position. If it is necessary to maintain an open airway, you should apply what is known as a trauma jaw thrust.

4.7. Calling for Help

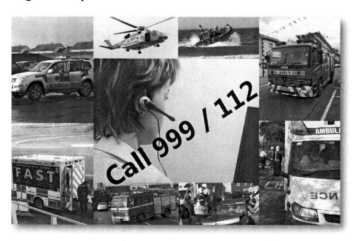

How hard can it be to call an ambulance? If you've never done it before, it can be a bit unnerving! The emergency numbers to remember are 999 or 112. Both numbers get you through to the operator and are free to call. While we are all familiar with 999 in Ireland and Britain, the 112 number is not as well known. It's been around for quite a while, but people sometimes choose to stick to the number they can remember, and if you are more comfortable with that then that's ok too. 112 is more or less the standard European emergency number, so it's worth noting if you go to mainland Europe. The advantage 112 has over 999 comes into play with mobile phones. While both numbers work on the mobile or landline, you can dial 112 on a mobile if you are out of credit. If you have to power up a phone and you don't know the pin number, by dialling 112, it will override the pin number and allow you make that emergency call, so it's a good number to know.

The emergency operator doesn't know if your house is on fire, if you're being burgled, if you're drowning, or if you're sick or injured. So when you dial 999 or 112, the first question the emergency operator will ask you will be what service you require. If you need an ambulance, just say so. However, there are situations where you may require multiple agencies. If for instance, you are first on scene at a road traffic collision or RTC for short, you may require the police to secure the area and perhaps the Fire Service if there is a danger of fire or to assist in extracting a patient. In some areas, when a call comes in to ambulance control relating to traffic accidents, they may automatically turn out a fire crew as part of their protocol or for health and safety reasons. Your priority is the patient's safety and well—being and your own safety, so if you think other agencies are warranted, describe the situation to the operator, and they will react accordingly.

Once you have described the nature of the emergency and the primary service you require, in this case you require an ambulance, the operator will redirect your call to that agency. You are now through to ambulance control. The call taker will ask a number of questions. These are from a list of standard questions used to extract the correct information in as little time as possible. First and foremost, you will be asked for your name and telephone number. You may have been asked for it already by the initial operator, but that's standard procedure. Your number will be checked as they are speaking to you to see if you are a genuine caller. When a caller gives their number, the emergency operator is already looking at it on caller identification, so if a false number is given, they can flag it.

All emergency calls are recorded in the event that if a problem arises, they have something to revert back to as poor mobile phone coverage can be a major issue and it can sometimes take several minutes to be re-connected to the caller. Every year, emergency services get turned out to thousands of hoax calls, resulting in delays getting resources to genuine emergencies. Although a reasonable number of these hoax callers are caught and prosecuted each year, the majority are never caught. So when you are asked for your name and number among other things, it's for a very good reason.

Information the call taker may look for

The Pre-Hospital Emergency Care Council (PHECC) of Ireland developed a Request Emergency Dispatch (RED) Card to make it easy for people to call the emergency services. This can be seen in the CPG's section on the bottom left-hand corner of three algorithms dealing with primary and secondary survey. They are similar in size to a credit card and designed to fit in your wallet.

1. First, you will be asked what service you require, and then your name and number.
2. Tell the call taker if you are a first-aider or a Responder, or an EMT or whatever.
3. Exact location: Give directions as best you can. If you're not familiar with the area, use landmarks or describe your surroundings. If a local appears, get them to give directions. If you have a GPS in your car or smart phone, give your coordinates, and the ambulance will find you.
4. Type and seriousness of incident, for example, is it a car crash or a collapse? How bad is it?
5. Number and condition of casualties: This will have a bearing on resources required.
6. Advise if there are hazards such as oil spillage, danger of electrocution, gas leak, etc.
7. Don't hang up until the operator tells you to.

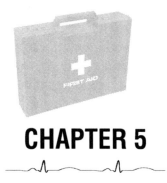

CHAPTER 5

5.1 Circulation

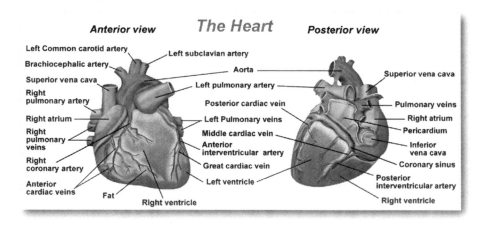

Circulation is the movement of blood around the body, pumped by the heart. This system is called the cardiovascular system. It contains about 5 litres (8 pints) of blood which your heart continuously recirculates. Each day, your heart beats about 100,000 times and pumps about 23,000 l (5,000 gallons) of blood. As described in the Anatomy and Physiology section in Chapter 3, the circulatory system is made up of three things: liquid (blood), a vessel (blood vessels), and a pump (the heart). The heart continually pumps the blood around the body, picking up oxygen as its travels from the lungs, transporting it through the blood vessels to all parts of the body. The cells of the body absorb the oxygen and nutrients from the blood and the waste produced, which includes carbon dioxide, is transported back to the lungs and is once again exchanged for more oxygen and the circle continues (Ref: Chapter 3). Anything that disrupts the smooth workings of this system is not good and needs to be addressed urgently, and we need to know how to fix it fast.

Coronary circulation is the circulation to the heart organ itself. The right and left coronary arteries branch from the ascending aorta and, through their branches, supply the heart muscle (myocardial) tissue. Venous blood collected by the cardiac veins (great, middle, small, and anterior) flows into the coronary sinus. The coronary sinus is one of the blood vessels which drain deoxygenated blood into the right atrium of the heart. Once the blood enters the right atrium, it can be pumped through the heart and lungs to acquire oxygen so that it can be returned to the circulatory system to supply oxygen to the cells. Delivery of oxygen-rich blood to the myocardial tissue occurs during the heart relaxation phase.

5.2. Heart Attack

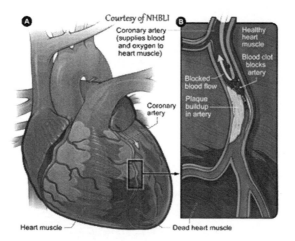

A heart attack or MI (myocardial infarction) as it is known for short in the medical world by definition is the interruption of blood supply to part of the heart, causing some heart cells to die. It occurs when one or more of the coronary arteries are completely blocked. Atherosclerosis and blood clots are the two primary causes of coronary artery blockage. Atherosclerosis is hardening of the arteries and is a common disorder. It occurs when fat, cholesterol, and other substances build up in the walls of the arteries and form hard structures called plaque. Over time, plaque can block the arteries and cause symptoms and problems throughout the body. Blood clots may form in these narrowed arteries and block the blood flow. Pieces of plaque can also break off and move to smaller blood vessels, blocking them. This blockage starves the tissues of blood and oxygen, which can result in damage or tissue death known as necrosis. This is a common cause of heart attack and stroke.

Blockage of a coronary artery causes immediate and severe pain. At first, the pain of a heart attack and that of angina pectoris are similar. Most people who suffer a heart attack describe the pain as crushing or as if their chest was caught in a vice followed by radiating pain. The classic heart attack is described as crushing central chest pain, radiating to the arm and neck, and that is how most people will describe it.

However, don't be fooled when someone says they have isolated jaw pain, muscular-type pain, or pain down the arm or back with no other symptoms. Indigestion or heartburn is another complaint that can be misinterpreted, although this is characterised by a burning pain behind the breast bone as a result of stomach acid moving up into the oesophagus, especially when you're lying down. This burning sensation in your chest may start in your upper abdomen and radiate all the way to your neck. This can be very confusing for the responder, especially if the patient says they don't normally get heartburn. The golden rule applies to this situation. If in doubt, treat as a heart attack!

Also when having a heart attack, the patient will present with shortness of breath and sweat profusely and become nauseated with an inclination to vomit. Heart attacks (MIs) are the leading cause of death for both men and women all over the world. It is estimated that approximately 25% of MIs are silent without chest pain or other symptoms, although this is more common among people with diabetes due to nerve degradation. Unlike angina, the pain of MI will not be relieved by the administration of a nitrate such as glyceryl trinitrate (*GTN*) and will persist unlike the pain of angina that rarely lasts more than five to ten minutes.

Risk factors such as previous cardiovascular disease and old age along with smoking, excessive alcohol consumption, and drug abuse are all well known. People who suffer from diabetes, high blood pressure, obesity, chronic kidney disease, heart failure, and chronic high stress levels are also high on the risk factor list.

Early recognition and understanding the symptoms of a heart attack is so important and can make the difference between the patient living or dying. The earlier you have EMS on scene, the faster they can stabilise the patient and minimise the amount of damage to the heart muscle as much as possible.

Early recognition

Persistent vice-like central chest pain

Pain may radiate to arms, face, jaw, neck, and back (particularly on the left side)

Rapid, weak, and/or irregular pulse

Profuse sweating, nausea, and dizziness

May have no previous history

Ashen colour and/or cyanosis (turning blue) of lips

Breathlessness, with or without chest discomfort

Patient may go unconscious

Treatment (Call 999/112)

If your patient is conscious, reassure them and make them comfortable. Make eye contact and talk to them. Remember, the patient will be anxious and frightened, and this only adds to the problem. Hence, if they are on the ground or sitting on a chair, don't stand over them as they may feel intimidated. Bend or kneel to their level. Talk to them calmly, constantly reassuring them. Don't lay them down flat as they will find it harder to breathe and may feel claustrophobic. It they are on the floor put them in a sitting position that makes them feel comfortable and able to breathe easily. Support their back with pillows, cushions, or whatever is available. Loosen any tight clothing (e.g., necktie or

top shirt button), and keep the patient calm. If cardiac chest pain is indicated, call for help (999/112). This patient needs to get to hospital. Get a SAMPLE history and make notes and record times of any interventions. To further understand symptoms, as part of your SAMPLE history, be sure to include OPQRST. This acronym is used to assess pain and will allow you to further understand specific complaints. This may not have been their first heart attack, and the patient may be on medication.

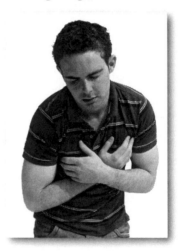

Trained Cardiac First Responders or CFR s for short (Ref: CPGs for Cardiac Chest Pain) can give oxygen (O2) in accordance with their appropriate guidelines. They can also give one 300 mg soluble aspirin dissolved in 100 ml of water, or if no water is available, the patient should be encouraged to chew it. Aspirin reduces the risk of further blockages in the coronary arteries by preventing the formation of further blood clots. Before you give aspirin, you need to find out if your patient is able to take it! If the patient has stomach ulcers, a bleeding disorder (haemophilia) or any known allergies to aspirin, do not give it. If your patient is less than sixteen years of age, *do not* give aspirin. Research has established a link between Reye's syndrome and the use of aspirin in the age group below eighteen. While the cause of Reye's syndrome and cure remain unknown, it attacks all body organs, with the liver and brain suffering most seriously. Because aspirin is a drug, you should note the time that you gave it and advise advanced life support (ALS). If you neglect to mention this, paramedics may also give aspirin and overdose the patient. Check that the packet isn't damaged and the tablet is in date. Most importantly, check that the strength is 300 mg. As oxygen is a drug, you must record this also. If your patient collapses and goes into cardiac arrest, be prepared to resuscitate. The steps of resuscitation and the use of an automated external defibrillator (AED) will be dealt with in detail under the heading of CPR/AED shortly (Ref: CPGs; Basic Life Support—Adult).

OPQRST

O— Onset: Ask the patient when did the pain or discomfort start?

P— Provocation: Ask what makes the pain or discomfort better or worse. If they take a deep breath or if they press on the chest, does it make things worse? What happens if they climb the stairs?

Q— Quality: Ask the patient what type of pain it is. Let them tell you in their own words how they feel and what's happening. Don't ask the patient a leading question. As an example, you shouldn't ask, does your chest feel like your car is parked on it? The correct way to ask would be something like, can you describe what the pain in your chest feels like? Remember, there are different types of pain, and if your patient can't answer that simple straightforward question, rephrase the question by saying, pain can be felt in many ways such as burning, sharp or stabbing, heavy, pressured, ripping, dull, or tingling. Does it resemble any of those I've listed?

R— Radiation: Once again, don't lead the patient. Simply ask, does the pain radiate or travel to other parts of your body? Let them answer for themselves without help. If they are coherent, allow them to describe where the pain is radiating from and where it's going.

S— Severity: To determine the severity of pain, we use a pain scale of 1 to 10. The question you will ask in this case is, on a scale of 1 to 10, with 10 being the worst pain you have ever experienced and 1 being no pain at all, how would you rate your pain? It's important to make a note of their score and the time you asked because you will ask this question several times more during your treatment. While their score may be high, don't use it to determine the seriousness of the problem. Use it to determine whether your treatment is working. For example, when you gave the patient GTN, did the pain subside? If their pain was 8 on the scale to start with and it's now 4, then your treatment is working.

T— Time: Ask if their pain is better or worse and how long it lasts since you started treatment. *Make notes.*

5.3. Angina Pectoris

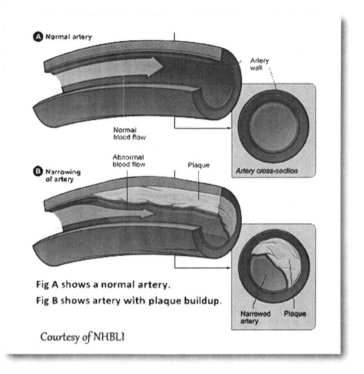

Fig A shows a normal artery.
Fig B shows artery with plaque buildup.

Courtesy of NHBLI

Angina pectoris or simply 'angina' is caused by an inadequate supply of oxygen-rich blood to the heart muscle. This inadequate blood supply is caused by narrowing of the coronary arteries as a result of atherosclerosis. Atherosclerosis causes layers of fat known as cholesterol to build up and coat the walls of the coronary arteries with the result that the supply of blood to the heart muscle is compromised. This is a progressive disease of the arteries with the accumulation of fatty deposits building up over many years. This process is known as hardening of the arteries. There may be no symptoms in the early stages and the person will be completely unaware of what's going on. The first indications may present under physical or emotional stress in the form of pain and discomfort when the heart muscle doesn't receive adequate blood to meet the increased oxygen needs during stress or exercise. Without treatment, atherosclerosis can lead to angina, heart attack, and cardiac arrest.

There are two types of angina, stable and unstable. The most common symptom of stable angina is pain or a feeling of discomfort or tightness in the chest, which can often spread to the jaw, back, shoulders, and arms. With stable angina, the pain is brought on by exertion and is relieved by rest. A person who has stable angina can live within certain boundaries with the help of medication. On the other hand, unstable angina may occur unpredictably at rest which may be a serious indicator of an impending heart attack. The symptoms of angina are similar to those of a heart attack. The difference is that the pain of angina rarely lasts more than ten minutes and is almost always relieved by taking GTN in the form of spray or tablet.

Treatment of angina

The treatment for angina is similar to that of a heart attack (Ref: CPGs for Cardiac Chest Pain). Take a SAMPLE history. This will provide you with the basic information about the patient's medical history. Always allow the patient to describe their symptoms because you will get a more honest picture. Prompting can lead to misdiagnosis, so don't put words in their mouth. Never attempt to diagnose a problem without ruling out all the other possibilities. The SAMPLE history 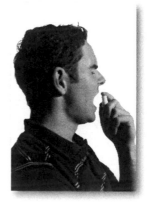 covers all relevant questions, and you can include the OPQRST to gather the remaining information.

Place the patient in the most comfortable resting position to reduce the workload on the heart. This is usually a semi-sitting position but may vary according to the patient. If the patient is on glyceryl trinitrate (GTN), assist them to take it. If the pump hasn't been used for a week or more, or is new, you should release one spray into the air away from both you and the patient. GTN is given under the tongue and comes in a pump spray bottle. One pump is a metered dose of 0.4 mg. GTN works by being converted in the body to a chemical called nitric oxide. This chemical is made naturally by the body and has the effect of making the veins and arteries relax and widen (dilate). When the blood vessels dilate in this way, there is more space inside them and hence less resistance. This makes it easier for the heart to pump blood around the body. Widening the veins also decreases the volume of blood that returns to the heart with each heartbeat. This makes it easier for the heart to pump that blood out again. As a result of both these actions, the heart does not need as much energy to pump the blood around the body and therefore needs less oxygen. GTN also widens the arteries within the heart itself, which increases the blood and oxygen supply to the heart muscle.

If they haven't taken it in the last five minutes, help them to take it. GTN usually relieves angina pain within five minutes. If the pain hasn't subsided after five minutes, help the patient to take a second dose. If the pain doesn't lessen five minutes after the second dose, you can assume the patient is having a heart attack.

If you are assisting the patient to take their own GTN, you shouldn't have to worry about side effects as they will already be aware of them. However, it's important for you to know what they are as certain reactions to the medication may confuse you. The usual side effects are headache, dizziness, weakness, nausea, flushing, fainting, increased heart rate (tachycardia), and decreased heart rate (bradycardia). Knowing the contraindications is also important. If you are a trained responder, and you know how to take the patient's blood pressure (BP), you should do so. If the patient's systolic BP is less than 90 mmHg (the 'top' number in blood pressure measurements), giving GTN will lower it even more and your patient will go unconscious.

You should also ask the patient if they have taken Viagra (Sildenafil citrate) in the last twenty-four hours. You may find this an embarrassing question to ask, but remember, people can die from embarrassment, so be sure to ask the question, but ask it discreetly. Sildenafil citrate is a vasodilator (i.e., a drug that dilates blood vessels), and consequently, it lowers the systolic blood pressure by an average of approximately 8 mmHg. The vasodilating effects of sildenafil citrate become potentially hazardous when combined with the vasodilating effects of nitrates such as GTN. Patients taking both nitrates and sildenafil are prone to develop severe hypotension (low blood pressure) and syncope (fainting.) Patients taking nitrates for their coronary artery disease, therefore, should *never* take sildenafil. Anyone who has taken Viagra or any related type of medication for erectile dysfunction during the past twenty-four hours should not take nitrates.

If it is safe for the patient to take GTN, record the time and the amount of doses given. Call 999 or 112 and get help. Give one 300 mg aspirin in a 100 ml of water after checking that your patient has no contraindications. Record the time and dose and pass this information on to EMS. Oxygen (O2) would also be appropriate if your level of training and CPGs or protocols allow it. Remember that O2 is a drug, so record this also. Keep the patient calm, but be prepared to resuscitate should they deteriorate and go into cardiac arrest.

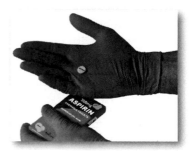

Lifestyle changes

Lifestyle changes will play a large role as part of the treatment of angina. Because heart disease is often the underlying cause of most forms of angina, you can reduce or prevent angina by working on reducing your heart disease risk factors. These risk factors include the following: Smoking, high blood pressure, high cholesterol, alcohol, stress, poor diet, and lack of exercise.

If you smoke, you should stop. This is often easier said than done, but there is help and support available to assist anyone who wants to stop. Blood pressure should be checked regularly, at least once a year. If it's high, it's treatable. High salt intake is one of the well-known contributors to high blood pressure. African-Americans are more likely to develop hypertension and to develop it at a younger age. Genetic research suggests that African-Americans seem to be more sensitive to salt. In people who have a gene that makes them salt-sensitive, just a half-teaspoon of salt can raise blood pressure by 5 mmHg. Diet and excessive weight can play a role, as well. Sodium, a major component of salt, can raise blood pressure by causing the body to retain fluid, which leads to a greater burden on the heart. The American Heart Association (AHA) recommends eating less than 1,500 mg of sodium per day. You'll need to check food labels and menus carefully. Processed foods contribute up to 75% of our sodium intake. Canned soups and lunch meats are prime suspects. High cholesterol can be managed by eating a healthy diet, getting regular exercise, giving up smoking, and avoiding stress. You don't need to quit drinking alcohol as long as you drink in moderation.

Excessive alcohol consumption can raise blood pressure, cause cardiac arrhythmias, and can be directly toxic to the heart muscle resulting in a cardiomyopathy where the heart becomes enlarged and weak. Increased stress can cause angina. Even too much coffee will have a temporarily effect, but one or two cups a day is acceptable according to the AHA. Stress can raise your blood pressure, which is a risk factor for angina as it can harm arteries and make them more likely to develop atherosclerosis. Some hormones that are released in response to stress can also cause narrowing of the arteries. Relaxation techniques may help you reduce stress.

A healthy diet and exercise will keep your weight in check and will reduce the amount of workload on your heart. Avoid consuming saturated fats and food stuffs that give rise to cholesterol. Include lots of fruits, cereals, rice, whole grain bread, vegetables, fibrous

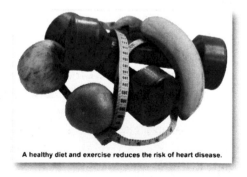

A healthy diet and exercise reduces the risk of heart disease.

foods, etc., in the diet. Fish is a necessary food item in an angina diet, especially oily fish like salmon, tuna, mackerel, etc. People who are meat lovers should opt for lean meat or chicken. It may be a good idea to consult a dietician whereby they will tailor-make a diet programme to suit the individual. There are also hundreds of good books on the subject of diet available. Moderate physical activity of at least thirty minutes a day can be very beneficial. Depending on the amount of exercise you do, simple activities such as walking, swimming, and cycling will keep the body in a good health. When you exercise, you sleep better and you are more alert during the day. You will also be more aerobically fit which will benefit your whole body. A person who suffers from angina should consult their doctor before undertaking any activities. They will advise on what activities are best for the patient.

5.4. Cardiac Arrest

Cardiac arrest is the sudden loss of cardiac function, when the heart abruptly stops beating. It occurs instantly or shortly after symptoms appear. In cardiac arrest, death results when the heart suddenly stops working properly. This is caused by abnormal, or irregular, heart rhythms called arrhythmias. The most common arrhythmia in 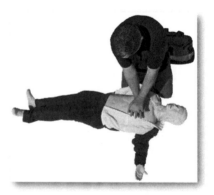 cardiac arrest is ventricular fibrillation (VF). This is when the heart's lower chambers suddenly start beating chaotically and don't pump blood. Another potentially life-threatening arrhythmia is known as ventricular tachycardia (VT). VT is an abnormal rapid heart rhythm originating from the lower pumping chambers of the heart (ventricles). The normal heart usually beats between 60 and 100 times per minute, with the atria contracting first, followed by the ventricles in a synchronised fashion.

In VT, the ventricles beat at a rapid rate, typically from 120 to 300 beats per minute, and are no longer coordinated with the atria. If the heart rate increases to more than 300 beats per minute and becomes totally uncoordinated, it progresses to VF. Death occurs within minutes after the heart stops.

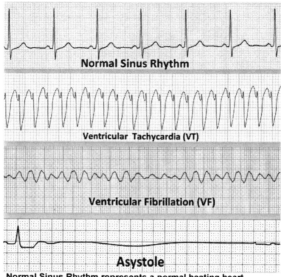

Normal Sinus Rhythm

Ventricular Tachycardia (VT)

Ventricular Fibrillation (VF)

Asystole

Normal Sinus Rhythm represents a normal beating heart.
Most sudden deaths are caused by VT and VF.
Asystole is a state of no cardiac activity.

On an electrocardiogram (ECG) monitor, the picture would have an almost flat-line appearance known as asystole because there is no longer cardiac output, meaning no electrical activity, or no contractions of the heart muscle or blood flow. Asystole is one of the conditions that may be used for a medical practitioner to certify clinical or legal death. Sinus rhythm, on the other hand, is the normal beating of the heart, as measured by an ECG monitor. On the monitor, this rhythm will have a regular pattern with certain generic features that serve as hallmarks for comparison against other normal ECGs.

Cardiac arrest may be reversed if cardiopulmonary resuscitation (CPR) is performed or a defibrillator is used to shock the heart and restore a normal heart rhythm within a few minutes. For every minute that defibrillation is delayed, the patient's chances of survival diminishes by 7%-10%. When the heart stops beating, blood stops flowing through the body. Without the circulation of blood, the cells of the body will die and the body's vital organs cannot receive a fresh supply of oxygen and nutrients nor can it eliminate waste products. Organs will start to deteriorate with some of the more sensitive organs deteriorating at a more rapid rate than others. Within four to six minutes of an arrest, brain damage begins, and within eight to ten minutes, brain damage may become irreversible. There are many causes of cardiac arrest. Medical emergencies such as diabetes, epilepsy, electrocution, poisoning, and allergic reactions are just some of the emergencies. Respiratory arrest if untreated will lead to cardiac arrest as will drowning and suffocation if treatment is not given. Trauma and shock as a result of massive blood loss is another cause.

5.5. CPR/AED

Cardiopulmonary resuscitation (CPR) is one of the simplest skills that one can learn, and it does save lives. It is probably oversimplifying the fact, but you can keep a person's heart and brain alive with just a pair of hands and a breath. Simply by pushing on the chest and blowing air into their lungs will help to prevent a victim's brain and vital organs from deteriorating.

Steps leading up to and including CPR

Taking scene safety into consideration, if you find a person who has collapsed, is not responding, and apparently has no pulse, what do you do? (Ref: CPGs Basic Life Support—Adult)

First, if it's safe to approach, check for a response by tapping the patient's shoulders, and in a raised voice near the victim's ear, say something like, 'Hello. Hello, can you hear me?' If there is no response, call for help. Next, tilt the victim's head back to open the airway. Check and see if the victim is breathing. Have a quick look in the mouth to make sure the airway is clear. Several things may block the airway depending on the circumstances. Food or sweets are the main culprits, but there is also vomitus, or even an allergic reaction may have caused swelling enough to occlude (block) the airway. In the case of small children, you may have a catalogue of foreign bodies such as small pieces of toys, etc. However, in most cases where a patient goes unconscious, the airway is compromised by a flaccid tongue, where the tongue goes limp and falls back in the throat blocking the trachea.

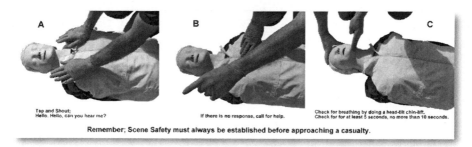

A — Tap and Shout; Hello. Hello, can you hear me?

B — If there is no response, call for help.

C — Check for breathing by doing a head-tilt chin-lift. Check for for at least 5 seconds, no more than 10 seconds.

Remember; Scene Safety must always be established before approaching a casualty.

Tilting the head back will lift the tongue away from the back of the throat. Dentures can sometimes be a problem. If they are flopping around in the patient's mouth, take them out. If they are a good well-fitting set, leave them there. Removing dentures will cause the face to cave in and you will find it difficult to do mouth to mouth. Getting a good seal with a pocket mask or bag valve mask (BVM) won't be as difficult. Check for a carotid pulse if you are trained to do so. Checking for breathing and pulse should take at least five but no more than ten seconds. If someone comes, ask them to dial 999 or 112, ask for an ambulance, and get an AED. If no one comes, you will have to make the call and get the AED yourself (if one is available). If the victim is unresponsive and not breathing, begin CPR. Remove all clothes from the victim's chest and start compressions.

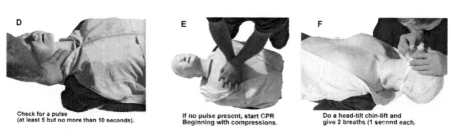

D — Check for a pulse (at least 5 but no more than 10 seconds).

E — If no pulse present, start CPR Beginning with compressions.

F — Do a head-tilt chin-lift and give 2 breaths (1 second each.

When giving compressions, push hard and fast (at least 100 compressions per minute) and allow for full chest recoil.

Compressions should be given at a depth of at least 2 inches (5cm) and at a rate of at least 100 per minute. After thirty compressions, do a head tilt, chin lift. This is done by placing one hand on the patient's forehead and the other on the bony part of the chin. Tilt the head back. This manoeuvre lifts the tongue away from the back of the throat providing an open airway. Pinch the victim's nose and cover their mouth with your mouth and give two breaths over one second each. Blow just enough to make the chest rise. If the chest doesn't rise, it may be because the head wasn't tilted back far enough and the airway wasn't open. If this happens, let the head go back to its neutral position and try a head tilt, chin lift again. If the second breath goes in, go back to doing chest compressions. In every cycle, you should only make two attempts at giving breaths, so regardless of whether you get two breaths or no breaths in, don't delay getting back to compressions. The correct timeframe for CPR is to give five cycles of thirty compressions and two breaths in two minutes.

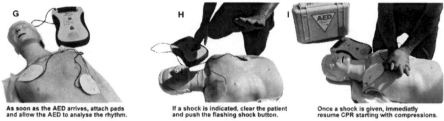

As soon as the AED arrives, attach pads and allow the AED to analyse the rhythm.

If a shock is indicated, clear the patient and push the flashing shock button.

Once a shock is given, immediatly resume CPR starting with compressions.

If the AED says no shock is indicated, resume CPR starting with compressions.

For Advanced Cardiac First Responders (CFR-A) and EFRs, when giving ventilations, you should consider oxygen therapy through a BVM if you have the appropriate assistance. A BVM is regarded as a two-person device unless you are well used to working on your own. One responder should position themselves at head using both hands to hold the mask in place while tilting the head back to open the airway, while a second responder squeezes the bag.

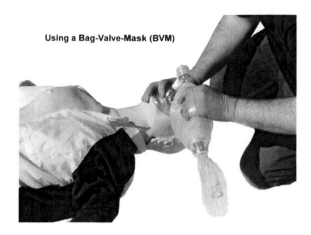

Using a Bag-Valve-Mask (BVM)

In the real world, we don't carry stopwatches in our first-aid kits, so, the speed at which we do CPR will vary. In the professional world, because of regular training and having to do CPR for real on a regular basis, the timing will be within the guidelines. However, for someone who has only practiced on a manikin during a course a few times may not get the appropriate timing anyway near correct. They may be too fast or too slow. For those of us who remember the Bee Gees pop group from the 1960s, they released a song called 'Staying Alive'. The British Heart Foundation even used it to promote hands-only CPR (http://www.youtube.com/watch?v=ILxjxfB4zNk). This song is quoted almost in every CPR course worldwide as it has exactly 100 beats per minute which also, coincidently, is the minimum number of compressions you need provide during CPR. I'm not suggesting that you sing while doing CPR, but you now at least have something that you can refer to in the back of your mind. If compressions are too fast, the heart doesn't get time to fill with blood; therefore, there is an insufficient amount of blood and oxygen flowing through the heart, brain, and other vital organs. If compressions are too slow, the same applies plus the heart isn't getting enough stimuli to generate electricity and build blood pressure.

Current AHA guidelines indicate that good compressions are more important than breaths. When you give good compressions, you build up blood pressure in your patient. When you stop compressions, blood flow also stops, and this cessation of blood flow leads to a quick drop in the blood pressure that had been built up during the previous set of compressions. Good CPR is delivering two breaths and getting back to compressions in less than ten seconds (seven to eight seconds would be excellent).

In the past, we have said that it is very rare that you will catch a disease from doing mouth to mouth and that still stands to a point. Cold sores or herpes is probably the most common thing. However, TB has raised its head in recent years. This will spread to the rescuer when the patient breathes out the TB bacteria and the rescuer breathes it in. If there is blood in or around the mouth, it's better not to attempt giving breaths unless you have a pocket mask.

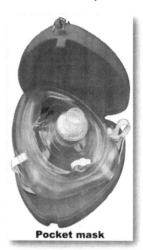

Pocket mask

Masks are made of firm plastic that fit over the victim's nose and mouth and come in sizes to suit adult, child, and infant and are simple to use. Because the mask covers both the nose and mouth, if the victim vomits or has any infections, you are much less likely to become infected. If your patient does vomit, turn their head sideways and clear the airway as best you can before continuing CPR. If your patient has a suspected spinal injury, suction is recommended as any movement of the head could be dangerous unless the patient is completely immobilised on a spinal board. If that's the case, then you roll the patient on the board to one side and clear the airway. Immobilisation of patients on spinal boards is only done by EFRs and practitioners who are trained and is a skill set that shouldn't be attempted by a first-aider. The main reason why a patient vomits during CPR is that the ventilations given are too strong. When you give breaths (ventilations), once you see chest rise, you should stop. Excessive ventilating will result in air entering the stomach causing the patient vomit and then aspirate. Aspirating is the act of inhaling fluid or a foreign body into the bronchi and lungs, often after vomiting.

Because compressions are the most important part of CPR, compression-only CPR for lay rescuers is now acceptable if you do not wish to give breaths. This means that the ratio of 30:2 changes to continuous compressions at a rate of at least 100 per minute. Keep doing this until help arrives. The science behind compression-only CPR tells us that as we do good deep compressions, an acceptable amount of passive air is drawn into the lungs. This is adequate enough to oxygenate the blood keeping the brain and other vital organs from deteriorating until EMS arrives. Remember that for every minute that goes by without CPR, the chance of survival diminishes by 10%, so if you are faced with a situation of having to perform CPR on a patient and you don't have a barrier device and you are a bit apprehensive about giving breaths, just do continuous compressions. Don't deprive the victim of their small window of opportunity for survival.

As soon as an AED arrives, *turn it on* and follow the prompts. Make sure the chest is clear of anything that may get in the way of applying the pads. If the chest is wet, wipe it quickly as it doesn't have to be completely dry. Defibrillator pads are extremely sticky, but if the chest is too wet or very hairy, they may not make contact with the skin. Most AEDs should have an add-on kit containing a disposable razor along with gloves, a pocket mask, alcohol wipes, and a spare set of pads. If the chest is very hairy, quickly shave the area where the pads go and attach them as fast as possible. If there are medicine patches in the way, remove them with a gloved hand and quickly wipe off any residue before attaching. Follow the pictures on the pads which will show you the correct position for each pad. Peel one pad and attach it before doing likewise with the second pad. Once the pads are in place, the AED will analyse the heart rhythm. Once the AED says 'analysing rhythm', no one should touch the patient. If the AED says 'shock indicated', the AED will charge up and the shock button will flash. Advise everyone to stay clear,

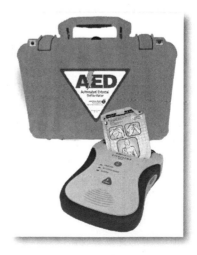

and when you are sure no one is touching the patient, press the flashing shock button to deliver the shock. Once the shock has been delivered, *immediately* continue CPR, starting with compressions. Don't wait for the AED to tell you start compressions after you have pushed the shock button. Once the shock has been delivered, it's safe to continue. Waiting for it to tell you to start will deprive the patient of at least six or eight vital compressions. After two minutes, the AED will automatically reanalyse the patient. Once again stay clear and let it do its work. If it says 'shock advised', continue as before and deliver the shock. If the AED says 'no shock indicated', continue the steps of CPR starting with compressions. Continue CPR, pausing only when the AED says analysing, until the patient starts to move or help arrives.

If the patient has been successfully defibrillated, their pulse will still be very weak and may take some time to strengthen. If the patient has a pulse but is not breathing effectively, rescuers should give breaths without chest compressions. This is called rescue breathing. For adults, give one breath every five to six seconds. For children and infants, you should give one breath every three to five seconds. If the patient starts to breathe adequately, leave the AED switched on with the pads attached to the patient as they may revert to cardiac arrest again. Place them in the recovery position (aka Safe Airway Position) and make sure they have an open and patent airway. Keep the patient warm and monitor their vital signs. If the patient goes into cardiac arrest again, roll them on to their back again and recommence CPR.

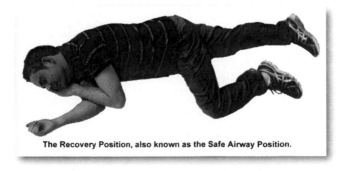

The Recovery Position, also known as the Safe Airway Position.

5.6. Management of Cardiac Arrest in a Pregnant Patient

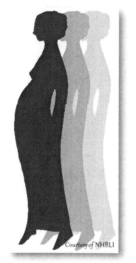

Significant physiological changes occur during pregnancy, for example, cardiac output, blood volume, minute ventilation (minute ventilation is the amount of air a person breathes in one minute), and oxygen consumption all increase. Furthermore, the gravid uterus (a uterus during pregnancy) can cause significant compression of iliac and abdominal vessels when the mother is in the supine position (lying down face up), resulting in reduced cardiac output and hypotension.

Courtesy of NHBLI

There are many causes of cardiac arrest in pregnant women. These include cardiac disease, pulmonary embolism, psychiatric disorders, and hypertensive disorders of pregnancy. Other causes include sepsis, haemorrhage, amniotic-fluid embolism, and ectopic pregnancy.

Many cardiovascular problems associated with pregnancy are caused by aortocaval compression. Aortocaval compression syndrome is compression of the abdominal aorta and inferior vena cava by the gravid uterus when a pregnant woman lies on her back. When treating a patient who is pregnant and that is V, P, or U on the AVPU scale, you should place the patient in the left lateral position or manually and gently displace the uterus to the left. If your CPGs allow, you should give high-flow oxygen guided by pulse oximetry. EMS including ALS should be informed as quickly as possible as obstetric and neonatal specialists should also be involved early in the event of resuscitation. Finally, try to identify and treat any underlying causes.

When dealing with a pregnant patient in cardiac arrest, BLS guidelines are slightly different but certainly not complicated. After twenty weeks of gestation, the pregnant woman's uterus can press down against the inferior vena cava and the aorta, impeding venous return and cardiac output. Uterine obstruction of venous return can cause pre-arrest hypotension or shock and, in the critically ill patient, may precipitate arrest. After cardiac arrest, the compromise in venous return and cardiac output by the gravid uterus limits the effectiveness of chest compressions. Therefore, the change (and only change) in the steps of CPR is that the pregnant patient is tilted slightly onto their left-hand side rather than laying them on their back before starting compressions.

According to the European Resuscitation Council, non-arrest studies show that left lateral tilt improves maternal blood pressure and cardiac output and stroke volume and improves fetal oxygenation and heart rate. Non-cardiac arrest data show that the gravid uterus can be shifted away from the cava in most cases by placing the patient in 15° of left lateral decubitus (lying down on left-hand side) position. Left lateral tilt is not easy to perform whilst maintaining good quality chest compressions. A variety of methods to achieve a left lateral tilt include placing the victim on the rescuer's knees, pillows, or blankets. Studies have shown that effective chest compressions decreased the more the patient was tilted.

The key steps to remember for BLS when dealing with a pregnant patient are first, immediately call for help (999/112) and advise EMS that you are dealing with a pregnant patient. Start basic life support according to standard guidelines. Ensure good quality chest compressions with minimal interruptions. Manually, displace the uterus to the left to remove caval compression. Add left lateral tilt if this is feasible—the optimal angle of tilt is unknown. Aim for between 15° and 30°. Even a small amount of tilt may be better than no tilt. The angle of tilt used needs to allow good quality chest compressions, and if needed, allow caesarean delivery of the fetus (Ref: CPGs for Basic Life Support—Adult for management).

Note: We will also deal with CPR in a later chapter under Respiratory Emergencies where we will discuss the differences in techniques when performing CPR in adult, child, and infant.

5.7. How an AED Works

For a clear understanding on how an AED works, it is important that the concept is broken down to a simple and understandable language. AEDs are lightweight, battery-operated, portable devices that are easy to use. Sticky pads with sensors (called electrodes) are attached to the chest of the person who is in sudden cardiac arrest (SCA). The electrodes send information about the person's heart rhythm to a computer in the AED. The computer analyses the heart rhythm to find out whether an electric shock is needed. If a shock is needed, the AED uses voice prompts to tell you when to give the shock, and the electrodes deliver it. Using an AED to shock the heart within minutes of the start of SCA may restore a normal heart rhythm.

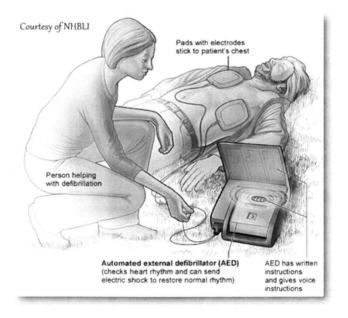

Courtesy of NHBLI

Pads with electrodes stick to patient's chest

Person helping with defibrillation

Automated external defibrillator (AED) (checks heart rhythm and can send electric shock to restore normal rhythm)

AED has written instructions and gives voice instructions

There are two shockable rhythms that the AED looks for. Ventricular Fibrillation (VF) is a cardiac condition in which the heart has adequate electrical energy, but it is disorganised. VF will prevent the heart muscle from contracting and pumping blood and is a shockable rhythm with an AED. Ventricular Tachycardia (VT) is a condition in which the heart is beating too fast. VT does not allow the heart's chambers to fill with enough blood, resulting in insufficient circulation to the body. VT is also a shockable rhythm with an AED. AEDs increase survival chances for the cardiac arrest patient. Used in conjunction with CPR, cardiac arrest (cessation of heart activity) can be managed until ALS can be provided and additional treatment is given.

5.8. Respiratory Arrest and Respiratory Distress

Respiratory arrest is the absence of respirations (i.e. apnoea). During both respiratory arrest and inadequate ventilation, the victim has cardiac output (*blood flow to the body*) detectable as a palpable central pulse. The heart rate may be slow, and cardiac arrest may develop if rescue breathing is not provided. The responder should be able to identify respiratory arrest. When respirations are absent or inadequate, the responder must immediately open the airway and give breaths to prevent cardiac arrest and hypoxic injury to the brain and other organs. It is important to note where children and infants are concerned that despite adequate oxygenation and ventilation, if the pulse rate is less than 60 beats per minute with signs of poor perfusion, you should start CPR.

The average adult breathes between twelve and twenty times per minute. A normal range for a child is between 15 and 30 breaths per minute (BPM) and between 25 and 50 BPM for an infant. Anything outside these ranges are classed as inadequate. Normal breathing is gentle and effortless with only slight movement of the chest as air is drawn into the lungs during inhalation providing the bloodstream with oxygen. Air is expelled during exhalation removing carbon dioxide. The combination of inhalation (chest rise) and exhalation (chest fall) is known as respiration. To evaluate quality breathing, look for normal chest rise and fall with a regular pattern. If you need to count the patient's respirations, don't tell them you're doing it as they will make a conscious effort to breathe as best they can. What you should do is tell the patient you are taking their pulse. Go through the motions of taking a radial pulse, but as you do so, hold the hand you are taking the pulse on gently on their chest. Now, you can monitor the breathing rate and observe a more natural chest rise and get a more accurate result.

Count the number of respirations for fifteen seconds and multiply by four to get the number of BPM. If you're unsure, count for the full minute. Most patients will gladly accept treatment, but they also have the right to refuse, so you must also work at gaining their trust and continue to reassure them.

When a patient is in respiratory distress, they have to work harder to breathe. Some obvious signs include increased respiratory rate and nasal flaring, which is the enlargement of the opening of the nostrils during breathing, although is seen more often in infants and younger children. Active accessory muscle use is another sign of respiratory distress because as the patient struggles to breathe, the neck muscles bulge, and the ribcage appears more prominent as the spaces between the ribs retract. The patient may be seen to bend forward in a standing position placing both hands outstretched on a table or other platform in what is known as the tripod position. They will have difficulty speaking in complete sentences. They will also be agitated and restless. Skin colour will be pale or cyanotic (blue), seesaw breathing, where the alternate use of chest and abdominal muscles are visible during breathing. Agonal breathing or gasping may be seen for a few minutes post cardiac arrest. At this stage, the patient is clinically dead. However, although the patient may struggle to breathe, they are still able to compensate for the problem and get enough oxygen to maintain mental responsiveness and muscle tone and to move air. Respiratory distress is treated by maintaining a clear airway, giving oxygen and putting the patient in a position of comfort. They may be having an asthma attack, a heart attack, or an allergic reaction to something. They may have a lung disease. If they are on medications such as bronchodilators, you may assist them to take it (Ref: CPGs Inadequate Respirations—Adult).

Respiratory arrest is the complete cessation of breathing. Respiratory arrest can lead to or be a sign of cardiac arrest which must be treated as a true emergency. If the patient has any chance of survival, you must act fast. If you can't definitely find a pulse within ten seconds, call for help and start CPR immediately, beginning with compressions. If the patient has an obvious pulse, you may give rescue breaths. For an adult, give one breath every five to six seconds. For a child, give one breath every three to five seconds. Remember to blow just enough to make the chest rise.

5.9. Barrier Devices

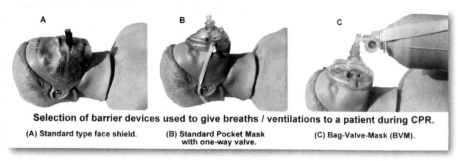

Selection of barrier devices used to give breaths / ventilations to a patient during CPR.

(A) Standard type face shield.   (B) Standard Pocket Mask   (C) Bag-Valve-Mask (BVM).
with one-way valve.

If mouth to mouth contact is not an option, a responder can deliver ventilations in three alternative ways. Mouth to mouth using a single use plastic face shield placed over the victim's mouth. These can be bought on a key ring for a few euro, or in some cases, they are given away free as promotional merchandise by medical suppliers. These are both cheap and effective. The pocket mask is the other option. As described earlier, they are made of firm plastic and fit over the victim's nose and mouth. The mask has a one-way valve fitted giving the rescuer control over the pressure required to inflate the lungs and achieve adequate chest rise. The third option is the BVM.

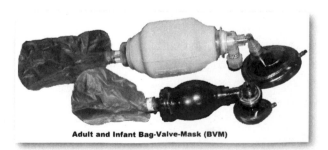

Adult and Infant Bag-Valve-Mask (BVM)

The BVM utilises room air rather than the rescuer having to give a breath. Using this device requires practice. As the name suggests, the device has three main parts. The mask fits over the mouth just like the pocket mask. The bag is attached to the mask with a one-way valve in between. When you squeeze the bag, the air is pushed out through the valve and into the patient through the mask. When you let the bag return to its normal shape, fresh air is drawn in through another one-way valve at the back. Oxygen can also be attached through a port on the bag and a reservoir bag is attached to the BVM allowing high flow oxygen of over 90% to be delivered to the patient. If you are not giving oxygen, be sure to remove the reservoir bag. Removing the reservoir bag allows room air to be drawn into the BVM giving your patient 21% oxygen. Although BVMs are used often by single responders, the preferred method is two rescuers. One rescuer positions themselves at the head of the patient and holds the mask with both hands to ensure a good facial seal while tilting the head to open the airway. The second rescuer positions themselves at the side and squeezes the bag. Facial hair, facial fractures, and loss of teeth or dentures are some of the problems the rescuer may encounter for both pocket mask and BVM. BVM ventilation is an essential emergency skill. This basic airway management technique allows for oxygenation and ventilation of patients until a more definitive airway can be established. This basic skill is also important in cases where endotracheal intubation, I-Gels or other definitive control of the airway is not possible. For the responder, basic BVM or pocket mask ventilation is most often the only option for airway management.

5.10. Stroke

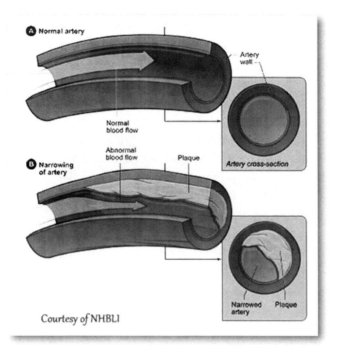

Courtesy of NHBLI

A stroke, also known as a cardiovascular accident (CVA), occurs when blood flow to the brain is interrupted by a blocked or burst blood vessel. It is one of the leading causes of death and long-term disability throughout the world. Stroke is a medical emergency, and without fast treatment, cells in the brain quickly begin to die resulting in serious disability or death. Time equals brain damage, and every second counts when seeking treatment for a stroke. When deprived of oxygen, brain cells begin dying within minutes. There are clot-busting drugs that can curb brain damage, but they have to be used within three hours of the initial stroke symptoms, and for that to happen, the patient needs to be in hospital. Once brain tissue has died, the body parts controlled by that area won't work properly. This is why stroke is a top cause of long-term disability. There are two main types of stroke, and they are not treated the same way. A CT scan can help doctors determine whether the symptoms are coming from a blocked blood vessel or a bleeding one. Additional tests may also be used to find the location of a blood clot or bleeding within the brain.

The most common type of stroke is known as an ischemic stroke. Nearly nine out of ten strokes fall into this category. The culprit is a blood clot that obstructs a blood vessel inside the brain. The clot may develop on the spot or travel through the blood from elsewhere in the body.

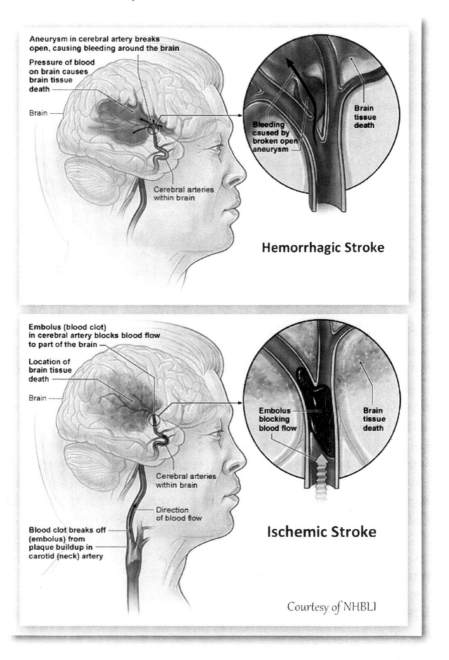

Haemorrhagic strokes are less common but far more likely to be fatal. They occur when a weakened blood vessel in the brain bursts. The result is bleeding inside the brain that can be difficult to stop.

A transient ischemic attack (TIA), often called a 'mini-stroke', is more like a close call. Blood flow is temporarily impaired to part of the brain, causing symptoms similar to an actual stroke. When the blood flows again, the symptoms disappear. TIAs usually only last about fifteen to twenty minutes and then subside. A TIA is a warning sign that a stroke may happen soon. It's critical, that the patient gets medical attention if they think they've had a TIA. There are therapies to reduce the risk of stroke. A TIA is a medical emergency and should be treated as such. The risk of that patient having a full-on stroke increases to 5% within the first forty-eight hours, 7%-8% within the first week, and 10%-15% within the first three months.

A common cause of stroke is atherosclerosis which means hardening of the arteries. Plaque made of fat, cholesterol, calcium, and other substances builds up in the arteries, leaving less space for blood to flow. A blood clot may lodge in this narrow space and cause an ischemic stroke. Atherosclerosis also makes it easier for a clot to form. Haemorrhagic strokes often result from uncontrolled high blood pressure that causes a weakened artery to burst. Certain chronic conditions increase the risk of stroke. These include high blood pressure, high cholesterol, diabetes, and obesity, and taking steps to control these conditions may reduce the risk. Smoking, using too much salt, not getting enough exercise, and heavy use of alcohol and drugs also increase the risk of stroke. People who have had a stroke or TIA can take steps to prevent a recurrence by limiting alcohol and salt intake, stop smoking, exercising and maintaining a healthy weight, and eating a healthier diet with more fish, vegetables, and whole grains. Learning to recognise the symptoms of TIA and reporting it quickly can be brain and even lifesaving.

Symptoms that can be treated

Hypertension or high blood pressure, heart disease, cigarette smoking, diabetes, elevated blood cholesterol, hyper/hypoglycaemia,

TIA, and underlying occlusive carotid artery disease referred to medically as Asymptomatic Carotid Bruit.

Signs of a stroke

Sudden numbness or weakness of the body, especially on one side; sudden vision changes in one or both eyes, or difficulty swallowing; sudden, severe headache with unknown cause; sudden problems with dizziness, walking, hearing, or balance; sudden confusion, nausea and vomiting, difficulty speaking, or understanding others. Call 999/112 immediately if you notice any of these symptoms.

Assessing a patient with stroke

Assessing a patient suspected of having a stroke is similar to assessing patients who present with any other complaints, and using an organised assessment approach will keep you focused and help you make a rapid diagnosis (Ref: CPG's Stroke). Strokes present in many ways, but be aware that these signs and symptoms can sometimes be confused with other conditions.

Consider other possibilities such as trauma or illnesses. Subdural or epidural bleeding is a collection of blood near the skull that presses on the brain. Bleeding like this is usually caused by trauma or a weakness in the blood vessels that causes them to rupture. The symptoms may not be rapidly apparent after trauma if it is a slow bleed. Headache is often associated with these conditions. As bleeding grows and continues to push on the brain, the symptoms of stroke will be similar in that the victim will have difficulty communicating and moving. Hypoglycaemia can cause the brain to lose proper function with loss of oxygen or glucose. Hypoglycaemia is when the blood glucose levels drop below the normal level. Similar symptoms to stroke can be hemiparesis (partial body paralysis). The difference is that a stroke patient may still be alert and attempting to communicate normally, whereas someone with low blood sugar almost always has an altered mental state. This condition can worsen, leading to seizures and postictal (the period following a seizure or convulsion; 'postictal drowsiness') states as well. Checking the patient's blood glucose level using a glucometer is essential to rule out a hypoglycaemic episode. Lesser common illnesses or diseases that mimic stroke are brain tumours, systemic (whole body) infections, and toxins in the body that will disturb metabolic functioning. It is important to get the patient's history before jumping to conclusions, but that may not always be possible.

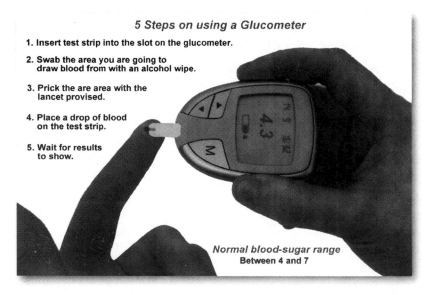

5 Steps on using a Glucometer

1. Insert test strip into the slot on the glucometer.

2. Swab the area you are going to draw blood from with an alcohol wipe.

3. Prick the are area with the lancet provised.

4. Place a drop of blood on the test strip.

5. Wait for results to show.

4.3

Normal blood-sugar range
Between 4 and 7

You may be in the situation whereby you are called to help someone who is lying on the street and not making any sense. Because of their altered level of consciousness (ALOC), you are unable to question them, and nobody seems to know them and no one has witnessed the event. There is no smell of alcohol and no signs of trauma, even though the person may have tripped and banged their head but have no bruises or cuts to give you a clue to why this happened. This example is designed to make the responder think outside the box. The obvious thing that stands out is the patient's ALOC. This is telling you that this person needs to go to hospital regardless. Once help is on the way, you can now try to assess the patient and form a general impression. A more straightforward scenario would be the call to a house to a person with ALOC; the whole neighbourhood knows this person and straight away, several neighbours and family members are telling you that this person has high blood pressure and has over the last six months had a few TIAs, sometimes referred to as mini strokes. It doesn't take a genius to work out what is most likely going on. Now you can see how difficult or easy it can be to make a diagnosis.

Treatment of stroke

For patients having a stroke, your initial assessment starts with airway, breathing, and circulation (Ref: CPG's Stroke). If they are conscious, talk to them. Reassure them and try to get a SAMPLE history. For stroke patients, the chief complaint may vary from confusion to slurred speech to unresponsiveness. Make sure help is on the way. If the patient is conscious, keep in mind their frustration, confusion, and embarrassment. Perform a focused physical exam using the FAST assessment or the Cincinnati Stroke Scale (CS Scale).

F.A.S.T. Assessment		
F	Facial weakness.	Can the patient smile? Have the eyes or face drooped?
A	Arm weakness.	Can the patient raise both arms and hold the position?
S	Speech problems.	Can the patient speak clearly and understand what you say?
T	Time.	If any of these symptoms are present, it's time to call 999 / 112.

If you do suspect stroke, as part of your physical examination, perform at least three key tests to confirm. These would involve checking facial expression, speech impairment, and arm drift (see FAST and CS Scale graphs). As a responder, assess the LOC using the AVPU scale. EMS will use the Glasgow Coma Scale (GCS) to calculate a patient's LOC as it is more comprehensive. Strokes can affect the body functions in several ways. The patient may have difficulty swallowing and are at risk of choking on their own saliva. If the patient is unresponsive with no gag reflex, an oropharyngeal airway (OPA) can be inserted to maintain a patent airway if you are trained in its use. Suction may also be necessary to prevent aspiration. If you conclude that the patient isn't capable of managing their own airway, put them in the recovery position. Check that their breathing is within the normal parameters and apply oxygen. Giving oxygen helps to limit the effects of hypoperfusion to the brain.

Cincinnati Stroke Scale		
Test	Normal	Abnormal
Facial Droop; Ask the patient to show their teeth or smile.	Both sides of the face are equal in appearance.	One side of the face does not move as well as the other.
Arm Drift; Ask the patient to close their eyes and hold out both arms palms up.	Both arms move equally and remain at the same level when raised.	One arm doesn't move or drifts down compared with the other side.
Speech; Ask the patient to say something or ask them a question.	Patient uses correct words without slurring.	Patient slurs words or uses inappropriate words, or is unable to speak.

If breathing is not adequate, you may have to provide rescue breaths. If the patient is responsive, check for a pulse and determine if it's fast or slow or strong or weak. If there is no pulse, start CPR beginning with compressions.

Glasgow Coma Scale					
Eye Opening		Best Verbal Response		Best Motor Response	
Spontaneous	4	Orientated conversation	5	Obeys commands	6
In response to speech	3	Confused conversation	4	Localizes pain	5
In response to pain	2	Inappropriate words	3	Withdraws to pain	4
No response	1	Incomprehensible sounds	2	Abnormal flexion	3
		No response	1	Abnormal extension	2
				No response	1
Score 14-15, Mild dysfunction.		Score 11-13, Moderate to severe dysfunction.		Score 10 or less is severe dysfunction.	

If the patient is in shock, be careful about rising arms or legs as this will increase blood flow to the brain and may aggravate a haemorrhage. Before concluding your focused history and physical exam, you should also, as part of your on-going assessment, obtain a set of baseline vitals. These are important to compare changes in the patient as time goes on. Pay attention to blood pressure, as in severe situations, the pressure build-up from bleeding into the brain can slow the pulse and cause respirations to be erratic. To compensate for poor perfusion in the brain, blood pressure will usually be raised significantly. Because the cause of altered mental status (AMS) sometimes can be unknown and it may still remain a mystery even when the patient gets to hospital, most of the interventions are based on the assessments the responder carried out and the history (vague as it may be) they managed to obtain. The best the responder can sometimes hope to achieve without knowing all the facts is to prevent the patient from getting worse. Maintain the ABCs, put them in the recovery position if appropriate, and administer oxygen according to your CPGs. It's worth remembering that although the patient may be unresponsive, they may still be able to hear you, so talk to them and reassure them. Tell them what you are doing in terms of treatment. Continue to reassess the patient and document any changes and interventions.

5.11. The Chain of Survival

The Chain of Survival was developed by the American Heart Association (AHA) to show the most appropriate sequence of actions required to help someone who has suffered sudden cardiac arrest (SCA). Without some form of organised sequence, things can fall apart under pressure, but by following the links in this chain, it will guide you step by step and give you the confidence knowing that you are doing the right thing at the right time. Each link is vital, and for the Chain to be effective, quick execution is critical. With each minute that passes, the likelihood of survival decreases by 7%-10%.

When you are confronted by a medical emergency as serious as SCA, unless you respond immediately, the patient has little chance of survival. The first link in the chain is Early Access. This simply means dialling 999 or 112, requesting EMS. Without activating this first link, everything else falls apart. The second link is Early CPR. This is the link that buys time and should be started as quickly as possible and maintained until an AED arrives. The third link is Early Defibrillation. This is a significant link as most victims in SCA are in ventricular fibrillation (VF) whereby the heart consequently immediately loses its ability to function as a pump. The heart beats with rapid, erratic electrical impulses causing the pumping chambers in the heart (the ventricles) to quiver uselessly, instead of pumping blood. The treatment for VF is defibrillation. AEDs deliver a brief electric shock to the heart, which enables the heart's natural pacemaker to regain control and establish a normal heart rhythm. It's worth noting that when CPR and defibrillation are provided within eight minutes of an episode, a person's chance of survival increases to 20% (see section on How an AED works). The fourth link in the Chain of Survival is advanced care. Paramedics or advanced paramedics (APs) provide this care, which can include basic life support, defibrillation, administration of cardiac drugs, and the insertion of advanced airways. This type of advanced care can help the heart in VF respond to defibrillation and maintain a normal rhythm after successful defibrillation. Finally, the fifth link in the chain is the coordinated care that the patient receives in the hospital.

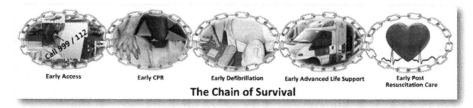

Early Access   Early CPR   Early Defibrillation   Early Advanced Life Support   Early Post Resuscitation Care

The Chain of Survival

The first three links can be carried out by anyone with a little training and can be done singularly or simultaneously. You may even assist on scene with the fourth link if EMS feels you are confident to do so. The Chain of Survival means exactly that, but unless someone activates the first link, the patient's chances of survival diminish rapidly.

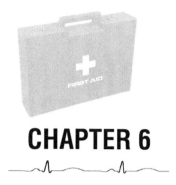

CHAPTER 6

6.1. Seizures

A seizure is a brief surge of abnormal electrical activity in the brain. It may affect only part of the brain (called a partial seizure) or may occur all over it (called a generalised seizure). Generalised seizures can be classified as a tonic, clonic, tonic-clonic, or absence on the basis of clinical symptoms. Tonic seizure is the rigid contracture of muscles, including respiratory muscles, which is usually brief. The clonic component is the rhythmic shaking that occurs and is longer. Together, a generalised tonic-clonic seizure (GTCS) is also called a grand mal seizure and is one of the most dramatic of all medical conditions.

A seizure may last from a few seconds to several minutes but rarely last more than fifteen minutes. It may be hard to tell if someone is having a seizure. Some seizures only cause a person to have staring spells that may go unnoticed. Specific symptoms depend on what part of the brain is involved. They occur suddenly and may include brief blackout followed by period of confusion, changes in behaviour such as picking at one's clothing, drooling or frothing at the mouth, eye movements, grunting and snorting, loss of bladder or bowel control, mood changes such as sudden anger, unexplainable fear, panic, joy, or laughter. Other specific symptoms include shaking of the entire body, sudden falling, tasting a bitter or metallic flavour, teeth clenching, temporary halt in breathing, and uncontrollable muscle spasms with twitching and jerking limbs.

Causes of seizures

Abnormal levels of sodium or glucose in the blood, choking, drug abuse, electric shock, epilepsy, fever (particularly in young children), head injury, heart disease, heat intolerance, high fever, use of illicit drugs, such as angel dust (PCP), cocaine, amphetamines, and kidney or liver failure. Other causes include low blood sugar, poisoning, stroke, toxaemia of pregnancy, uraemia related to kidney failure, very high blood pressure (malignant hypertension), venomous bites and stings, withdrawal from alcohol after prolonged periods of heavy drinking, withdrawal from certain drugs, such as painkillers and sleeping pills and benzodiazepines such as valium. Most symptoms of epilepsy also apply to seizures.

6.2. What causes epilepsy?

Epilepsy is a brain disorder in which a person has repeated seizures (convulsions) over time. In more than half of all cases, no cause can be found. This is sometimes called idiopathic epilepsy. The person with epilepsy is apparently healthy in every respect, and there is no underlying illness, disease, or damage causing them to have seizures. Anything that damages or injures the brain can result in epilepsy. Some of the

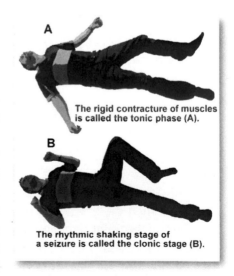

The rigid contracture of muscles is called the tonic phase (A).

The rhythmic shaking stage of a seizure is called the clonic stage (B).

common causes are stroke or TIA, dementia, such as Alzheimer's disease, traumatic brain injury, infections, including brain abscess, meningitis, and encephalitis (inflammation of the brain), and AIDS, brain problems that are present at birth (congenital brain defect), brain injury that occurs during or near birth, metabolism disorders that a child may be born with (such as phenylketonuria or PKU for short), brain tumour (rare), abnormal blood vessels in the brain, and other illness that damage or destroy brain tissue. In some individuals, the existing seizure threshold may be lowered if the brain is subject to unusual stimulation, such as, certain frequencies of flickering light and some drugs.

In most cases, epilepsy is treated with medication. Over the years, new drugs for epilepsy have become available which allow many people with epilepsy to live virtually seizure free lives.

6.3. Treatment of Seizures and Epilepsy

Most seizures stop by themselves and will be well over when EMS arrives, but keep in mind that seizures that last more than five minutes can become major emergencies where the patient may have trouble breathing or they may hurt themselves during the event. When a seizure occurs, the main goal is to protect the person from injury, and this should be the main focus of your treatment. Try to prevent a fall. Lay the person on the ground in a safe area. If the patient is on the ground, clear the area of furniture or other sharp objects. Try to protect the person's head and don't put anything in their mouth. Loosen any tight clothing, particularly around the patient's neck. (Ref: CPG's Seizure/Convulsion—Adult and Seizure/Convulsion—Paediatric)

During a seizure, the patient generally does not breathe and may turn blue. At this stage, you can't do anything about their airway, but once the seizure has stopped, it is essential to ensure the patient's airway is open and clear, so put them in the recovery position (AKA the safe airway position) as soon as possible and use the head tilt, chin lift method to open the airway. Oxygen should be given to prevent the possibility of recurrent seizure if there is a hypoxic component to the source of the convulsion.

Patients who have had a seizure may have excess oral secretions, and opening the airway will allow this to drain. The patient may have bitten their tongue during the fit, so be sure to wear gloves as their saliva may have blood mixed with it. When the patient stops fitting, although they may appear to be unconscious, they can still hear you, (this is called the postictal state), so talk to them and reassure them. During a seizure, the patient may lose bladder and bowel control and will be highly embarrassed when they recover, so bare this in mind. Reassurance is everything. Let the patient know of your awareness and understanding of what happens during a seizure and that what happens during the event is out of their control and can't be helped. Look for a medical bracelet as it may have specific information. Stay with the patient until they recover and medical help arrives and try to get a medical history. If they haven't recovered sufficiently, try to get information from bystanders if possible. Don't put pressure on them to move or get up. Allow them the time to gather their thoughts and recover properly. If the patient stops breathing after the seizure, call 999/112 and begin CPR.

If a baby or child has a seizure during a high fever, cool the child slowly with tepid water. Do not place the child in a cold bath. Seizures can be frightening for parents or even the responder, and they can vary as with adults from simple momentary staring spells to generalised seizures where the entire body stiffens and shakes severely, but they are not generally serious. During a seizure, a child may lose consciousness, and their eyes will roll back. Their teeth will clinch, and it is very important that nothing is placed between their teeth. It is also important for the rescuer that they don't attempt to put a finger in the patient's mouth as they will bite down, locking their jaw resulting in possible dislocation of the victims jaw and injury to the rescuer's finger. It's important to time the seizure from the beginning to the end of convulsions. A seizure lasting more than five minutes will be treated differently than a shorter one. When they recover to the stage where they can breathe properly, put them in the recovery position. If the child stops breathing after the seizure, call 999/112 and begin CPR.

6.4. Shock

Shock is defined as failure of the circulatory system to adequately supply the cells of the body with oxygen. As discussed in the section explaining the cardiovascular system, the circulatory system is made up of three things: liquid, a vessel, and a pump. The liquid being blood, the vessel being the blood vessels, and the pump being the heart. There are lots of possible causes to circulatory failure, but the three primary causes are dealt with here. These are pump failure, vessel failure, and fluid loss.

Pump Failure

If the heart can't pump enough blood to supply the body's needs, cardiogenic shock occurs. A heart that has been weakened as a result of myocardial infarction (MI) can result in inadequate perfusion causing blood to back up in the blood vessels of the lungs resulting in congestive heart failure (CHF).

Vessel failure

Capillary dilation is the expansion of up to three or four times the normal size of the small blood vessels we call capillaries. This causes blood to pool in these small vessels instead of circulating throughout the system in the normal way. When pooling in the capillaries occurs, the rest of the body including the heart and other vital organs is deprived of blood resulting in a significant drop in blood pressure causing the body to go into shock. When shock occurs in this fashion, blood pressure may drop so fast that you are unable to feel a radial or a carotid pulse. Three types of shock are caused by capillary expansion. These are shock brought about by fainting, anaphylactic shock, and spinal shock. The least serious being fainting. This is a short-term condition and is the body's response to a major psychological or emotional stress which corrects itself once the patient is put in the horizontal position.

Anaphylaxis is an allergic reaction caused by your body's immune system over-reacting to the presence of a foreign body. An anaphylactic reaction is quickly reversible with an injection of adrenaline (also called epinephrine). This will be dealt with in detail later.

Fluid loss

Our third type of shock is hypovolaemic shock. This is due to insufficient blood volume, either from haemorrhage from an internal or external wound or loss of fluid from widespread vasodilation so that normal blood volume cannot maintain tissue perfusion. Symptoms are like those of cardiogenic shock. To compensate for fluid loss, the heart has to pump faster to maintain pressure in the blood vessels, but as blood continues to leak out, pressure continues to drop and the heart eventually stops pumping because there is nothing to pump, resulting in heart failure and death. In the case of an external bleed such as an arterial bleed or any other bleed that is visible, because you can see it, you can make every effort to treat it and stop the blood flow, whereas with an internal bleed, there isn't much you can do, and by the time one realises what's happening, it's often too late. The average adult has approximately 5 litres (approx. 8.80 pints) of blood and 40% or greater is usually considered the maximum amount of blood that an adult can lose before the body can no longer compensate. In an 80 kg (around 12 ½ stone) adult, this would be about 2.24 litres (approx. 3.94 pints).

Spinal shock

When a spinal cord injury is caused due to trauma, the body goes into a state known as spinal shock. This injury allows the capillaries to expand and blood pools in the lower extremities. Vital organs including the brain, lungs, and heart are deprived of blood resulting in shock. It is characterised by sensory, motor, and reflex loss occurring below the level of injury. While spinal shock begins within a few minutes of the injury, it may take several hours before the full effects occur. Spinal shock can last for four to six weeks following injury, but in some cases, can last for several months. Clinical presentation of spinal shock involves changes in skeletal muscles, sensory response, breathing, heart, blood vessels, vasomotor response, body temperature, gastrointestinal (GI) tract, urinary bladder, and genitalia. Immediate medical care within the first few hours following injury is critical to the patient's recovery, so prompt evaluation, immobilisation, and transportation of the patient by EMS is paramount.

Hypoglycaemia (insulin shock)

Hypoglycaemia means low blood sugar and is also referred to as insulin shock. This is a medical emergency that requires prompt treatment. Insulin shock can happen quickly, and if not diagnosed and corrected by administration of some form of sugar, the patient could die. As part of a diabetic's routine, apart from taking their insulin, regular exercise and eating are important, and a simple thing like exercising too vigorously or going for long periods without eating can cause the blood sugar level to drop dramatically resulting in insulin shock. The signs and symptoms are similar to other types of shock. Early or mild symptoms include sweating, shakiness, increased heart rate, and anxiety. As blood sugar decreases, the patient will feel weak, tired, or dizzy. They may experience blurred vision, confusion, and difficulty in speaking. Inevitably, they will become comatose and eventually die. One of the biggest mistakes made by responders dealing with insulin shock is misinterpretation of the signs. The patient presenting with slurred speech, confusion and staggering, or indeed falling over due to dizziness can appear to be intoxicated.

Septic shock

Septic shock is a potentially lethal drop in blood pressure due to the presence of bacteria in the blood. It may progress to cause 'adult respiratory distress syndrome,' in which fluid collects in the lungs, causing breathing to become very shallow and laboured. Septic shock can lead to multiple organ failure, including respiratory failure, and may cause rapid death. The first sign of shock is often confusion and a decreased level of consciousness (LOC) with the extremities warm to the touch. As time progresses, the extremities become cool, pale and bluish with fever giving way to lower than normal temperatures. Other symptoms include rapid heartbeat, shallow, rapid breathing, and decreased urination. During an infection, certain types of bacteria can produce and release complex molecules called endotoxins that may provoke a dramatic response by the body's immune system. Endotoxins when released into the bloodstream are particularly dangerous, because they become widely dispersed and affect the blood vessels themselves. Arteries and the smaller arterioles open wider, increasing the total volume of the circulatory system. At the same time, the walls of the blood vessels become leaky, allowing fluid to seep out into the tissues, lowering the amount of fluid left in circulation. This combination of increased systemic volume and decreased fluid causes a dramatic decrease in blood pressure and reduces the blood flow to the organs. Other changes brought on by immune response may cause coagulation of the blood in the extremities, which can further decrease circulation through the organs. Common places where an infection might start include the bowel (usually seen with peritonitis), the kidneys (upper urinary tract infection or pyelonephritis), the lining of the brain (meningitis), the liver or the gall bladder, the lungs (bacterial pneumonia) and the skin (cellulitis). In children, sepsis may accompany infection of the bone (osteomyelitis). In hospitalised patients, common sites of infection include intravenous lines, surgical wounds, surgical drains, and bedsores (decubitus ulcers).

6.5. Treatment for Shock

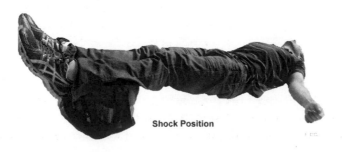

Shock Position

Although we have discussed several types of shock, the treatment in all cases is more or less the same. The key points are correct patient position, maintaining the patient's ABC's, treating the cause, and keeping them warm. Using these points can prevent shock from getting worse. As shock is a medical emergency, it is important to call EMS as soon as possible. Provided there are no injuries, lay the patient on their back on a blanket with their legs elevated about 12-15 inches. This will help the blood to drain back to the core to the vital organs. If the patient has a head injury, do not raise the legs. If the patient has chest pain or has difficulty breathing, raise them into a semi-reclining position. Check airway, breathing, and circulation at least every five minutes. Some of the causes of shock are beyond the responder's capability, but one common cause is bleeding. External bleeding can be controlled by elevation of a limb and by applying direct or indirect pressure to the wound. Preventing further blood loss will greatly improve the patient's chances of survival. Keep the patient warm, and if you are outdoors, protect them from the elements. Don't give anything to eat or drink, but if there is a long delay before EMS arrives, you may moisten a small sponge or clean cloth such as a rolled bandage for them to suck on. Keep monitoring the patient and prepare if necessary to resuscitate.

6.6. Anaphylactic Shock

Anaphylaxis is an allergic reaction caused by your body's immune system overreacting to the presence of a foreign body. It responds to something harmless as if it is a threat. After being exposed to a substance such as bee sting venom, the person's immune system becomes sensitised to it. On a later exposure to that allergen, an allergic reaction may occur. Anaphylaxis symptoms usually occur within minutes of exposure to an allergen. Sometimes, however, anaphylaxis can occur a half-hour or longer after exposure. It is severe and involves the whole body. This may in severe cases eventually lead to lack of oxygen to the brain as the airway constricts even more resulting in a rapid drop in blood pressure causing respiratory failure. The victim will then fall unconscious and eventually suffer a heart attack followed by cardiac arrest.

When in anaphylactic shock, the blood vessels leak, bronchial tissues swell, and blood pressure drops, causing the victim to choke and collapse. The most common causes of anaphylactic shock are peanuts, tree nuts such as almonds, walnuts, cashews, Brazil nuts, fish, shellfish, dairy products, eggs, soya, wasp or bee stings, natural latex (rubber), penicillin, and other drugs. An anaphylactic reaction is quickly reversible with an injection of adrenaline (also called epinephrine). People who know they suffer from this condition sometimes carry medication in the form of an auto-injector (such as an EpiPen® or Anapen®).

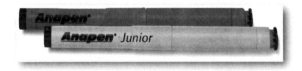

Signs and symptoms

The symptoms of a mild to moderate allergic reaction can include tingling in the mouth or a tingling sensation on the skin, particularly to the extremities such as the fingertips, swelling of the lips, face and eyes, hives along with itching, flushed or pale skin (almost always present with anaphylaxis), dizziness or fainting, a feeling of warmth. Other less severe symptoms are diarrhoea, nausea, vomiting, and cramping.

A severe allergic reaction can include difficult or noisy breathing, swelling of the tongue which can cause wheezing and trouble breathing, swelling in the throat (the sensation of a lump in your throat), difficulty talking and or hoarse voice, wheezing or persistent coughing, loss of consciousness, a weak, rapid pulse, and a feeling of impending doom. Young children may appear pale and floppy.

6.7. Treatment for Anaphylactic Shock

First, if the patient is conscious and can communicate, ask them if they are allergic to anything and if they are carrying medication such as an auto-injector. If there is a family member, friend, or work colleague present, they should be able to give you the information you need. Talk to the patient and reassure them. Explain what you are doing. This will help to decrease their anxiety level. If the patient can't communicate with you and the symptoms suggest anaphylaxis, call EMS immediately. This may be a first time attack and will have taken the patient completely by surprise resulting in panic causing further complications.

Whatever the circumstances, even if you are not sure, you must act fast and call EMS to arrange rapid transport to hospital. Better safe than sorry! The patient should be kept quiet and still. This should slow down the spread of the poison. The more they panic and move about, the faster the poison will travel through the body. Keeping the patient as calm as possible will buy them some time until EMS arrives. Elevating the person's legs (shock treatment position) may help in some cases. Check if the person is wearing a medical alert bracelet or carrying an auto-injector. If so, hand it to them and let them use it. If the person's condition progresses to the point of respiratory or cardiac arrest, begin mouth to mouth resuscitation or CPR.

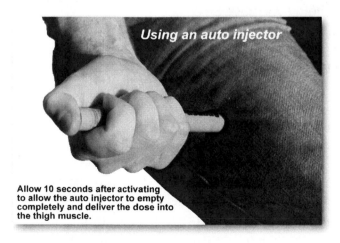

Using an auto injector

Allow 10 seconds after activating to allow the auto injector to empty completely and deliver the dose into the thigh muscle.

Duration of an anaphylactic episode

When the patient gets the appropriate and timely treatment, they can improve within a few hours and recover completely.

However, if they had already advanced to the more serious stage before intervention, it may take a few days before full recovery. If untreated, anaphylaxis can cause death within minutes to hours. Unfortunately, even with treatment, some people die of anaphylaxis.

Prevention of an anaphylactic episode

Anaphylaxis can be prevented by avoiding the allergens that trigger your symptoms. People with food allergies should always check the list of ingredients on food labels. If you are a person who eats out regularly, it's always prudent to ask the waiter or waitress to check with the chef or cook about food ingredients before eating at a café or restaurant. If you are allergic to bee stings, take extra care when gardening. Certain perfumes, deodorants, and hair sprays attract insects. If you have a history of anaphylaxis, wear a medical alert bracelet or necklace. This will help others to quickly recognise your problem and get you the help you need. Ask your doctor if it's appropriate for you to carry an auto-injector. Tell your family, friends, and co-workers of your situation, and if you are carrying an auto-injector, tell them where you store it and how to respond should you have an episode.

6.8. Diabetic Emergencies

(Hypoglycaemia/Hyperglycaemia)

Diabetes is caused as a result of the body's inability to process the natural sugar that is carried by the blood to the cells of the body. In order to survive, the body cells need sugar as well as oxygen as it is an important nutrient. Under normal circumstances, the body produces insulin which enables sugar (glucose) carried by the blood to enter the individual cells so that it can be used up as fuel. If the body can't produce enough insulin, the cells will starve and the brain will fail to function normally. The severity of the fuel starvation will determine the victim's level of response and what action needs to be taken. Insulin shock as discussed earlier in this chapter and diabetic coma are the two things that give great cause for worry, and emergency medical assistance should always be a priority.

Insulin shock occurs when there's enough insulin in the body but not enough sugar in the blood (hypoglycaemia). Insulin shock can occur rapidly, and if the victim doesn't get sugar literally within a few minutes, they could die. Sometimes the symptoms are misinterpreted as the person will appear to be drunk or confused due to light-headedness. They may not have taken their insulin or if they did, they may not have eaten to keep up their energy level. They may also have over exerted themselves either through physical work or strenuous exercise. This in itself will burn energy rapidly, and without replacing that energy, that person could quickly show signs of insulin shock. The important thing for the diabetic is to know what their body needs, make a plan, and stick to it. Take regular exercise, eat regularly, and take their medications on time. The next part of the plan should be to check their glucose levels regularly using their glucometer. More frequent testing will give a better indication of their sugar (glucose) levels and should help them to be in control.

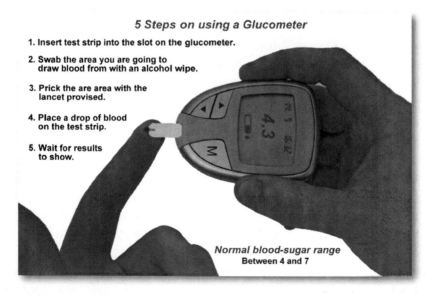

5 Steps on using a Glucometer

1. Insert test strip into the slot on the glucometer.

2. Swab the area you are going to draw blood from with an alcohol wipe.

3. Prick the are area with the lancet provised.

4. Place a drop of blood on the test strip.

5. Wait for results to show.

Normal blood-sugar range
Between 4 and 7

Diabetic coma (Ketoacidosis coma) occurs as a result of too much sugar in the body (hyperglycaemia) and not enough insulin to process it. This is more common in people with type 1 diabetes and is triggered by a build-up of chemicals called ketones which are very acidic and cause the blood in turn to become too acidic. Diabetic coma is usually the result of the patient going for several days without insulin, and when there is not enough insulin circulating, the body cannot use glucose for energy. Instead, fat is broken down and then converted to ketones in the liver. The ketones can build up excessively when there is insufficient insulin in the body. This can sometimes be misinterpreted as the person will have the appearance of having a heavy cold or flu.

Signs and symptoms

The signs and symptoms differ in both cases.

In the case of insulin shock, the patient will be quite pale with cool but moist skin. The pulse will be weak but rapid. They may complain of headache or dizziness. Breathing is usually within the normal range, and they may appear confused or may even be unconscious. The onset of symptoms of insulin shock is rapid.

In the case of diabetic coma, the patient will have a history of diabetes. The skin will feel warm and dry, and they will have a weak and rapid pulse. Breathing is usually deep and rapid with a distinct fruity smell from the patient's breath. Unlike insulin shock, the onset of the symptoms of diabetic coma is slow (usually over a period of several days).

Treatment

The treatment for any diabetic emergency depends on the level of consciousness. (Ref: CPG's Glycaemic Emergency—Adult, OFA, EFR) Establishing the LOC using the AVPU scale is the simplest method. Regardless whether they are A or V on the scale, you should at least be able to get a history and ascertain the cause of the onset and treat accordingly. However, although a patient may be conscious, they may also be confused to the point that they can't understand you or give you definitive answers. Regardless, we always treat any glycaemic incident as an emergency, so call EMS and ensure that help is on the way.

If you are unsure as to whether you are dealing with a hyper or a hypo incident and your patient's LOC is at a level whereby they can swallow in safety, give them a sugary drink as you will do no further harm to the patient. For the insulin shock patient, it may improve their condition, and in relation to the diabetic coma patient, you won't raise sugar level enough to do any further harm. If the patient is unconscious, do not attempt to give them anything to drink or eat as you may cause them to choke. Roll them on their side into the recovery or safe airway position and ensure they have a clear airway. Cover the patient with a blanket and monitor them until help arrives. When EMS arrives, they will administer 1 mg of glucagon intramuscularly if necessary to reverse the effect.

Sugar can be given in the form of a cup of tea (not too hot) with several spoons of sugar or just plain sugared water. You can also give any of the brand-named orange, cola, or glucose drinks as they are also high in sugar content. Never use diet drinks to treat a glycaemic emergency as they have no sugar content. Sugar can also be given to the conscious patient in the form of chocolate or sweets.

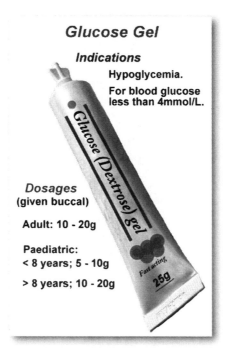

If you have glucose (dextrose) gel, for an adult or child over eight years of age, you should give 10-20 g buccal (inside the cheek). For a child less than eight years old, give 5-10 g. This is generally given by squeezing the gel either onto a gloved finger or tongue depressor and rubbing it inside the person's cheek. Glucose gel is an over-the-counter medication consisting primarily of dextrose and water. It is generally available in 25 g tubes, normally in packets of three. Dextrose is a completely pure glucose and more concentrated than regular table sugar. Table sugar (Sucrose) is half glucose and half fructose (fruit sugar).

The side effect of glucose gel is that if given too quickly, it may cause vomiting to patients below the age of five. It is also not recommended for children below two years of age.

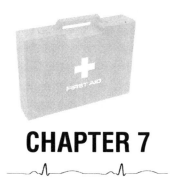

CHAPTER 7

7.1. A Brief Biology of the Blood

Blood is a complex mixture of plasma, white and red blood cells, and platelets. The plasma is the liquid component which makes up more than half the blood's volume. It consists of mostly water containing dissolved salts (electrolytes) and proteins. One of the main proteins in plasma is albumin which helps to keep fluid from leaking out of the blood vessels and into the tissues. Other proteins in plasma include antibodies (immunoglobulin) which fight against bacteria, viruses, and cancer cells. Plasma prevents blood vessels from collapsing and clogging and helps maintain blood pressure and circulation. It also plays a part in maintaining the body's temperature.

Red cells (erythrocytes) make up approximately 40% of the blood's volume. Red cells contain haemoglobin which gives it its colour and enables it to deliver oxygen from the lungs to all body tissues. The body's cells use the oxygen to produce energy, and the waste product, carbon dioxide, is transported back to the lungs for disposal. If there is a low red cell count (anaemia), it means that less oxygen is being carried, and we become weak and tired. If the red blood count is too high (polycythaemia), the blood can become thick increasing the risk of blood clots and in turn increasing the risk of stroke and heart attack. White cells (leukocytes) are fewer in number than red cells. There are 660 red cells for every one white cell. The primary responsibility for white cells is to defend the body against infection. When the white blood cell count is too low (leucopenia), infection is more likely to occur. When the white cell count is too high (leukocytosis), this may be an indication of a disease such as infection or leukaemia. Finally, we have platelets, also known as thrombocytes, which are smaller than red or white blood cells and fewer in number than red cells with a ratio of one platelet to twenty red cells. Platelets help the clotting process by gathering wherever the bleed is and clump together to form a plug in order to seal the puncture in the blood vessel.

Blood accounts for about 7% of the average human body weight. The blood volume of an average adult is approximately 5 litres (approx. 8.80pints). If the heart is beating between 60 and 80 BPM, it will pump between 4½ and 6 litres of blood through the entire circulatory system in one minute. If you exert yourself by running, for example, depending on your fitness level, your heart rate will obviously increase and your blood will circulate faster and may only take half the time for those 5 litres to travel throughout the system. The message to take forward from this is, if someone has a serious bleed, unless they get immediate treatment, they could bleed to death in anywhere between one and four minutes.

7.2. Description of Wounds and Bleeding

The nature and variety of wounds that one could encounter are many, but regardless of how minor or catastrophic they are, the treatment is basically the same. The bleeding must be stopped! The three types of bleeding are arterial, described as bright red and spurting; venous, described as dark red with a steady flow; and capillary, described as brick red and oozing.

The heart, arteries, veins, and capillaries are the main components of the blood's transport system. Think of it in simplistic terms as if it was the heating system in your home. Imagine the arteries, veins, and capillaries as the piping and heart as the pump that circulates the water through all those pipes. The big difference is if your plumbing springs a leak, your house can get flooded because there's always a reserve water supply to keep the system full and the water will continue to pour out at the same rate until someone turns off the supply and repairs the leak, whereas if your patient have a bleed, they only have around 5 litres in their system and no reserve, so it makes a lot of sense that the faster you stop the bleed, the better the outcome for your patient.

Understanding Wounds

Shallow cuts in most areas of the body rarely bleed much and will stop bleeding on their own, whereas a cut to the scalp, however, can bleed a lot due to the venous nature of that area and can look a lot worse than it really is. Initially, wounds can be painful, but the pain tends to lessen after a day. Pain that worsens a day or more after an injury is often a sign of infection. The infected wound may in due course become red and swollen and may ooze pus. If a nerve is affected, the patient may complain of 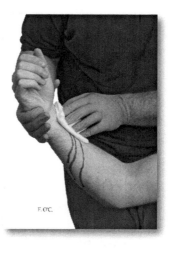 numbness. If a foreign object remains inside the wound, the area near the object will be painful to the touch.

If the wound is minor, the aim of the first-aider should be to prevent infection. Infection can develop when a wound is contaminated with dirt and bacteria. The longer the wound remains contaminated, the greater the risk of infection. Deep wounds that contain foreign objects such as glass, splinters, grit, or fragments of clothing will almost always become infected. Remember that any break in the skin will not only allow blood and other fluids to leak out, it will also allow germs to enter the body.

With a minor wound such as a scratch or graze, your main function here is infection control. Gently clean away any visible dirt or grit that may have bedded itself. Ideally, you should clean the wound under warm running water while gently swabbing it with a clean gauze wipe. Cotton wool swabs aren't really the best as sometimes the wool fibres can bed into the wound and remain there. If you feel you must use a cleaning agent to remove more stubborn dirt, you may use a mild soap along with warm running water but *do not* use harsher agents such as alcohol, iodine, or peroxide as these solutions can damage tissue and impair the wound's capability to heal. Bottled still water can be got in any shop these days and should be kept in mind as an alternative for cleaning if you have to provide first aid on the street and you don't have a kit with you.

If the wound is severe, it may be difficult to deal with, but your priority here is to stop the bleeding as quickly as possible in order to prevent the onset of shock. Obviously, infection control is important, but one can only do their best in certain circumstances. For example, you may be somewhere sometime whereby you don't have access to a first-aid kit, so you may have to improvise using whatever is available. Whenever possible, use BSI (gloves etc.) to avoid cross infection between yourself and your casualty. Be aware that gloves can puncture or tear, so check them often and replace them if necessary and dispose of them appropriately. If you have more than one patient, be sure to change gloves when you change patients and wash your hands as soon as you get the opportunity.

If you have any break in the skin such as a cut or graze, be sure to cover it up before you treat someone. Washing your hands whenever possible is a good practice. If you get blood spatter on your skin, wash it off as soon as you can and discard contaminated clothing once you are finished dealing with your patient. If you are washing contaminated clothing at home, keep them in a sealed plastic bag until you put them in your washing machine. You don't want other people handling them. Some closed wounds such as bruising or contusions could indicate an underlying injury, and first-aiders need to be aware of the cause or mechanism of injury (MOI) as this may alert you to a more serious condition, such as internal bleeding. We only mention three types of bleeding when teaching basic first aid so as not to complicate things for the beginner, and although internal bleeding does get a mention, it's never addressed in great depth. For the advanced learner, internal bleeding is known as the fourth type of bleed which we will deal with to a certain depth as part of wounds and bleeding.

7.3. Treatment of Wounds and Bleeding

Incised palm wound: We have already discussed treatment for minor wounds such as scratches and grazes and the importance of hygiene, so now, let's move on to the more serious stuff. The visible bleed in most cases is the easy to deal with. So let's start with that. Take as an example, the housewife who was preparing dinner and a sharp kitchen knife slips and cuts deep into the palm of her hand. This is a serious cut which will bleed considerably and requires immediate attention. There is also the danger of shock if enough blood is lost. Instinctively, the casualty will cover the wound with a tea towel or whatever is at hand as it will give a little comfort and also hide the sight of blood. This is a good start to the treatment as it slows the blood flow. The nature of this wound is what we call an incised (clean cut) wound, and although it may be deep, it will pull together perfectly and should heal well in time leaving only a small scar.

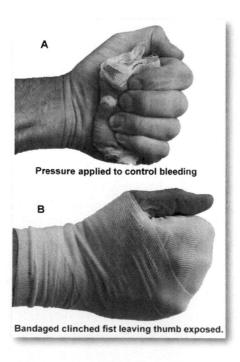

A

Pressure applied to control bleeding

B

Bandaged clinched fist leaving thumb exposed.

Your job as a first-aider is to stop the bleed, prevent infection, and immobilise the injured limb. First, sit the patient down, introduce yourself if you are a stranger, and reassure them. Tell them what you are doing and why, as it helps them to deal with the situation and trust you. Apply a sterile padded dressing onto the wound. Then place a 3 or 4 inch (7.5-10 cm) crepe roller bandage or equivalent on top of the dressing and ask the casualty to make a fist and lightly squeeze the bandage. This will put pressure on the wound and help slow down or stop the bleeding. Next, you have two choices. You can either wrap the fist in a triangular bandage or use a 2 or 3 inch (5-7.5 cm) crepe bandage to wrap the fist in place. What you want to achieve is to keep an acceptable amount of pressure on the wound by keeping a closed fist on the roller bandage. How you decide to do it is up to you, once you do it properly. Do not over tighten the dressing as you don't want to obstruct circulation. Leave the thumb exposed. If blood seeps through the dressing, apply a second dressing. Do not attempt to remove the first one as you will interfere with the clotting process. Finally, apply an elevation sling so that the fisted hand is raised to the height of the opposite shoulder. This will also slow the blood flow as the injury

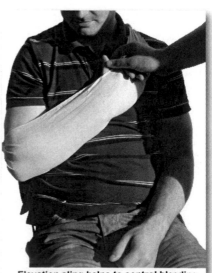

Elevation sling helps to control bleeding from wounds to the hand or forearm.

is now secured higher than the heart. Arrange transport to hospital as this wound will require stitching and treatment for infection and should be examined to make sure that no damage was done to nerves or tendons. The patient may complain of loss or movement or sensation if the nerves or tendons are severed, so it's important not to delay advanced treatment. As a way of remembering the four main stages of treatment, we use the acronym PEEP which stands for Posture, Elevation, Examination, and Pad and Bandage. Posture means to sit or lay the casualty down. Elevation means to raise the injured limb (if possible). Examination simply means to expose and examine, and finally, pad and bandage means to apply direct or indirect pressure and apply a suitable dressing. I deliberately started with this particular injury as the treatment has a certain level of difficulty and requires thought to achieve a result.

Injuries to the Upper and Lower Arm

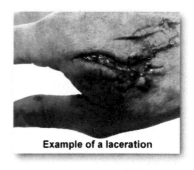

Example of a laceration

Injuries to the upper and lower arm are by nature easier to bandage, as are the legs, so let's look at dealing with a laceration which is a tear or rip in the skin. This type of injury may be as a result of contact with jagged metal or a protruding nail from discarded wood or contact with broken glass to name but a few examples. This is a common accident in the construction industry and indeed to a lesser degree in the home. The aim as always is to stop the bleed and prevent infection. This is brought about by PEEP. If the injury is to the arm, sit your patient down and examine the wound for any foreign objects such as dirt or debris. Avoid touching the wound directly. Clean it as best you can, and then place a padded dressing directly on the wound and apply pressure on the dressing to stop the bleeding. Then secure the padding in position using an appropriate size roller bandage. Roll the bandage around the limb making sure you cover the entire pad.

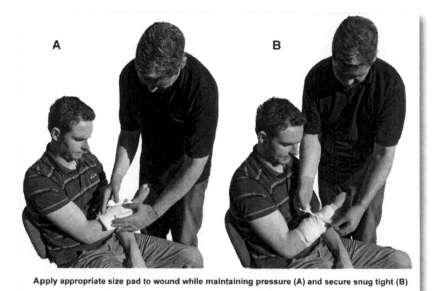

Apply appropriate size pad to wound while maintaining pressure (A) and secure snug tight (B)

If there is an object stuck in the wound such as a piece of metal or glass, etc., do not remove it as this may lead to more aggressive bleeding as the object may be lodged in a vein or artery. In this case, secure the imbedded object in the position you found it in and build around it to protect it from movement. This can be done by placing roller bandages at either side of the object, or if the object is small such as a splinter or nail, a doughnut-shape pad can be made using a triangular bandage and securing it in position.

Do not press down on the object as you may push it further in and cause more damage. If the imbedded object is too large and you are unable to pad around it, bandage around it. If the wound is in the leg, the treatment is the same. The only difference being that you should lay your patient down before you start treatment. Don't forget to raise the injured leg as this will help slow the blood flow and help to minimise swelling. A pillow or cushion or two should be enough. If you suspect a fracture, try not to move the limb too much. Rough handling may cause the bone to splinter or separate leading to other complications whereby the bone may protrude through the skin (open fracture). We will deal with this under fractures, sprains, and strains later.

Wound at a Joint Crease

Occasionally, you may have to deal with a cut at a joint crease. These are found at the back of the knee or the inside of the elbow. These joint creases are also found on the palm side of the fingers and under the toes, but bleeding wouldn't be as severe and the complications would be more limited to tendons and nerves. Major blood vessels pass across the inside of the knee and elbow, and if cut, it will bleed profusely. If treatment isn't immediate, the patient may lose a substantial amount of blood and could go into shock.

Your gold standard first part of treatment is scene safety followed by BSI. Get those gloves on before you attempt to start the treatment! Tell the casualty what you are going to do and why. Lay or, if appropriate, sit the patient down. Expose and examine the wound and clean away any loose dirt or debris that might cause infection. If any debris is imbedded and won't wash away easily, don't attempt to poke at it. Place a padded dressing on the wound and bend the joint so that it puts pressure on the pad keeping it in place. Lift and support the limb. Check circulation and sensation regularly (at least every eight to ten minutes). We have already discussed this in an earlier chapter, but to recap, what we want to see is a nice pink healthy colour below the injury. By squeezing the nail bed, the colour under the nail will turn pale and should return to its natural colour within three seconds. If you know how to, you could also do a pulse check. These are good indicators that circulation is present. If the patient complains of numbness or pins and needles, it could be an indicator that circulation is impaired. If this is the case or if your CSM check shows deficits, release the pressure on the wound to restore normal blood flow to the extremity of the limb. Make your patient as comfortable as possible, and if necessary, cover them with a coat or blanket. As with all serious injuries, especially where excessive bleeding is concerned, arrange for transport to hospital.

7.4. Varicose Vein Bleeds

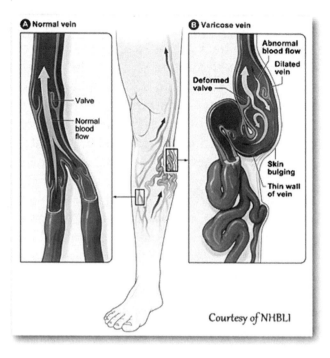

Courtesy of NHBLI

Varicose vein bleeds can be very serious, and it's worth understanding what varicose veins are by definition and why early treatment is important. Recognising varicose veins is easy. They may look like a snakelike bulge under the skin and are dark purple or blue in colour because they contain deoxygenated blood. Remember, arteries distribute oxygenated blood throughout the body, while veins carry deoxygenated blood to the heart. Pulmonary arteries and veins function differently. The exact cause of varicose veins is unknown, but the onset is mainly due to a weakness in the walls of veins close to the surface of the skin. This weakness causes the veins to lose their elasticity over time, causing them to stretch and widen allowing the valve cusps (one way valves) in the vein to separate. In a normal vein, the blood can only travel in one direction because tiny valves (cusps) open allowing blood to flow toward the heart and close to prevent blood from flowing backward. To return blood to your heart, the veins in your legs must work against gravity, and muscle contractions in the lower legs act as a pump and the elasticity in the walls of the vein help the blood return to the heart. When a vein is varicose, the cusps can't close and blood that should be moving toward the heart tends to flow backwards. This results in pooling. Any vein can become varicose, but those most commonly affected are the veins in the legs and feet as standing and walking increases pressure in the veins in these areas. Some pregnant women develop varicose veins, although veins that develop during pregnancy generally improve without medical intervention within three to twelve months after childbirth. Usually, there is no pain, but this is not always the case. When pain occurs, it can be in the form of a slight burning or throbbing sensation. Muscle cramping and swelling of the lower legs is common, and they can become itchy around one or more vein. Skin ulcers near the ankle can be an indication of a serious vascular disease and should be addressed by your doctor.

Varicose veins, because they have no protection and the walls are thin, can be ruptured quite easily. Even a simple knock can cause serious bleeding, and if not addressed urgently, the patient can go into shock. As a responder or first-aider, your priority is to control the bleed and minimise shock. First, BSI! Lay the casualty down on their back. If they are indoors on a carpeted floor, that's OK, but if it's a tiled or concrete floor or if they are outdoors, organise a blanket, quilt or a coat to put under them as soon as you have control of the bleed. Raise the leg well above the body as this will slow down the bleeding. A chair would be good as it will give you a base to work from, or you could kneel down at the patient's feet and place the heel of the injured leg on your shoulder. Quickly expose the bleeding site and apply padding over the wound. Apply direct firm pressure on the padding. If you do not have padded dressings to hand, use a clean tea towel or hand towel, face cloth, or whatever is at hand. Your priority is haemorrhage control, so don't get hung up on what or what not to use. Use whatever is available once it's clean. Cover this dressing with a roller bandage and try to apply firm but even pressure as you roll the bandage around the leg.

Be aware that circulation was poor even before the injury happened, and you don't want to be the cause of making it worse by over squeezing the bandage. The key here is firm even pressure over the entire bandaged area. You may be in a situation where you don't have roller bandages! If this is the case, just keep firm pressure on the padding with your gloved hand. If blood seeps through the padding, as with all wounds, do not remove any dressings. Simply put more padding on top and maintain pressure. Cover the patient with a blanket, if necessary. Because this injury needs medical attention, you should call an ambulance and keep the leg elevated and maintain pressure on the wound until help arrives.

Many factors may raise the risk for varicose veins, including family history, older age, gender, pregnancy, overweight or obesity, and lack of movement. Having family members who have varicose veins may raise your risk for the condition. About half of all people who have varicose veins have a family history of them. Getting older may raise your risk for varicose veins. The normal wear and tear of aging may cause the valves in your veins to weaken and not work well. Women tend to get varicose veins more often than men. Hormonal changes that occur during puberty, pregnancy, and menopause (or with the use of birth control pills) may raise a woman's risk for varicose veins. During pregnancy, the growing fetus puts pressure on the veins in the mother's legs. Varicose veins that occur during pregnancy usually get better within three to twelve months of delivery. Being overweight or obese can put extra pressure on your veins. This can lead to varicose veins. Standing or sitting for a long time, especially with your legs bent or crossed, may raise your risk for varicose veins. This is because staying in one position for a long time may force your veins to work harder to pump blood to your heart.

Lifestyle changes often are the first treatment for varicose veins. These changes can prevent varicose veins from getting worse, reduce pain, and delay the formation of other varicose veins. Lifestyle changes should include avoiding standing or sitting for longer periods without taking a break. When sitting, avoid crossing your legs. Keep your legs raised when sitting, resting, or sleeping. When you can, raise your legs above the level of your heart. Do physical activities to get your legs moving and improve muscle tone. This helps blood move through your veins. If you're overweight or obese, try to lose weight. This will improve blood flow and ease the pressure on your veins. Avoid wearing tight clothes, especially those that are tight around your waist, groin (upper thighs), and legs. Tight clothes can make varicose veins worse. Avoid wearing high heels for long periods. Lower heeled shoes can help tone your calf muscles. Toned muscles help blood move through the veins. A doctor may recommend compression stockings. These stockings create gentle pressure up the leg. This pressure keeps blood from pooling and decreases swelling in the legs.

7.5. Internal Bleeding

Internal bleeding is the most serious type of bleed because initially, there are little or no symptoms that you can read into, and when the symptoms do show, the patient may be in a serious condition. Internal bleeding can be due to trauma or can be spontaneous. An aneurysm, for example, is a balloon-like bulge or weakening of an artery wall which puts pressure on surrounding structures and may eventually rupture.

Cerebral aneurysm

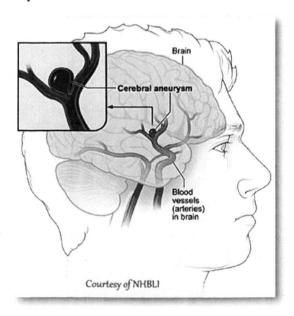

Courtesy of NHBLI

Aneurysms in the arteries of the brain are called cerebral or brain aneurysms. Brain aneurysms are also called berry aneurysms because they're often the size of a small berry. Most brain aneurysms don't cause any symptoms until they become large, begin to leak blood, or rupture (burst). A ruptured brain aneurysm can cause a stroke. When blood haemorrhages into the brain, it is known as a subarachnoid haemorrhage. Blood in the subarachnoid space increases pressure on the brain, cutting off oxygen-rich blood from the affected area resulting in stroke. The subarachnoid space normally contains cerebrospinal fluid (CSF). A subarachnoid haemorrhage is a bleed into this space. Survival rate from this type of haemorrhage is in the region of about 50%. The symptoms are headache and visual problems and should be acted on quickly. The patient may present with only one or both symptoms, and it may be difficult for the responder to interpret what's going on. If in doubt, call an ambulance. Don't wait just because people are pressuring you to hold on to see if the symptoms go away. This type of pressure from a relative is common as it is a form of denial on their part that something serious may be wrong. You must get the message across quickly but tactfully that in your opinion this is a medical emergency and time is important. Reassure those around you that it is in the victim's best interest to be assessed in a hospital without further delay so that they can either confirm your diagnosis or rule it out.

Aortic aneurysms

The aorta is the largest artery in the body. It extends from the left chamber (ventricle) of the heart and goes through the chest, down through the belly, or midsection of the body (abdomen), and into the pelvis (groin). In the groin, it divides into two vessels that supply blood to the lower trunk and both legs. In the chest, the aorta is called the thoracic aorta; in the abdomen, it's known as the abdominal aorta.

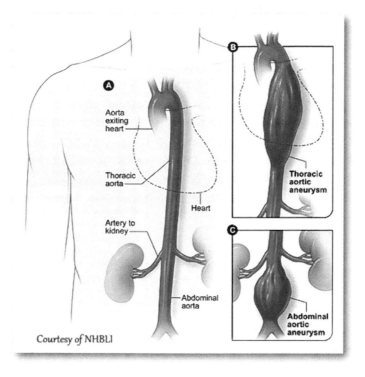

Courtesy of NHBLI

We already know the effects of an aneurysm in the brain, but if a patient has an aortic aneurysm, the chances of survival are at best about 30% if the patient was hospitalised before or during the event, and as low as 10% for an out of hospital event. The most common cause of aortic aneurysm is atherosclerosis (hardening of the arteries). Three-quarters of aneurysms develop in the abdominal aorta with the remainder developing in the thoracic aorta. The good news is that with the advent of computer tomography (CT), more and more thoracic aneurysms are being detected than in the past. Before the aneurism ruptures, there may be no warning signs or symptoms; however, when the event occurs, the symptoms can be both severe and many. These may be sudden intense pain in the back of the abdomen, radiating to the buttocks, the groin, and legs. The abdomen may become rigid followed by a throbbing sensation. Other symptoms (which can be related to any form of spontaneous or traumatic internal bleed) are anxiety, nausea and vomiting, dizziness, trembling, rapid weak pulse, rapid shallow breathing, and extreme thirst. Skin will feel cold and clammy and will be pale in colour. If bleeding is ongoing, the patient' skin colour will turn ashen, and there will be cyanosis (blue) on the lips and earlobes from lack of oxygenated blood. In dark-skinned people, check the mucus membranes (gums, lips or around the eyes). Note also that in dark skinned victims, cyanosis may present as whitish grey around the lips and gums and not blue as you might expect. The conjunctivae may present as grey or bluish. Cyanosed yellow skinned people on the other hand may present with a greyish-greenish skin tone. The patient may show signs of dizziness or could go unconscious. It is also worth noting that natural light is better for assessment of cyanosis. Fluorescent lighting for example may alter the true skin colour giving it a bluish tint.

Peripheral aneurysms

Aneurysms that occur in arteries other than the aorta and the brain arteries are called peripheral aneurysms. Common locations for peripheral aneurysms include the popliteal femoral and carotid arteries. The popliteal arteries run down the back of the thighs, behind the knees. The femoral arteries are the main arteries in the groin. The carotid arteries are the two main arteries on each side of your neck.

Peripheral aneurysms aren't as likely to rupture or dissect as aortic aneurysms. However, blood clots can form in peripheral aneurysms. If a blood clot breaks away from the aneurysm, it can block blood flow through the artery. If a peripheral aneurysm is large, it can press on a nearby nerve or vein and cause pain, numbness, or swelling.

7.6. Treatment for Internal Bleeding

So what can the responder do in these situations? The first and most important thing you can do is call the ambulance service as quickly as possible (999 or 112). While you are waiting for them to arrive, talk to your patient and reassure them. Lay them on the ground and raise their legs off the ground. This will allow the blood to flow back to the body. Do not give anything to drink. If the patient insists that they are very thirsty, moisten their lips with a damp sponge or pad, and this should take away the craving. It's important not to upset your patient. Loosen any tight clothing that may restrict their breathing. This will mainly be a necktie and or top button of a shirt, no more. Cover them with a blanket to keep them warm. Monitor their ABCs and LOC (AVPU scale). It will be very helpful to the emergency services if you can obtain a SAMPLE history. If you know how to take a radial pulse, do so and check it about every two minutes. Note if it's strong or weak, fast or slow, and how many beats per minute. By comparing your latest pulse check with the previous ones, you will know how your patient is doing. For example, if during the last check, the patient had a pulse rate of 75 strong beats per minute and now you find it has changed to 90 weak beats per minute, you know now that your patient is getting worse. Write everything down. Each time you take a pulse, write down the time, number of beats, and strength. If you feel that you are out of your depth or unsure of anything, phone back the ambulance service, and they will help you and give you an estimated time of arrival (ETA) for the ambulance. If you ask the call taker to talk you through or clarify things you are not sure of, put your phone on loudspeaker and they will assist you in your assessment or treatment. That way you won't feel alone. These are just two examples of internal bleeding caused by a spontaneous rupture, but the treatment used in dealing with these catastrophic events is exactly the same treatment given for all types of internal bleeding although some may not be as immediately life-threatening as others as we will now deal with.

We have dealt with symptoms. Now, let's deal with signs associated with internal bleeding in specific areas. Depending on the site of the bleed, signs may vary, but a discharge of blood from a body opening (orifice) is very obvious, so let's match the site where blood shows to the source of the problem to find the cause.

The obvious sign of bright red frothy blood being coughed up by a patient suggests bleeding in the lungs (haemoptysis). This could be a sign of pulmonary embolism, a bacterial infection, or even lung cancer. Bleeding in the lungs from pneumonia is rare, but it does happen.

Pulmonary contusion (bruising of the lungs) caused by blunt force trauma to the chest may be obvious after examination and palpation, but if there is blood in the lung and the patient coughs, you will see this frothy spittle in the mouth.

If your patient vomits blood and the colour is dark red or reddish brown looking like coffee grounds, this may be a sign of bleeding within the digestive system (gastrointestinal tract). This bleeding may be as a result of cancer in the digestive tract or a viral infection.

If your patient is bleeding from the nose and the blood is bright red in colour, it may be as a result of a rupture of a blood vessel in the nostril. This can be caused by sneezing, blowing, or picking the nose or indeed high blood pressure. If the blood is thin and watery, it may be an indication of a head injury, that is, a fractured skull. The watery appearance means that the blood is mixed with cerebrospinal fluid (CSF). We will deal with nose bleeding in depth in a later section.

Blood from the ear that is bright red in colour may indicate an injury to the inner or outer ear, or it could signify a perforated eardrum. If the blood is thin and watery, it may be an indication of a head injury. If there is a skull fracture, it is not unknown for this watery blood to appear in both ear and nose.

Bleeding from the anus or rectal bleeding (haematochezia) is commonly dealt with by EMS but not so common, in fact rare to the first-aider or responder. Once again, colour of blood can indicate where the bleed is coming from. If the blood is bright red, it usually means bleeding is coming from the rectum or low in the colon, whereas dark red or maroon colour usually means that the bleed is higher in the colon or in the small bowel. A black or tarry (melena) stool usually means that the blood is coming from the stomach. Rectal bleeding can be caused by a number if things such as ulcers, large polyps, diverticulitis, anal fissure, inflammatory bowel disease, or colon cancer. Aspirin can be another cause of rectal bleeding.

Vaginal bleeding can be from menstruation, ectopic pregnancy, miscarriage, pelvic inflammatory disease, sexual abuse, uterine fibroids, and cancer of the cervix, uterus, or ovaries. The colour will vary between bright and dark red.

Blood in the urine (haematuria) can be present in one or two ways: blood that is visible to the naked eye and blood that can only be identified under a microscope. Both can be serious. Certain foods such as beetroot and berries can colour the urine to give it a blood-like appearance which is normal, but if blood does appear for no known reason, it should be addressed as soon as possible. Blood in the urine may be caused by trauma to the kidney, kidney stones, or kidney disease. It could also be a sign of a urinary tract infection, cystitis, sexually transmitted disease, enlarged prostate gland, prostate, or kidney or bladder cancer.

7.7. Nosebleed

Nosebleeds (epistaxis) can be quite dramatic but in truth, most can be dealt with without having to call EMS. So, who gets nosebleeds? The simple answer is that anyone can have a nosebleed. Nosebleeds can start at the front (anterior) or the back (posterior) of the nasal passage. Anterior bleeds mainly come from the lower septum which is the cartilage that gives the nose its shape. There are many tiny and delicate blood vessels in this part of the nose which are easily damaged. Bleeds in this area are normally caused by picking or scratching the nose with a sharp fingernail or blowing too hard. A cold or flu or the overuse of nasal decongestants can also bring about a nosebleed in this area as can a dryness caused by dry air in hot climates or stuffy hot rooms where there is no fresh airflow. Use of drugs such as sniffing cocaine can also cause nosebleed. A bang to the nose is another cause. Anterior nosebleeds are more common among children and can be treated quite easily.

Nosebleeds that start at the back (posterior) of the nose are more serious. Unlike anterior bleeds, posterior nosebleeds are more common in adults than children and tend to be heavier requiring medical intervention. A posterior nosebleed originates in branches of the arteries that feed the nasal cavity between the roof of the mouth and the brain. Bleeding from the back of the nose can be caused by high blood pressure, a growth or tumour in the nasal cavity, certain medication such as aspirin or blood-thinning medicines (anticoagulants) such as warfarin, or perhaps the patient may have had recent nasal surgery. It could also be an indicator of a blood clotting abnormality such as haemophilia which affects the blood's ability to clot. Keep in mind what we have previously discussed that if the blood is thin and watery, there is a danger of head injury.

Treatment for nosebleeds

This is one of the times where the patient does all the work and you're there to give advice and to monitor the situation. Sit the casualty down. Get them to lean forward and tilt the head slightly downwards. If the patient keeps their head in the neutral position, the blood will run back the throat and into the stomach causing the patient to feel ill and perhaps vomit. Get the patient to pinch the nose just below the bony prominence and keep the pressure on for ten minutes. The patient should be 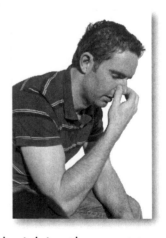 encouraged to breathe through their mouth. Advise them not to spit, cough, speak, sniff, or swallow. Reassure your patient. Release the pressure after ten minutes to see if the bleeding has stopped. If it hasn't stopped, reapply pressure and keep the nose pinched for a further ten minutes. If the bleeding has stopped, advise the patient to rest for a while and not to blow their nose because they will disturb the clots that have formed and it will bleed again. If the bleed is severe and still bleeding after twenty minutes, pinch the nose again and arrange for transport to hospital.

7.8. Crush Injury

Crush injuries can be serious and life-threatening and are defined as compression of extremities or other parts of the body between two solid objects. This injury can become complicated if open wounds, fractures, or poor circulation are involved. These injuries mainly occur as a result of accidents where people are trapped for long periods in cars, trucks, tractors, and agricultural machinery and to a lesser degree in the construction industry.

Whenever we hear about earthquakes, we automatically visualise jagged cracked and open roads and collapsed buildings. Collapsed buildings are the main source of casualties that suffer from crush injuries, and because of the volume of casualties involved and the initial available resources, not to mention the time involved in locating casualties, fatalities are inevitable.

Nearly all injuries sustained by crushing are internal with bruising being the only obvious sign. If the chest is crushed, it is likely that ribs may be broken with the added possibility of a punctured lung (pneumothorax). When several ribs are broken, this is known as a flail chest and with this comes difficulty in breathing with the added problem of respiratory arrest leading to shock and eventually, cardiac arrest, because the protection provided by the ribcage which allows room for the lungs to fill is gone and the casualty can't draw a proper breath. Crushing of the abdominal area may involve the liver, intestines, kidneys, or spleen. A ruptured spleen or liver will result in massive internal bleeding, and a ruptured intestine will cause the contents to leak into the abdominal cavity causing infection (peritonitis).

If the patient has been trapped for any length of time, they may have damage to body tissue and especially to muscles. The big dangers to be aware of are that shock may develop rapidly as the pressure is removed, and tissue fluid leaks into the injured area and also, toxic substances that build up around the crush site may cause kidney failure if suddenly released into the circulation. This is known as crush syndrome and not only is it serious, it can be fatal.

Treatment for crush injuries

Lessons to learn when dealing with a crush injury apart from knowing what to do is what not to do! First, consider scene safety, and only when it is safe to approach, do so, but as you approach, let the MOI also tell its story. You can learn a lot by looking at the scene, and be more informed as to what treatment and resources you need. Like any other trauma casualty, check and establish that their ABCs are intact. Keep the casualty calm and still and reassure them. The event may 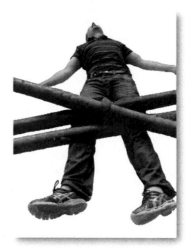 throw you at first sight, and your reaction will be picked up quickly by your patient. In short, if you get excited, your patient will get even more excited and may start to panic. If your patient sees you being calm and confident, they will be more at ease. Phone EMS as soon as possible and give brief details of the incident. This information will also help the ambulance crew to prepare en route. If the casualty was trapped for less than fifteen minutes and you are able to release them safely, do so as quickly as possible. If the casualty is bleeding, place a padded dressing on the wound and apply pressure. Secure the dressing with a bandage. There may be a fracture (break) in the same area as the bleed with the possibility that a piece of bone may be sticking out through the wound (open fracture). Build up around the bone with roller bandages or padding until there is enough for you to bandage over the wound without pressing on the bone. Remember to check circulation before and after you apply the dressing. Do not bandage too tightly as the wound area may swell. Immobilise the injured limb exactly the same way as you would a closed fracture. Keep the patient warm and be prepared to treat for shock.

If your casualty has been trapped for more than fifteen minutes, do not attempt to remove them. Call EMS and advise them of the situation. Monitor their vital signs (ABCs and AVPU scale and pulse) and make notes. Talk to your patient and reassure them. Cover them with a blanket and do not give anything to drink.

7.9. Eye Injuries

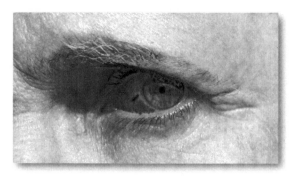

Our eyes are very sensitive and even a minute piece of dust can be very irritating. When we have an accident involving the eye, it must be taken seriously until proven otherwise. The cornea is a clear, dome-shaped surface that covers the front of the eye. When something such as dust or grit gets in our eyes, we rub them. It's difficult not to because it's an automatic reflex, but this action only irritates the eye and can cause even more damage. Injuries to the outer surface of the cornea can be caused by scratches and scrapes (abrasions), ill-fitting or overuse of contact lenses, and chemical irritation from some shampoos, cosmetics, or contact lens solutions. Over exposure to sunlight can burn the eyes, and it is advisable to wear sunglasses when exposed to sunlight for long periods.

Because your eyelids close quickly in a reflex reaction, burns as a result of splashes from hot liquids, corrosive chemicals, or flame may be confined to the eyelids themselves. The level of pain and appearance of the eyelids will depend on the severity of the injury, but be aware that the eye itself may be burned also.

People who use arc-welders use shields to protect their eyes but occasionally get flashes from accidently looking at what they are welding. Imagine looking directly into a camera flash. You're blinded for a few seconds and then it wears off. Not so with a weld flash. You may be blind or partially blind for several minutes, but although your sight returns, your eyes will feel like someone has thrown a fist of salt in them, and this sensation could last for two or three days. Because of the sensation, you will involuntarily rub the eyes making them worse. They will continuously weep as if you are crying all the time, and closing your eyes to sleep is difficult as it feels like there is grit under the eyelids. Bright lights will aggravate the eyes also, and the victim should wear dark glasses when going out into sunlight. The only cure for this is time (usually two or three days) and prescribed eye drops from your GP (general practitioner) to keep them from drying out and crusting and also to prevent infection setting in.

Other injuries can come from particles hitting the eye at high speed such as splinters of metal, glass, or masonry. Splinters of metal and glass in particular may penetrate the cornea and bed deep in the eye, resulting in serious injury or even blindness. There is always a danger of scaring and or infection from a foreign body either scratching or penetrating the eye, and without the appropriate treatment, the injury, if ignored, may lead to permanent damage.

Treatment for Eye Injuries

Treatment for eye injuries as with any other treatment depends on the severity of the injury. If possible, wash your hands with soap and water before you treat the patient.

A burn to the eyelids can be treated by cooling the burn with a sterile solution poured onto gauze and gently patting the affected area. You may only have water to work with, but cooling the burn is the priority and first-aiders often have to improvise. A chemical burn should be treated as quickly as possible by flushing the eyes with cold water. You may have to physically keep the eyelids open in order to flush them out as the victim may find it impossible to cooperate with you because of the pain. Because you are dealing with chemicals, it is important that you wear gloves and take all necessary precautions to protect yourself from accidental contamination. When flushing out an eye, it is important to have the affected eye lower than the good eye. This allows the contaminant to drain away from the unaffected eye creating less of a risk of accidental damage. If both eyes are affected, lay the victim down flat and flush out each eye in quick rotation getting the patient to turn their head from one side to the other to allow drainage. For example, if you are flushing the left eye, have the patient turn their head to the left and vice versa. Don't spend too long on either eye. Rotate every few seconds, but don't stop, keep flushing. Don't forget to communicate with your patient and reassure them. Tell them you understand that they are in pain, but what you're doing is for their good and encourage them to trust you. If the burn is very serious, call EMS as quickly as possible and keep flushing the eye or eyes for ten to fifteen minutes or until EMS arrives. If the burn is minor, as before, cool it with a cold damp gauze or clean cloth and arrange for someone to drive them to hospital to have it checked out at the earliest convenience.

A piece of dirt or grit that enters the eye can normally be removed with a moist piece of gauze or flushed out with water, but if you cannot dislodge the object or it appears to be stuck in the eye, do not persist in trying to remove it as you may do more harm than good. Have it removed professionally. Scratches, scrapes, and cuts to the eye can get infected quite easily, and apart from that, because of the complexity of the eye, any injury of that nature should get expert treatment. It's so easy to think that a small scratch is nothing to worry about but your sight is a gift and it can be taken away in a flash. To avoid infection and to stop your patient rubbing the eye, close the affected eye and cover it with a clean bandage. Explain to your patient that they shouldn't move the good eye as both eyes follow each other and movement will only aggravate the injury. It will make things easier for them if you cover the good eye as well as this will prevent movement, but explain your actions as you don't want to frighten the patient into thinking that things are worse than they are. If there is a foreign body embedded in the eye and is protruding in a way that it may be knocked out accidently, if it is long, say for example three or four inches, it may be difficult to stabilise. Find something like a clean paper or plastic disposable cup and cover the affected eye with it and tape or bandage it in place. It may be necessary to cut the cup to an appropriate size, but be sure that you allow enough free space so that the end of the cup doesn't make contact with the foreign body. Remove the end if necessary. Again, to avoid movement, cover the good eye with a pad and tape it in place. Be aware that paper cups are far more stable then plastic.

For someone that has received a blow to the eye, apply a cold compress such as an icepack or a bag of frozen peas wrapped in a triangular bandage or tea towel directly over the eye without putting pressure on the eye itself. Monitor the injury, and if there is bruising, bleeding, or pain when the eye moves or any change in their vision, have it seen to as soon as possible.

7.10. Impalement

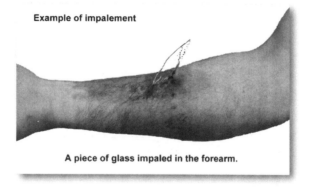

Example of impalement

A piece of glass impaled in the forearm.

An impaled object is something that punctures and lodges in the body. The first picture that comes to mind for some people is someone falling from a height and impaling themselves on a railing. Although it is a good example, and it does happen, thankfully it's not a regular occurrence. If you do happen to witness such an event, it won't be pretty, and the outcome depending on the height of the fall and area of the body impaled may not be good. You may be looking at fractured limbs, spinal damage, paralysis, perforated organs, entrance, and perhaps exit wounds and so on. The list of possibilities is endless, but if you were unfortunate enough to attend such an event, there are still options open to you to be able to help the victim.

Once again you must look at scene safety. Look to where the victim fell from and from what height. Is it safe to approach? It's obvious that the injuries are serious, so call EMS, give the location, and tell them what you see. They will in turn contact police and fire service because manpower will be an issue and cutting equipment may be required. The area will have to be secured for everyone's safety and the incident will have to be investigated. The fall may be accidental or may be as a result of a suicide attempt or perhaps someone pushed the victim out of a window or off a balcony. If the latter is true, the area is now a crime scene. While you are waiting for help to arrive, you may be able to support the person's weight, but that may be all you can do. You may think you're not doing a lot but promptly calling EMS and supporting the victim may save their life.

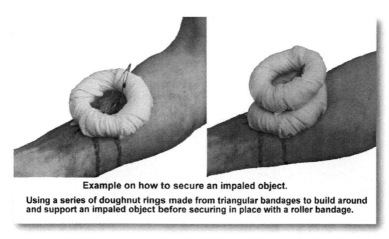

Example on how to secure an impaled object.
Using a series of doughnut rings made from triangular bandages to build around and support an impaled object before securing in place with a roller bandage.

Less dramatic but equally life-threatening would be, for example, the impalement of something like a knife, a large piece of glass, or metal. Once again, scene safety is paramount. Read the scene. Are these injuries accidental, or the result of a struggle or fight? Is the perpetrator still there? If so, keep away until the police or ambulance arrives. Don't play the hero! If it's safe to approach, use BSI (gloves) and check ABCs and LOC (AVPU scale). Do not attempt to remove the impaled object unless it's absolutely necessary. You only remove an impaled object if the victim needs CPR and the object is in the way, or, if the object is obstructing the airway to the point that the victim can't breathe.

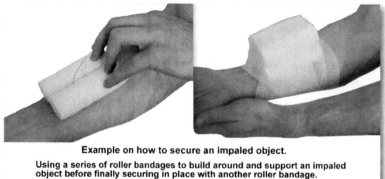

Example on how to secure an impaled object.
Using a series of roller bandages to build around and support an impaled object before finally securing in place with another roller bandage.

When an object becomes impaled, it creates a puncture wound, but it also tamponades (applies pressure) the wound thereby controlling the bleed. If you must remove the object, follow the steps on bleeding control, but remember, once you remove the object, the wound will haemorrhage so have your padding ready in advance. Assuming the patient is on the ground, the first step after removing the object is to plug the hole by applying direct pressure

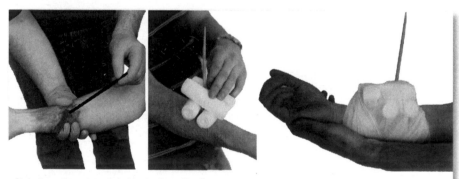

Stabalise a large impaled object using roller bandages or equivalent as building blocks around the object. Secure in place with an appropriate size roller bandage and seek medical assistance.

on a sterile gauze pad. If the pad soaks through with blood, add another layer on top but never take off the original gauze. Removing a blood soaked pad from a wound removes vital clotting agents causing the bleed to resume. Fast flowing rivers by nature never freeze because of the rapid flow rate, but calm lakes can freeze over quite easily because there is little or no movement of water. Blood works in the exact same way. If blood is allowed to flow freely from a wound, it can't and won't clot; therefore, the healing process cannot begin, but by stopping the flow, it will start to coagulate and the healing process begins.

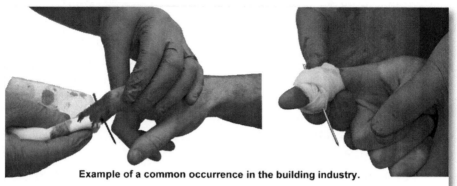

Example of a common occurrence in the building industry.

When something like a nail penetrates a finger and becomes impaled, stabalise the object in situ using a small roller bandage and seek medical assistance.   Check Distal CSM's.

If it's not necessary to remove the impaled object, but the victim is in further danger because of their location, it may be prudent to secure the object. Use bandages or whatever is at hand to build around it and secure it as best you can. If the object can be shortened without doing more damage, it will be more stable and easier to secure. If it is a sizable object, say for example, a spear-shaped object such as an iron bar which is 2 or 3 feet long, it will, without doubt, wobble and add to the seriousness of the injury depending on where it is impaled in the body. If moving the victim is the only option, it may take more than rolls of bandages to secure the object; hence, use a towel or a bed sheet to build around it forming a cone shape with a wide base resting on and around the puncture point. One person should take charge of the object and try to keep its movement to a minimum while others concentrate on moving the victim as gently as possible. Keep the victim warm and check their vitals every few minutes and try to control the bleeding. If the impalement site is a limb, elevate it above the heart if it is possible. At this stage, you have done as much as you can until EMS arrives.

7.11. Abdominal Wounds

Abdominal injuries are caused by blunt or penetrating trauma or occasionally both and can involve internal bleeding or the exposure of internal organs to air. Car crashes and falls are the two main causes of blunt trauma which has a relatively high mortality rate of between 10% and 30%. A few common examples of penetrating trauma would be stab wounds, gunshot injuries, or crush injuries where organs and major blood vessels may be ruptured, punctured, or lacerated. The thing to worry about with gunshot wounds is the damage caused by the energy from the bullet. Has it fragmented causing multiple injuries or has it exited the body leaving an exit wound? Eviscerations occur when the abdominal wall is open and an organ, usually the small intestine, protrudes. These injuries have two life-threatening dangers which are infection and haemorrhage. The thing about gunshot and stab wounds without being flippant is that you can see them. Seeing the injury is half the battle, and you can plan your treatment accordingly, but blunt force trauma is a whole different ballgame.

When dealing with penetrating trauma, the first action is scene safety followed by BSI. Read the scene for clues and look at the MOI. This will give you an idea of the level of treatment and resources required. Call EMS and give as much information as possible (nature of incident, location, and condition of patient) in the shortest of time. Make the patient comfortable, introduce yourself, and reassure them that help is on the way. Tell them what you are doing. While waiting for the ambulance, there are many things you can do. The priority would be to stop the bleeding by applying direct pressure on a padded bandage on the wound as quickly as possible and secure it in place. As with all bleeding, if blood seeps through the pad, put another pad over it and secure it as before. Monitor their vital signs (AVPU, ABCs, and get a SAMPLE history). If the victim is unconscious, talk to them as if they were alert; they may hear you. *Do not* say anything negative within earshot of a patient as they may hear you and it may affect the patient's outcome. Try to get a history from bystanders. Make notes! Be prepared to resuscitate. If you are trained to administer oxygen, do so.

When dealing with blunt force trauma, it can get complicated and misleading. For example, a patient with blunt force trauma may have no pain and there may be no outward signs of injury. This may lead you into thinking that the patient has only minor injuries or none at all. We've all seen people walking away from car crashes and genuinely having no injuries, but it's not always the case. People have been known to walk away feeling fine, calling a friend for help or a drive home, and die later as a result of internal injuries. Another thing that throws the responder into false security is the patient with fractured collarbone or ribs. This is their chief complaint. The pain is so severe that it makes the responder concentrate on the obvious and treat the injury the patient is complaining about. Meanwhile, the patient may be bleeding to death because the injuries to the abdomen went unrecognised. This is sometimes referred to as a distraction injury, but to be fair to the responder or first-aider, this is something that can occasionally throw even the professional medic at first until further examinations are done.

Always look at the mechanism of injury for clues. The typical example of such an injury is a car crash. Scene size up and MOI in this case will tell you a lot. When a car that hits a solid object, the energy of the speeding vehicle is converted into the work of stopping it by the crushing of the car's exterior. A sudden impact or deceleration causes three separate actions. Take for example a car hits a solid object at 50 mph. Although the car has stopped, the driver will still continue to travel forward toward the steering wheel at 50 mph. When the car hits the wall and the driver hits the steering wheel or the passenger hits the dashboard or windscreen, the organs will continue forward at the same speed initially and depending on their mobility within the body may tear or rupture. The same applies to a person who falls from a height. We have all heard the story 'it wasn't the fall that killed him, it was the sudden stop at the bottom'! Once again we have the speed of the fall. The speed will depend on the height. For example, the person who falls 10 feet will have fallen at a slower rate and will have fewer injuries than the person who falls 100 ft. In all incidents where deceleration is involved, by calculating the person's weight, the height of the fall, and speed before impact, the severity of the injuries can be reasonably determined, but let's keep things simple and at an appropriate level for the first-aider and responder. If you study the MOI and the severity of the damage to a vehicle, for example, it will speak for itself and you should have enough information to act accordingly.

Assessing your patient is not that simple in this instance. It is very difficult to diagnose abdominal injuries outside of the hospital setting. A patient who is bleeding internally may present with signs of shock with or without any obvious signs of blood loss. Your primary survey should be a quick visual examination and palpation (feeling with your hands). Study the torso for any deformities, contusions, abrasions, or punctures (DCAP). Look also for distension or evisceration. An evisceration is the protruding of internal organs (usually the small intestine) through a wound in the abdomen.

You may find your patient lying supine or on their side with their knees drawn toward their chest, with shallow breathing. This is their way of avoiding movement and at the same time giving them some comfort. They may be holding (guarding) their abdomen. Be aware of other complaints that the patient may have such as shoulder pain. This could be referred pain. A good example of referred pain that we are all aware of is the classic pain down the arm when one is having a heart attack. While the event is happening in one place, the symptom shows up somewhere else. This also applies with abdominal injuries. Shoulder pain in this situation could be signs of very serious injuries. If your patient complains of left posterior (rear) shoulder pain, it may indicate damage to the spleen. If they complain of right posterior shoulder pain, it could be an indication of injury to the liver. If the abdomen is distended (swollen), it should be taken as a sign that there is severe haemorrhaging within the abdominal wall. This is a serious and life-threatening situation and warrants immediate transport to the nearest hospital.

When treating a patient with abdominal injuries, first remember scene safety followed by BSI. Check the patient's ABCs and then call EMS. Give as much information as possible (nature of incident, location, and condition of patient) in the shortest of time. Let the patient within reason find their own comfort position. Be aware that abdominal trauma cannot be stabilised in an out-of-hospital setting and your patient may deteriorate anytime, so be prepared to treat for shock or even resuscitation. Start by securing the ABCs. If you can give oxygen, do so at 100% or 15 litres per minute using a non-rebreather mask. Talk to the patient and reassure them. He or she may not be in a position to talk to you, so if there are family members or bystanders around, try to get information such as the patient's name, approximate age, and, if possible, a medical history. If there were witnesses to the accident, they may provide vital information as to how the accident happened. For example, they may have seen the patient driving in a strange manner or pass out before the impact. Make notes as soon as you can. Include times of interventions, if possible.

When treating an evisceration, remove all clothing from around the wound. Do not try to push the intestine back into the abdomen. Cover the wound with a large sterile gauze dressing soaked in normal saline solution. If you don't have saline, ordinary water will do. Cover the moistened dressing with a sterile occlusive dressing. (An occlusive dressing is an air/water-tight trauma dressing.) This will prevent the moistened dressing from drying out. If the intestine dries out, it will become irreversibly damaged. If you do not have an occlusive dressing, you can improvise by using kitchen foil or cling film. As a last resort, you could cut a clean plastic bag to the appropriate size and secure it over the dressing with tape. Get a SAMPLE history and monitor the patient's vital signs until EMS arrives.

7.12. Pneumothorax

A pneumothorax is a build-up of air in the pleural cavity which results in the collapsing of the lung. The pleural cavity is the space situated between the pleura, which are two thin membranes that both cover the lungs and cushion them during respiration and also line the chest cavity. This cavity produces a small amount of fluid (pleural fluid) which acts as a lubricant allowing the pleura to slide against each other during respiration while at the same time keeping them tightly together. When air enters the pleura, it separates them, and the more air that enters the cavity, the more it expands the pleural space and in turn reduces the lung's ability to expand on inhalation resulting in its collapse. When the lung collapses, the patient's oxygen intake is reduced causing that person to become hypoxic.

There are different types of pneumothorax.

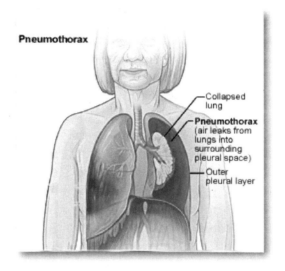

Closed pneumothorax

A closed pneumothorax, whereby the chest wall is intact and the injury happens within, is often referred to as a simple pneumothorax. An example of this would be if someone were to sustain an injury to the chest resulting in fractured ribs. If a sharp part of a broken (fractured) rib punctures a lung, the air will leak into the pleural space and build up, reducing lung capacity and eventually collapsing the lung. Road traffic accidents and collisions can also cause the lung to rupture having made heavy contact with the steering wheel. What usually happens in this case is, when the driver realises that impact is inevitable, as they brace for impact, they take a deep breath and the lung ruptures like a balloon on impact. When this happens, the patient will complain of chest pain and breathing difficulties. All that a responder or advanced first-aider can do is to call EMS, and if your CPGs allow you to give oxygen, you should give 100% O2 (15 litres per minute) using a non-rebreather mask. You may also have to assist their breathing by using a pocket mask to give breaths (positive-pressure ventilation (PPV)). Remember that you can attach oxygen to a pocket mask which will greatly improve oxygenation during PPV.

Spontaneous pneumothorax

A spontaneous pneumothorax can occur in a healthy person (usually men) without warning. These people are usually tall, thin, fit muscular young men who have been born with blebs which are a type of blister-like defect in the lung. As the name suggests, the lung can collapse without warning leaving the victim with an acute shortage of breath (dyspnoea) depending on the level of collapse. This needs careful monitoring and hospitalisation as soon as possible as this can progress to what is called a tension pneumothorax. When this happens, the pressure (tension) in the chest cavity pushes the lung and heart to the other side. This is caused by a build-up of air in the pleura. When the patient inhales, air gets into the pleural space through the hole in the lung and can't get out when they exhale; so, the more they inhale, the bigger the build-up. This is recognised by distended neck veins, caused by obstructed veins (superior and inferior venae cavae), and deviation of the trachea (wind pipe) to the opposite side which is a late sign. To the untrained eye, the veins in the neck will be very pronounced and easily spotted, and when you look at the person face to face, the trachea (windpipe) will appear bent. The absence of breath-sounds on one side is also a sign, but this is only detectable using a stethoscope. Blood pressure will also be low and the patient may go into shock. The treatment for this is out of the scope of practice for a responder apart from keeping the patient calm, calling the emergency services quickly and arranging rapid transport to hospital whereby a large bore needle must be inserted in the chest to let the air out before repairing the lung.

Open pneumothorax

An open pneumothorax, often referred to as a sucking chest wound, is the result of penetration of the chest wall by a foreign object. When we inhale normally, the pressure of air that moves into the lungs equalises with atmospheric pressure before we exhale. When the chest wall is punctured, air enters through the wound into the thoracic cavity, and the bigger the wound, the more air will get in. If the hole in the chest is bigger than an adult's thumb, more air will enter the thoracic cavity than what will be inhaled into the lungs through the trachea resulting in poor tidal volume. The end result will be a complete collapse of the lung.

The patient in this instance will complain of breathing difficulties and chest pain that gets worse when breathing. There will be tenderness around the affected area of the chest with a possibility of subcutaneous emphysema which is recognised as a smooth bulging of the skin that when palpated produces a crackling sensation as gas is pushed through the tissue.

The treatment for such an injury is well within the boundaries of an advanced first-aider or responder. The first thing is to apply direct pressure over the wound with a gloved hand to prevent more air getting in. Call EMS as soon as possible. The next step is to apply an occlusive dressing. This can be made on scene if you don't have a commercial dressing available. What is needed is a square of plastic or tinfoil relevant to the size of the hole in the chest. If, for example, the hole is about an inch (25 mm) long or in diameter, the piece of plastic or foil should be around 4 inches (10 cm) square. This square is then placed over the wound and taped in place on three sides only (usually the top and two sides). The remaining side is left open to act as a flutter valve which prevents more air getting in on inhalation but allows air to escape if pressure in the cavity raises. Sometimes when we work outside of our comfort zone, we imagine we do not have everything we need for every event, but first aid is about improvisation. When making up an occlusive dressing, you have an abundance of stuff at your disposal whether you know it or not. The plastic packaging of a non-rebreather mask although not sterile can be cut to size as can a surgical glove. Sit the patient in a comfortable position unless there is a question of spinal injury. This will allow the wound to drain if necessary. Monitor the patient's airway and give 100% oxygen using a non-rebreather mask if your guidelines allow. If the patient should go into respiratory arrest, you will need to breathe for them. This must be done gently as you will only push more air into the thoracic cavity. When you give breaths, give just enough to see visible chest rise. Give breaths slowly, taking one to two seconds for each breath.

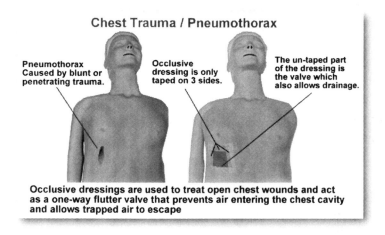

Chest Trauma / Pneumothorax

Pneumothorax Caused by blunt or penetrating trauma.

Occlusive dressing is only taped on 3 sides.

The un-taped part of the dressing is the valve which also allows drainage.

Occlusive dressings are used to treat open chest wounds and act as a one-way flutter valve that prevents air entering the chest cavity and allows trapped air to escape

Haemothorax and Hemopneumothorax

The last two types of pneumothorax are haemothorax, which refers to blood in the pleural cavity as a result of blunt trauma or damaged blood vessel, and hemopneumothorax, which is a combination of blood and air in the pleural cavity. Treatment for this is similar to all the others in this section which includes, giving 100% oxygen, PPV using a pocket mask, if necessary, and monitoring the patient for signs of shock. Finally and most importantly, call EMS.

7.13 Childbirth

Childbirth is one of the most natural processes in the world. The normal gestation from the period of development in the uterus from conception until birth is approximately thirty-eight to forty weeks. When babies are born before the thirty-seventh week, they are considered to be premature, whereas babies that are born after the fortieth week are considered post-mature. About 99% of the time and nature being what it is, babies are born without any fuss or complications, and it is one of the most memorable events in the life of 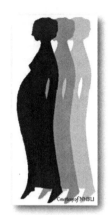 any mother. However, things can go wrong, and it's that 1% that we must always be aware of and prepared for. In this section, I would like to deal with the more common things that occur during the pregnancy and at the birth that can be dealt with within the first-aider or responder's level of training.

Many physiological changes occur during pregnancy. Plasma volume increases by as much as 50% resulting in increased cardiac output, but red blood cell volume only increases by 20%-30%, and because of this dilution of the blood, the imbalance creates what is referred to as physiologic anaemia (most noticeable during the sixth and seventh month). Other changes such as an increase in heart rate between 15 and 20 beats per minute (BPM), the normal or marginally increased breathing rate, and a lower than normal blood pressure are also associated with a normal pregnancy. Mood swings due to hormonal changes can also occur during pregnancy. While we have just mentioned that lower than normal blood pressure is part of the norm, one of the most common problems associated with pregnancy which statistics put at 6% and 8% of pregnancies is high blood pressure, and this has to be addressed so that there is no doubt as to complications that can arise both for the expectant mother and the unborn child.

High blood pressure in pregnancy

What Is High Blood Pressure?

Blood pressure is the amount of force exerted by the blood against the walls of the arteries. A person's blood pressure is considered high when the readings are greater than 140 mmHg systolic (the top number in the blood pressure reading) or 90 mmHg diastolic (the bottom number). In general, high blood pressure, or hypertension, contributes to the development of coronary heart disease, stroke, heart failure, and kidney disease.

What Are the Effects of High Blood Pressure in Pregnancy?

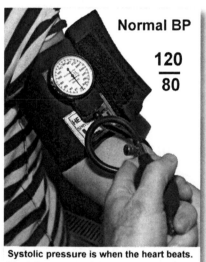

Normal BP

120
—
80

Systolic pressure is when the heart beats.
Diastolic pressure is when the heart relaxes.
The top number is always the Systolic pressure.

Although many pregnant women with high blood pressure have healthy babies without serious problems, high blood pressure can be dangerous for both the mother and the fetus. Women with pre-existing, or chronic, high blood pressure are more likely to have certain complications during pregnancy than those with normal blood pressure. However, some women develop high blood pressure while they are pregnant (often called gestational hypertension). The effects of high blood pressure range from mild to severe. High blood pressure can harm the mother's kidneys and other organs, and it can cause low birth weight and early delivery. In the most serious cases, the mother develops preeclampsia or 'toxaemia of pregnancy' which can threaten the lives of both the mother and the fetus.

What Is Preeclampsia?

Preeclampsia is a condition that typically starts after the twentieth week of pregnancy and is related to increased blood pressure and protein in the mother's urine (as a result of kidney problems). Preeclampsia affects the placenta, and it can affect the mother's kidney, liver, and brain. When preeclampsia causes seizures, the condition is known as eclampsia, the second leading cause of maternal death in the US. Preeclampsia is also a leading cause of fetal complications, which include low birth weight, premature birth, and stillbirth. There is no proven way to prevent preeclampsia. Most women who develop signs of preeclampsia, however, are closely monitored to lessen or avoid related problems. The only way to 'cure' preeclampsia is to deliver the baby.

How Common Is High Blood Pressure and Preeclampsia in Pregnancy?

The problem of high blood pressure occurs in 6%-8% of all pregnancies, about 70% of which are first-time pregnancies. The rate of preeclampsia has increased by nearly one-third, due in part to a rise in the numbers of older mothers and of multiple births, where preeclampsia occurs more frequently. For example, in the United States, according to the National High Blood Pressure Education Program, in 1998, birth rates among women between the age thirty and forty-four and the number of births to women aged forty-five and older were at the highest levels in three decades, according to the National Center for Health Statistics. Furthermore, between 1980 and 1998, rates of twin births increased about 50% overall and 1,000% among women aged forty-five to forty-nine; rates of triplet and other higher-order multiple births jumped more than 400% overall, and 1,000% among women in their forties.

Who Is More Likely to Develop Preeclampsia?

- Women with chronic hypertension (high blood pressure before becoming pregnant).
- Women who developed high blood pressure or preeclampsia during a previous pregnancy, especially if these conditions occurred early in the pregnancy.
- Women who are obese prior to pregnancy.
- Pregnant women below the age of twenty or above the age of forty.
- Women who are pregnant with more than one baby.
- Women with diabetes, kidney disease, rheumatoid arthritis, lupus, or scleroderma (Scleroderma is a disease that involves the build-up of scar-like tissue in the skin).

How Is Preeclampsia Detected?

Unfortunately, there is no single test to predict or diagnose preeclampsia. Key signs are increased blood pressure and protein in the urine (proteinuria). Other symptoms that seem to occur with preeclampsia include persistent headaches, blurred vision or sensitivity to light and abdominal pain. All of these sensations can be caused by other disorders; they can also occur in healthy pregnancies. Regular visits to the doctor help him or her to track the patient's blood pressure and level of protein in the urine, to order and analyse blood tests that detect signs of preeclampsia, and to monitor fetal development more closely.

How can women with high blood pressure prevent problems during pregnancy?

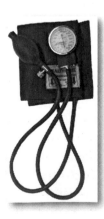

If you are thinking about having a baby and you have high blood pressure, talk first to your doctor or nurse. Taking steps to control your blood pressure before and during pregnancy and getting regular prenatal care go a long way toward ensuring your well-being and your baby's health.

Before becoming pregnant,

- Be sure your blood pressure is under control. Lifestyle changes such as limiting your salt intake, participating in regular physical activity, and losing weight if you are overweight can be helpful.

- Discuss with your doctor how hypertension might affect you and your baby during pregnancy, and what you can do to prevent or lessen problems.

- If you take medicines for your blood pressure, ask your doctor whether you should change/reduce the amount you take or stop taking them during pregnancy. Experts currently recommend avoiding angiotensin-converting enzyme (ACE) inhibitors and Angiotensin II (AII) receptor antagonists during pregnancy; other blood pressure medications may be OK for you to use. Do not, however, stop or change your medicines unless your doctor tells you to do so.

While you are pregnant,

- Obtain regular prenatal medical care.
- Avoid alcohol and tobacco.
- Talk to your doctor about any over-the-counter medications you are taking or are thinking about taking.

Does hypertension or preeclampsia during pregnancy cause long-term heart and blood vessel problems?

The effects of high blood pressure during pregnancy vary depending on the disorder and other factors. According to the National High Blood Pressure Education Program (NHBPEP), preeclampsia does not in general increase a woman's risk for developing chronic hypertension or other heart-related problems. The NHBPEP also reports that in women with normal blood pressure who develop preeclampsia after the twentieth week of their first pregnancy, short-term complications including increased blood pressure usually go away within about six weeks after delivery.

Some women, however, may be more likely to develop high blood pressure or other heart disease later in life. More research is needed to determine the long-term health effects of hypertensive disorders in pregnancy and to develop better methods for identifying, diagnosing, and treating women at risk for these conditions. Even though high blood pressure and related disorders during pregnancy can be serious, most women with high blood pressure and those who develop preeclampsia have successful pregnancies. Obtaining early and regular prenatal care is the most important thing you can do for you and your baby.

Onset of Labour

The onset of labour is defined as regular, painful uterine contractions resulting in progressive cervical effacement (process by which the cervix prepares for delivery) and dilatation which we can break down into three stages.

The first stage of labour is known as the latent stage (present but not visible). This is the longest stage with the least intensity. This stage begins with mild irregular uterine contractions which accomplish a number of things such as causing the cervix (neck of the womb/uterus) to soften and shorten as well as dilate in order to help the baby descend into the birth canal. At the onset, these contractions can be several minutes apart and feel like mild irregular cramps in the lower abdomen and should be timed from the start of one to the start of the other. These contractions continue to get stronger, more painful, and more frequent more so during the second stage, resulting in full or complete cervical dilation which is about 10 cm (4 inches). On a first pregnancy, complete dilation can take as long twelve to fourteen hours and sometimes much longer, whereas subsequent labours can be much shorter. Also occurring at this stage is what is often referred to as 'the breaking of the waters,' whereby the mucus plug which protected the uterus from infection is expelled allowing the amniotic fluid that surrounded the baby in the womb to leak out, although this isn't necessarily always an indicator of impending birth as the amniotic sack can rupture anytime during or even before labour.

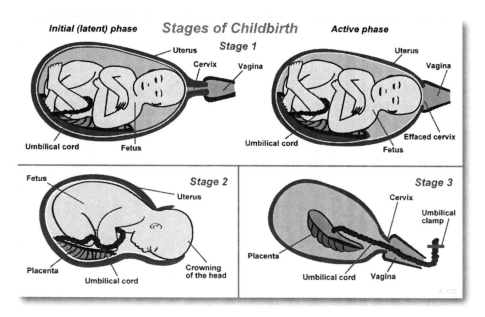

The second stage begins once the cervix is fully dilated whereby the baby's head presses down on the pelvic floor creating a strong urge to push. Those who have had previous pregnancies will normally at this stage deliver within a few minutes as there will be less resistance within the soft tissues of the pelvic floor having been already stretched during a previous delivery; however, if this is a first birth, the delivery may take anywhere from thirty minutes to two hours. In a normal delivery, the baby's head will appear first. When the head remains visible, it is referred to as crowning. Controlled breathing is essential, and the mother will already be aware of this from prenatal classes and should be encouraged to pant as this will help her to concentrate. At this stage, the mother will experience what will feel like a stinging or burning sensation as the head stretches the vaginal opening. At this point, the mother should be advised to stop pushing because continuing to push and bear down will lead to tearing or the need for an episiotomy which is an incision made by a doctor to enlarge the vaginal opening. Situations where this procedure is necessary are when the baby is in distress, if the birth canal can't facilitate delivery of the baby without causing a jagged rip of the perineum due to not having enough time to stretch slowly and naturally, if the baby's head is too large, if a forceps or vacuum delivery is required, if there are other complications such as a breech, or if the mother can't control the pushing. If the mother can control the urge to push when the baby crowns, the pain will subside due to the pressure exerted on the vaginal tissue which causes the vaginal nerves to block giving an anaesthetic effect. At this point, the mother should rest to allow the vaginal opening to stretch fully before continuing. The baby's head can remain in the crowning position for as little as a few seconds, or up to a couple of contractions. In some cases, the mother will use their own hand to control the delivery of the baby's head. Once the head is fully delivered, the rest of the baby will follow quickly. Once the baby has been delivered, we move on to stage three.

This stage is defined by the time period between the delivery of the baby and the delivery of the placenta, umbilical cord, and embryonic membrane. The placenta develops in the uterus during pregnancy. It provides oxygen and nutrients and removes waste products from the baby's blood. It attaches to the wall of the uterus, and the baby's umbilical cord arises from it. In most pregnancies, the placenta attaches at the top or side of the uterus.

Once the baby has been born, contractions although not as uncomfortable, will continue to occur. The wall of the uterus will by this time have reduced greatly in size causing the placenta to lose its grip and be expelled. It should be noted that the delivery of the placenta can occur sometimes in ten minutes or less, but occasionally it can take up to thirty minutes. Postpartum (after delivery) contractions help to reduce blood flow and help the uterus clot, aiding in the prevention of possible blood loss.

Management of emergency childbirth

For a responder of any level, being involved in an out-of-hospital delivery of a baby is a very rare event, but should you ever be called upon to assist, it's essential that you know what to do, or at least know the basics. The first thing to remember is that childbirth is a natural event and nature generally takes care of itself. In truth, the responder will probably get far more excited than the woman who is about to give birth, but if you know what to expect, you will be able to assist in a more professional manner. You have two things to focus on from the beginning, and they are, keep the patient calm, and above all, keep yourself calm. You are there to help the mother deliver the baby and not raise her blood pressure any higher than it may be already. (For guidance, see CPGs for Pre-Hospital Emergency Childbirth EFR)

There are a number of questions you will need to ask which will tell you if you have time or not to get her to hospital. Is there what we call a bloody show? This is the result of the mucus plug being mixed with blood and expelled from the cervix signalling the start of labour. Have her waters broken? This usually happens toward the end of stage one, although occasionally it may not happen until the actual birth. How far apart are the contractions? The rule is generally, if greater than five minutes, it is safe to transport (depending on where you live) but less than two minutes indicates that delivery will be very soon and you should prepare. Is there an urge for bowel movement? This happens when the baby's head is in the birth canal and pressing on the rectum. Under no circumstances should you allow the woman go to the toilet. This is a definitive indicator that she is about to give birth. Is there crowning? This indicates that birth is imminent. Has she given birth before? If so, the delivery will be faster. Have you notified the emergency services and or midwife for an estimated time of arrival (ETA)?

Try to get the mother to adopt a comfortable position (semi-recumbent position), but remember, if it's her second pregnancy, this will be all over in a very short time. If you have an obstetrics kit (maternity pack), prepare it for use. Wash your hands (often). Wear gloves to avoid cross infection. Remember there will be blood present, and you need to be protected from any blood-borne diseases that the mother may have. Glasses or eye protection should be worn also to protect from spatters entering the eye. Because you are not in a sterile environment, you should make every effort to keep everything as clean as possible. However, this is not an easy task as childbirth isn't as glamorous and clinical as it is shown in the movies; in fact, it's quite messy! Make sure the mother is lying on clean sheets and that there is a protector such as a plastic sheet underneath the sheet or towel to protect the bed or whatever she is lying on. Have someone bring fresh, clean towels, and have a warm soft blanket or bath towel ready when the baby arrives. Talk to the mother and keep reassuring her. If you have a partner with you, ask them to contact EMS and update them on what's happening. Encourage the mother to pant (breathe rapidly in short gasps) and advise her not to push too strongly but gently during contractions.

In order to find out if the baby is crowning, you must look at the vagina during contractions. Avoid touching except during delivery. If the head is visible during a contraction, there is no time for transporting and you should prepare for delivery. The mother should lie on her back and the hips should be elevated slightly by placing a pillow or folded blanket or blankets underneath her buttocks and covering them with a clean towel or sheet. Ask the mother to draw her knees up and open her legs. Once the head is visible, support it gently by placing your hand underneath to act as a pillow while it continues to deliver. Do not physically hold the head as it will need to move later. Ideally, the head should deliver slowly both to avoid tearing of the vagina and to avoid undue stress to the baby. Once the head is clear, tell the mother to stop pushing and pant for a few seconds as this will help her to regain control. The head position at this stage will be facing the mother's anus.

Now that the head is delivered, the body will rotate sideways and the head will turn in order to realign itself with the body. Do not attempt to pull the baby. Once it turns on its side, the nearest shoulder (anterior) will deliver first to avoid being caught behind the pubic bone, and this will be quickly followed by the other shoulder. Once both shoulders are free, the rest of the body will be delivered spontaneously. Be sure to continue to support the newborn's head while at the same time catching the body in a clean towel as it is fully delivered, and remember that he or she will be very slippery. Once the baby is delivered, wrap it in a warm towel and place him or her on the bed between the mother's legs and clean the mouth and nose first before drying the rest of the body. If you have a suction bulb, suction the nostrils and mouth a few times to clear away any mucus and amniotic fluid, but be careful not to go too far into the mouth or nose.

Remember that newborns are only nasal breathers, so be sure the nostrils are clear. If you don't have a suction bulb, just clean away what you can see with a soft cloth or gauze. If you discover that the baby isn't breathing, tap the soles of the feet with your finger in a flicking motion or rub its back as this will stimulate breathing. Drying with a towel will also stimulate breathing. You may also need to suction a few more times to ensure that the nose is clear. It would be rare that you would have to resuscitate a newborn during a normal birth, but it does happen. Place the newborn on its side on mother's abdomen keeping the head lower than the body as this will help to drain any remaining secretions. Cover them both with a clean blanket or towel as this will help to maintain heat while you wait for the delivery of the placenta. Note the time when the baby was born as this is important information for the birth certificate.

Delivery of the placenta can take up to half an hour, and you should never be tempted to help it along by pulling on the cord. It will deliver naturally, but in its own time. When the placenta finally does deliver, place it in a bowl or clean plastic container or plastic bag and place it beside the baby at the same level or slightly higher to prevent blood from the baby flowing back into the placenta. You can also tie off the umbilical cord with clean gauze. This can also be done before the placenta is delivered once the cord itself stops pulsating. Leave it to the ambulance crew, doctor, or midwife to actually cut the cord as they will have sterilized equipment which will reduce the risk of infection.

Once the placenta is delivered, bleeding should stop within a few minutes. If bleeding doesn't appear to ease, gently massage the uterus by placing one hand on the abdomen near the bellybutton at the top of the uterus while placing the other hand above the pubic bone to support the lower part of the uterus. In a kneading motion, massage the uterus until bleeding stops and the uterus feels firm which generally takes about five minutes or so to work. This is a job you could consider giving to the woman's partner or husband! It's not unusual for a mother to lose as much as half a litre of blood during a normal birth. However, because of the large increase in plasma volume during the pregnancy, the body is able to handle the loss without any complications.

Complications

Occasionally, the amniotic sack fails to rupture. If this is the case when the baby's head starts to appear, tear it with your fingers and move it away from the baby's mouth and head. Another important issue that can arise at this stage is that the umbilical cord may be wrapped around the neck. If this happens to be the case, try to slip the cord over the baby's shoulder but do not attempt to pull it. If you are unsuccessful in your attempts, try to reduce the pressure on the cord until the baby is born. Your partner should make EMS aware of this situation if they haven't yet arrived as this is a life-threatening situation.

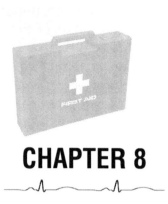

CHAPTER 8

8.1. Associated Musculoskeletal Injuries

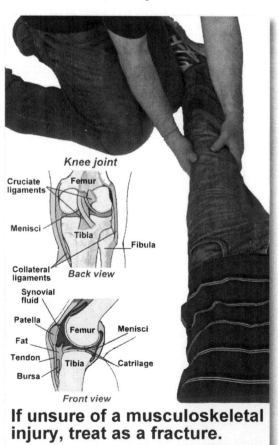

Knee joint

Cruciate ligaments
Femur
Menisci
Tibia
Fibula
Collateral ligaments
Back view

Synovial fluid
Patella
Femur
Menisci
Fat
Tendon
Tibia
Catrilage
Bursa
Front view

If unsure of a musculoskeletal injury, treat as a fracture.

Musculoskeletal Injuries are mainly caused by direct and indirect force and twisting force. To briefly explain these types of injuries, let's take an example, and include the mechanisms of injury for each one. When a car hits a person crossing the road resulting in a fractured (broken) leg, the injury is caused by the direct force of the car's bumper striking the leg. Take the example of a footballer tackling his opponent during a game. The opponent receives a heavy push and falls over on his shoulder while running. The shoulder is strong enough to take the force, but the energy is transmitted to the clavicle (collarbone) indirectly resulting in a fracture to the clavicle. A typical example of a twisting force injury which is quite common is the runner taking part in a marathon. After a few miles, he or she stumbles into a pothole and turns their ankle causing severe injury. At a glance, it's difficult to determine the difference between a sprain, a strain, a dislocation, or a break, so let's break down the types of injuries so there can be no misunderstandings. A fracture is a crack or break in a bone. Generally, it takes a considerable amount of force to break a bone, but not so where the elderly are concerned as bones tend to get brittle with age. Fractures can also occur where a person suffers from brittle bone disease. A greenstick fracture happens in growing bones. In this instance, when direct force is applied, a child's bone will crack, bend, or split.

There are two types of fractures. A closed fracture sometimes called a simple fracture is a break where the surrounding skin is intact, and an open or compound fracture is usually accompanied by a wound caused by the bone breaking through the skin. Sprains and strains are referred to as soft tissue injuries. Sprains are caused by stretching or tearing ligaments or other tissues at a joint. These injuries are usually caused by sudden twists or stretching of a joint beyond its normal motion. A strain is an injury to a muscle or tendon caused by overexertion. In severe cases, muscles or tendons may be torn and muscle fibres stretched. Finally, we have a dislocation which is a partial or full displacement of bones at a joint. This injury can be associated with torn ligaments or can be caused by strong force due to wrenching.

When dealing with a fracture or any type of muscle or skeletal injury, the responder must apply the steps of patient assessment (see, assessing the casualty) in order to determine whether the fracture is stable or unstable.

Stable and unstable fractures

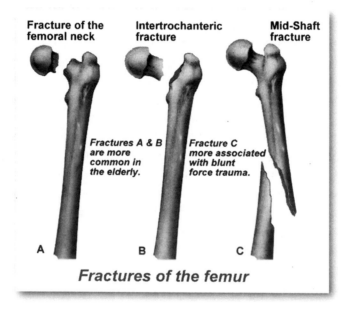

Fractures of the femur

A stable fracture, as the name suggests, is generally easy to manage, mainly because the ends of the broken bone are still aligned and can't move or may only be cracked. The shoulder, wrist, hip, or ankles are the most common areas where these injuries occur. By gentle management, you as a first-aider or responder should be able to treat this kind of break without further injury to the casualty.

An unstable fracture, however, can be more difficult to manage. This is because the ends of the broken bone have the potential to move out of position and damage nerves, puncture and protrude through the skin, puncture major blood vessels, or penetrate organs.

Treatment of a closed fracture

Before you start any treatment, check that the scene is safe for you to approach. Glove up (BSI) before you touch the patient. Study the MOI and the position of the patient as you approach. There is a lot of information right there in front of you if you take a few seconds to analyse it. Introduce yourself and talk to your patient in a calm manner. Tell them you are there to help them and that you are a trained first-aider or responder. This helps to give the casualty confidence in you, and you will find that they tend to open up and cooperate with you in return. Even if your casualty is unconscious, you should still talk to them. If they are conscious and can speak to you, let them tell their story. This helps them to come to terms with their injury, especially if they are very young or very old. Listening to them may also give you more information on how the accident happened which can often determine the type of treatment given. Remember that the obvious injury may not always be the only injury and that is why we study the mechanism as well as collect as much information as possible about the injury in order to diagnose and treat the patient correctly.

Start your treatment by establishing the patient's ABC's are intact. Obviously, if the patient is alert and talking to you, they have a clear airway, and they are breathing, so just note the quality and rate. Limb fractures aren't life-threatening as such unless they are associated with a heavily bleeding open wound, so regardless of the pain and deformity, always secure the patient's ABC's first before moving on. Never hesitate in cutting clothes away from the injury site when it comes to examination. If it's necessary, get it done, but do this gently without moving the limb unnecessarily as you may only cause more injury and pain. When examining, start at the top of the limb and work your way down using both hands (either side of the limb) in a gentle but firm manner. Look and palpate for DCAP-BTLS and compare the injured limb with the uninjured one. Explain your actions to the patient and ask them where it hurts the most. If there are no deformities and you can't see any outward signs of injury, ask the patient to move the limb cautiously. If an injury exists, the patient will react accordingly and will refuse to move the limb. All limb injuries in an out of hospital setting are treated in the same way regardless of their severity for good reason. First, unless the fracture is obvious, it can be difficult to determine the difference between sprains, strains, and fractures without an X-Ray. Secondly, and most important if you wrongly diagnosed the injury as a sprain and it was a fracture, the patient may take your word for it and delay or refuse to get hospital treatment, so the rule is, if you are unsure, treat as a fracture. Call EMS (999/112) and give the relevant information about the injury and don't hang up until the operator tells you to. If you are worried or unsure about what to do, ask the emergency operator, and they will tell you what you should do. These operators are trained specially to give advice over the phone. There's no shame in asking for advice, and in certain circumstances, it may work out better for the patient. We all ask our peers occasionally when we have doubts about treatments or medications. It's normal and it keeps us out of trouble. If we as professionals do it routinely, then there is no reason why you as a first-aider or responder shouldn't. The advantages nowadays of having a mobile phone is that when faced with a situation that you aren't sure about, you can put your phone on loudspeaker, place it on the ground near you and have a two-way conversation with the emergency call taker where they can talk you through the treatment. You also have the added bonus of not feeling alone.

Advise your casualty not to move. If you have help with you, get them to hold the injured limb until you can immobilise it, or if you are alone, support it with your hands until the patient is happy enough to let you continue.

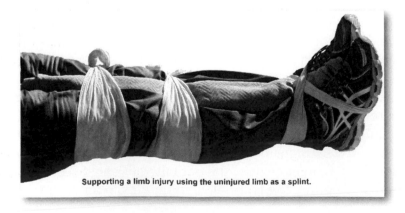

Supporting a limb injury using the uninjured limb as a splint.

If the fracture is in a lower limb, strap the uninjured limb to the injured one. Always move the uninjured limb to the injured one, never the other way around. Secure both limbs together using triangular bandages or whatever soft material you have available. Place a towel or light blanket between the legs to cushion the injury. A bed sheet or similar material could be torn into wide strips and used to tie both limbs together above and below the injury making sure the knots are tied at the uninjured side. If the leg is bent at an angle preventing you from immobilising it, you may have to apply traction to straighten it. By applying gentle traction, it overcomes the pull of the muscles and will help reduce the pain and bleeding. To apply traction to a lower limb, you need two people. One to pull the leg steadily in the straight line of the bone and hold it until the second person immobilises it. If

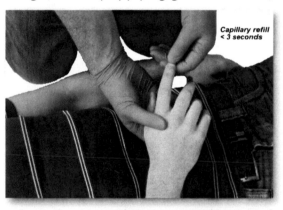

Capillary refill
< 3 seconds

your patient can't tolerate the pain, stop what you are doing and wait for help to arrive. The emergency services will apply a vacuum splint to immobilise the injured limb in the position it's in. The reason we like to immobilise fractures is to prevent closed fractures becoming open fractures by preventing movement of broken bone ends. It also helps to reduce pain and potential damage to soft tissues. Always check capillary refill and sensation, but in relation to movement, when the injury is between the foot and the body or the hand and the body, it will be more than enough evidence that nerves and muscles are working if the patient can wiggle their fingers or toes. (This is known as a modified CSM check.) Check for a pulse below the injury (distal). In a lower limb fracture, it is usually the lower leg bones namely the tibia (shin bone) or the fibula (splint bone) or both that fracture. The femur is one of the largest and strongest bones in the body. The femur is the thigh bone which extends from the hip joint down to the knee joint. Because the femur is such a strong bone, it can take tremendous force to fracture it. A fracture to the femur is usually caused by blunt force trauma as a result of a fall from a height or car accident.

Immobilising an upper limb fracture is done by securing the limb against the trunk. In most cases, when upper limb fractures occur, it is usually the radius or ulna or both that are affected. A humerus (upper arm bone) fracture often referred to as a mid-shaft fracture isn't as common due to its strength. Another injury known as a distal humerus fracture can occur during a fall whereby the person lands directly on the elbow or is hit directly by a hard object such as a baseball bat. Alternatively, if a person falls with an outstretched arm where the elbow is locked straight, the ulna is driven backwards into the distal humerus causing it to fracture. Occasionally, some of the wrist bones (carpels) will also fracture during this type of fall.

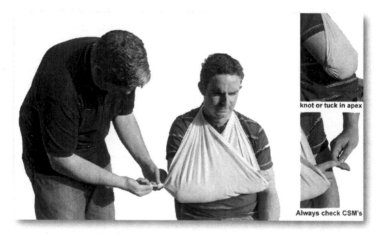

knot or tuck in apex

Always check CSM's

The danger associated with a mid-shaft fracture to the humerus is that nerves, and in particular, the radial nerve may become trapped if the bone separates. The nerve injury is nearly always temporary, but the patient may notice some weakness to the muscles in the hand and wrist and may also feel a sensation on the back of the hand.

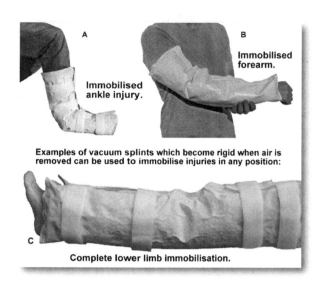

Examples of vacuum splints which become rigid when air is removed can be used to immobilise injuries in any position:

Complete lower limb immobilisation.

When immobilising an upper limb, sit the patient down. As we have already mentioned, talk to the patient and explain your actions. Ask the patient to support the injured arm with their other hand. Using a triangular bandage to make a sling, tie a knot in the point. This will form a pocket or cup. Slide the elbow into the pocket and pass the two ends over the patient's neck and tie it off making sure the wrist is higher than elbow. To prevent any movement, using a second triangular bandage, fold it into what we call a broad-fold bandage (about 3 or 4 inches wide) and tie it around the upper injured arm and chest. Check CSMs (modified version) every ten minutes, but bear in mind, you only want to see slow gentle movement of the fingers as proof that nerves and muscles are intact. If circulation is impaired, loosen any bandages that may be causing the problem. It's possible that the area around the injury has swollen even more since bandaging and this may be restricting circulation. Remember to document your actions.

It's worth a mention that sometimes, we may be in a place where we do not have the luxury of a first-aid kit. When this happens, we improvise, overcome, and adapt. A neck scarf, for example, makes an ideal sling. If the casualty was wearing a coat or jacket, you could button or zip it up to a comfortable height placing the wrist of the injured arm inside and have the patient cup the injured elbow with the palm of the other hand for support.

Treatment of an open limb fracture

Immobilising an open fracture is basically the same as immobilising a closed fracture. However, the work that must be done before you get around to actually immobilising the limb can be challenging. When dealing with an open fracture, the first two things that should concern you as a first-aider or responder are infection awareness and bleeding control. Once again, glove up (BSI). You must always be cautious when coming into contact with any form of bodily fluids. If the break in the skin is small and blood is only weeping through, clean around the wound with a gauze pad, or any type of sterile dressing, but do it quickly. Do not use cotton wool as fibres can stick to the wound and remain there unnoticed. Once the wound has been cleaned, apply a clean sterile pad and secure it in place with a snug-tight bandage. Do not over tighten the bandage as the limb will swell and circulation may become impaired. As with a closed fracture, if it's a lower limb (leg), bring the good leg to the injured one and secure both limbs together above and below the injury site using triangular bandages or equivalent. Place some form of padding between the legs to act as a cushion before securing. Check for CSMs (modified version) and a pulse every 10 minutes.

If the wound is bleeding profusely and the bone is protruding, you may not have time to clean it. Quickly build up as many padded dressings as it takes around bone until you can bandage over the pads to form a cushion over the bone. Do not over tighten the bandage as the limb will swell. The amount of padding used should be enough to control the bleeding, but if blood starts to seep through, simply apply more padding on top of the existing dressing and secure with another bandage. The dressing doesn't have to look pretty, and there are no prizes for best dressed limb! Just do the best you can with what you have and do no harm. If you have to use more dressings, re-check CSMs (modified version) and pulse again. Do not try to realign the bone or push it back as you will only add to the damage. Likewise, if you are dealing with an upper limb, once you have stopped the bleeding and protected the protruding bone, immobilise as you would a closed fracture. Cover the patient with a blanket and be prepared to treat for shock. Contact EMS as soon as possible to arrange transport to hospital. When dealing with a closed or open fracture, the less movement, the better for the casualty. You should only move the casualty if they or you are in imminent danger.

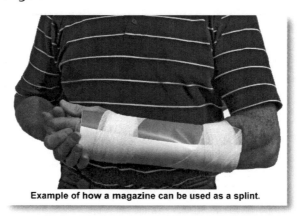

Example of how a magazine can be used as a splint.

So far we have only mentioned immobilising the injury using the good limb or trunk as support. However, a variety of splints exist that are user friendly and can be really useful to have in a first-aid kit. SAM splints, for example, are made from a lightweight aluminium covered by a thin layer of closed-cell foam. It is an ideal splint for any kind of limb fracture as it can be moulded to support the injury with little or no effort. It comes in a range of sizes from 3¾ inches used for finger injuries to 36 inches which is the more common size found in every trauma kit and used for limb fractures. Weighing just 4 ounces (100g), it is available in either flatfold or rolls and can be cut with a regular household scissors to any size required. Once the SAM splint is bent into a curve shape, it becomes extremely strong and rigid and will support any limb fracture. It is widely used throughout the world by Fire an Ambulance services, Sea and Cliff rescue, the Military and the various voluntary first aid organisations. It's waterproof, latex-free and reusable and not affected by extreme temperatures. It is a very cost-effective product and can be secured by tape or roller bandage. Cardboard splints are also widely used. This product is cheap and effective and gets its strength from the corrugation makeup of the card. Once folded around the fracture, it can be secured in the same manner as the SAM splint. You can also make these splints at no cost from strong corrugated cardboard boxes from the supermarket by cutting them to various sizes. By rolling a newspaper or magazine, it will also become rigid and will also work as a splint. Remember when using a splint of any type, make sure it's long enough to allow you to secure it above and below the injury and always check CSMs before and after splinting.

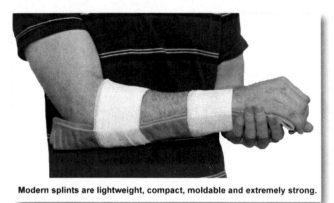

Modern splints are lightweight, compact, moldable and extremely strong.

Shoulder girdle injuries

The shoulder is made up of three bones: the clavicle (collarbone), the scapula (shoulder blade), and the humerus (upper arm bone). Shoulder blade (scapula) fractures are rare, and when they do occur, it's usually as a result of high energy trauma such as a fall onto the back from a height or vehicle accidents.

Collarbone (clavicle) fractures, however, are without doubt more common. The majority of clavicle fractures are caused by falls from horses or motorbikes or bicycles either directly on to the shoulder or as a result of falling on outstretched arms. This injury is also common in the sports industry and in particular where collisions occur during contact sports such as football and rugby.

Symptoms of a clavicle fracture are immediate with severe pain along the collar bone accompanied by swelling which will be visible within a short time of the occurrence. Where the fracture occurred if the broken ends are displaced, a lump may be visible and the patient may also feel pins and needles in the arm and hand. There is the possibility that the fracture may not heal properly if the bone ends are not correctly aligned leading to deformity. Although this is rare, every effort should be made to have this type of injury looked at professionally. An X-ray will confirm whether or not the bone ends are aligned.

The treatment for this injury is to immobilise the arm using a sling made from a triangular bandage making sure the wrist is higher than the elbow. A second triangular bandage should be folded into what we call a broad-fold bandage or swath (about 4 inches or 10 cm wide). This should be wrapped around the injured arm and chest and tied off away from the injury site, preferably to the opposite side of the injury under the arm and slightly to the back. If you are dealing with a large person, you may have to use two swaths by joining them together. You may also find the need to place padding between the sling knot and the shoulder and also between the swath knot and the patient's side to give comfort.

Shoulder dislocations are another common injury, and the causes are basically the same as that of a fractured clavicle. The shoulder joint can dislocate forward, backward, or downward. A common type of shoulder dislocation is when the shoulder slips forward. If you fall with outstretched arms or get shouldered during a football or rugby game, you are just as likely to have a dislocation or have a fracture. The shoulder joint is what we call a ball and socket joint. When we have a dislocation in this area, the head of the humerus (upper arm bone) which is ball shaped pulls free from the socket which is part of the scapula (shoulder blade). For some people, this is a reoccurring injury. First-aiders or responders should never attempt to relocate a dislocation due to the danger of trapping nerves or blood vessels. This injury is usually X-rayed firstly for confirmation before being rectified under anaesthetic in a hospital setting. Because the shoulder is such a mobile joint, the risk of injury is always there, and the level of injury is sometimes determined by luck or lack of it.

Sometimes, the shoulder may only partially dislocate during these types of falls or collisions but ligaments may be torn in the process. With a full dislocation, the casualty will experience severe pain with loss of mobility and sensation and the shoulder will look deformed. Because of the tension from the ligaments, the head of the humerus will be trapped in its new but unnatural position and unable to slip back into its socket without medical intervention. When ligaments get torn, the shoulder will feel loose as if it is slipping in and out of the joint. This is known as subluxation. Previous injuries to the shoulder may increase the risk of subluxation as associated tissues such as tendons and shoulder muscles may have been stretched or torn. If this remains untreated, the shoulder joint will wear out over time and will require surgery to repair the damage. The recovery time may be anywhere from three months to a year depending on the amount of damage. Regular physiotherapy will be the key factor in the recovery process.

First-aid treatment for this injury is the same as that for a clavicle fracture with one exception, if the patient cannot move their arm into position to sling it due to the severity of the pain or because it's locked in position and further movement will be too much for the patient to bear and may only do more damage, support it in the position you found it in, use padding to cushion it, and immobilise it without further movement. Wrap an icepack in a towel and place it on the injury to help reduce the swelling and organise transport to a hospital.

Elbow injuries

Elbow injuries can become complicated injuries if they are treated roughly. The humerus (upper arm bone) can fracture just above the elbow as a result of a fall on to the hand. This must be treated as an unstable fracture as the bone ends may damage nerves and blood vessels. For this reason, it is important that the injured arm is not moved and should be splinted in the position you find it. Once you have immobilised the elbow, if the patient's injury isn't significant, that is to say if a shoulder injury isn't also involved, you may be able to move the limb to the patient's side. Remember, after immobilising it, if the pain is too severe or the limb won't move from the shoulder without causing further distress to the patient, leave it in the position you found it. This may or may not ease the pain, but it will make things easier for stretchering and transportation by the emergency services. If the elbow is bent in an unusual angle, splint it in that position. A pillow is a very effective splint for this type of injury. When using a pillow, gently wrap it around the elbow and secure it with tape. Use more padding to keep the entire limb in the position found. If you do not have the luxury of splints or pillows and the patient's fracture is confined to the elbow area, it may be possible to move the limb to the patient's side without too much hardship. If this is the case, place something like a towel or small blanket to act as padding between the entire limb and torso. Secure the limb to the torso using three broadly folded triangular bandages tying one at the wrist and hip area, then one above and below the elbow. Tie all three bandages firmly at the opposite side of the torso. If it's possible to apply an icepack, do so as it will help to keep down the swelling. Always check CSM's before and especially after you immobilise an injury. Keep the patient warm and reassured.

Wrist injuries

Falling with outstretched hands on the palm or any strong force that may push the hand backwards can sprain, dislocate, or fracture the wrist. A Colles' fracture is a wrist fracture involving a break of the end of the radius bone of the forearm also known as a distal radius fracture. The radius is the larger of the two bones of the forearm and is located on the thumb side of the arm. Sometimes, the other bone of the forearm (the ulna) is also broken. This is located on the little finger side of the arm. When this happens, it is called a distal ulna fracture. A broken wrist usually causes immediate (acute) pain, tenderness, bruising, and swelling as well as difficulty in bending it. It may also appear deformed to some degree. Ignoring or delaying treatment can have serious complications including permanent loss of hand function.

The wrist itself is made up of several small bones. One in particular called the scaphoid bone is located at the base of the thumb just above the radius where the thumb bends. The scaphoid bone can break under the same mechanisms of injury and occasionally both the radius and scaphoid are fractured at the same time. However, if only the scaphoid fractures, it can be less obvious and can be misdiagnosed as a sprain as there will be no deformity or other outward signs such as bruising apart from pain, and it is usually because the pain becomes so severe that only then after being X-rayed will the break be confirmed.

When treating a wrist injury, sit your patient down. Wear BSI and clean and cover any wounds with sterile dressings before immobilising the injury. Place a chunky roller bandage or soft padding into the patient's palm before you immobilise as this will give them something to grip and fill the space rather than leaving an empty closed fist. It will also help to keep the hand in a slightly open and comfortable position and prevent the hand from cramping. It is also important that you are able to check CSMs afterwards, and if the fist is in a clinched position and covered, you will be prevented from doing so thereby you are not able to monitor your patient correctly. If you are using a splint, be sure it's long enough to support the wrist, hand, and fingers and that you also pad between the splint and the limb as padding provides comfort. Remember, when securing the limb to the splint, make sure that you secure above and below the wrist to prevent movement. Elevate the injury above the level of the heart using a triangular bandage to form an elevation sling as this will help to ease the pain and help to control the swelling, and apply an icepack to the wrist. If this injury was only a sprain or you weren't sure, you would treat it in exactly the same way as a precaution.

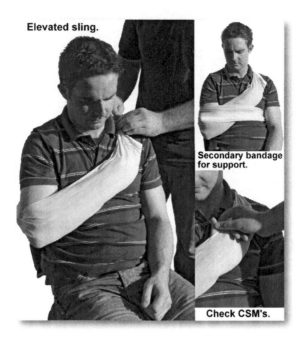

Elevated sling.

Secondary bandage for support.

Check CSM's.

Hand and finger injuries

Hand and finger injuries are also a common occurrence because we use our hands every minute of every day and occasionally expose them to all sorts of danger. Crush injuries or having a heavy object strike the hand directly will often result in one or more fractures. A common injury among children and occasionally among adults is slamming the car or room door trapping the fingers between the door and frame. Even catching a fast object such as a baseball in full flight can do serious damage like straining or tearing tendons. Boxers can also have the occasional mishap. Knuckles, and in particular the small finger knuckle, can be easily damaged as it has less protection.

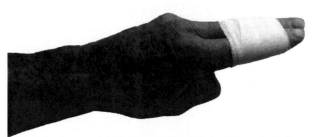

Finger fractures are splinted by securing the injured finger to the finger next to it.
A small amount of padding may be put between the fingers if available.

Because the hand is a complicated area with lots of moving parts, any injury must be treated seriously. Tendons are tissues that connect muscle to bone and when muscles contract, tendons pull on the bones. This causes parts of the body such as the fingers to move. Tendons are like elastic bands and are always to a lesser or greater extent under tension; hence, when one is severed, the ends will pull apart making it impossible to heal without surgical intervention. The muscles that move the fingers and thumb are located in the forearm. Long tendons extend from these muscles through the wrist and attach to the small bones of the fingers and thumb. The tendons on the top or back of the hand are known as extensor tendons which allow the fingers to straighten. The tendons on the palm side are known as the flexor tendons which allow the fingers to bend. When a tendon is cut either at the wrist, palm or along the finger, it is not possible to bend the finger joints. If the cut is deep, it is more likely that a flexor tendon will be severed as these tendons are close to the skin surface and have little protection. Sometimes, flexor tendons may only be partially cut or torn, and although it can still be possible to bend the finger to some degree, it is difficult to diagnose and must be treated with the same urgency as a full tear as it could tear completely. Blood vessels may be cut depriving the finger or fingers of a blood supply. This will require immediate surgery. Nerve damage may also be involved to some degree. This will result in numbness either to the front, back, or both sides of the finger depending on the severity and location of the cut.

When an object such as a baseball strikes the tip of the finger with force and speed, the tendon can be torn away from the bone. The force of the strike may even pull away a piece of the bone. When this happens, the finger or thumb will look bent and will not be able to be straightened. This is known as extensor tendon injury or mallet finger (aka Baseball finger). Treatment for this can be with or without surgery depending on the severity. Symptoms include pain, tenderness, and swelling. The finger will appear noticeably drooped and occasionally, blood will collect under the nail. When blood is present under the nail bed or the nail becomes detached, it may be a sign of a compound fracture. In some cases, the patient may find it difficult to hold a finger or even the hand straight without help from the other hand. A cut on the palm side of the hand, especially on the creases where the fingers bend, shouldn't be taken lightly, especially if the patient finds difficulty with movement or sensation.

Treatment for this type of injury starts by gloving up (BSI) to prevent cross contamination if there is blood involved. Apply a padded dressing directly on the wound and secure it snugly but not too tight. If the patient is wearing a ring or rings, remove them as the hand or fingers will start to swell and circulation to the tip of the ringed finger will be compromised. Elevate the hand to reduce swelling. This will also help to control any bleeding. Place a chunky roller bandage or soft padding into the palm to give the patient something to grip but large enough to prevent them from making a full fist. This will help also when you are bandaging the hand as it will prevent the fist from over clinching and possibly cutting off circulation. Keep in mind that you want to be able to check circulation sensation and movement (CSMs) occasionally, so ensure that the fingertips are exposed. If the tip of one or two of the fingers has to be covered because of the injury, do so but expose the others and use them as a CSM guide. Support the hand using an elevated sling, and if necessary, tie a broad-fold bandage around the patient's chest to secure the limb. Check CSMs when you have secured the limb to ensure that you haven't over tightened anything. Apply ice to the injury and arrange for transport to hospital.

Ring removal using the elastic from a pocket mask or oxygen mask

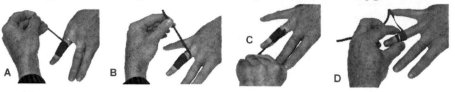

Starting above the nail, wrap the elastic tight around the swollen finger until you reach the ring (A). Slip the end under the ring (B) then pull the elastic back towards the fingernail unwinding as you go (C) until the ring is free (D).

If you are in a situation whereby a finger is swelling and there is a danger that a ring may become an issue, here is something you could try. Using the elastic from a pocket mask or a non-rebreather mask, wrap it tightly around the finger, starting at the middle phalanx (below the knuckle) and gradually bring it spirally over the knuckle until it reaches the ring. Pass the end of the elastic under the ring then unwind the elastic slowly pulling the ring with the elastic as you go. The ring should slip down the finger which is compressed by the elastic and slip off.

Ribcage injuries

Injuries to the ribcage area are not uncommon. The more common causes of fractures are vehicle accidents, falls, and impact injuries during sports. An elderly person with brittle bone disease such as osteoporosis or cancer can sometimes fracture a rib by coughing hard. Regardless whether a rib is cracked or broken it's still a painful injury and will take a month or two to heal. One of the problems that can arise from multiple rib fractures is that the patient is afraid to breathe normally due to the severity of the pain. Deep adequate breathing is essential to keep the lungs clear and healthy in order to avoid complications. If you don't breathe deep enough, mucous and moisture can build up in the lungs and lead to an infection such as pneumonia. The sharp end of a broken rib can puncture a lung (pneumothorax) and cause it to collapse as can a break in one of the first three ribs at the top of your ribcage. The sharp end of a broken rib could rupture the aorta or another major blood vessel. If a break occurs in the lower rib, the broken ends can cause serious damage to the spleen, liver, or kidneys. A history of the accident along with a physical examination will help you diagnose the problem.

When assessing the injury, apply a small amount of pressure to another part of the rib. If this causes pain to the injured area, it is a good indicator that at the very least there is bruising and also a strong possibility of a crack or fracture. If you suspect a fracture or fractures to the front or back of the ribcage, place your hand on either side of the chest and apply gentle inward pressure. If your patient can tolerate the pressure or there is no pain, it is a good indicator that there is no break. If it hurts every time the patient takes a breath, you shouldn't dismiss it as it is also an indicator of some form of rib damage.

Treatment for rib fractures

Make the patient as comfortable as possible by allowing them to pick their own position of comfort where they are able to breathe easier. Place a pillow against the injured rib or ribs and secure it in place. The pillow will act as a splint and will support the injury. Don't allow your patient to move around too mush as this will aggravate the injury. If you are trained to administer oxygen, do so and arrange for transport to hospital.

If three or more ribs are broken in at least two places, it is known as a flail chest. The key sign of flail chest is 'paradoxical movement', which means the natural movement of the ribcage during breathing is in reverse. For example, the injured area of ribcage sinks in when the person inhales, instead of lifting outwards. A flail chest creates breathing problems that can worsen progressively as it decreases the intake of oxygen and restricts the removal of carbon dioxide because the patient isn't able to inhale and exhale properly. Breathing is the bigger issue here. To stabilise the injured area, place a pillow firmly on the flail section. Your hand will do if a pillow or soft cushion isn't immediately available. Remember to glove up beforehand as there may be blood if a sharp piece of bone managed to penetrate the chest wall. At the very least, there will be perspiration, and avoiding contact with body fluids of any kind is what keeps you as a first-aider safe.

You may have to assist your patient with breathing. There are two ways we can achieve this. First, if you are trained to use a BVM, you can give one breath every five to six seconds. If you are certified in the administration of oxygen (O2), connect it and administer it through your BVM. The second way to assist breathing would be by using a pocket mask. Mouth to mouth is a last resort. Monitor the patient's ABCs and arrange for transport to hospital. If you are using a BVM without oxygen, remember to remove the reservoir bag from the end of the unit. This will allow atmospheric air to be pulled in while using it. You only attach the reservoir bag when using supplementary oxygen.

Pelvic fracture

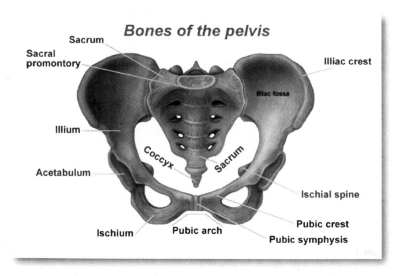

Bones of the pelvis

A pelvic fracture is a very serious and potentially life-threatening injury and must be treated with the greatest of care. The pelvis is a butterfly-shaped group of bones located at the base of the spine formed by three fused bones: the ilium, ischium, and pubis. On the lateral (side) surface of the hip bone is a bowl-shaped depression known as the acetabulum (hip socket), and together with the ball-shaped head of the femur, they make up the hip joint. The pelvis is a ring-shaped structure where digestive and reproductive organs are located, as are a complex series of nerves and major blood vessels that supply the legs. The pelvis is also an anchor point for muscles that travel down each leg and upwards into the trunk. The pelvic ring can often break in more than one place making the injury even more unstable. One specific kind of pelvic fracture is known as an 'open book' fracture. This is often the result of a heavy impact to the groin (pubis), a common motorcycling accident injury. In this kind of injury, the left and right halves of the pelvis are separated at the front and rear, the front opening more than the rear, that is, like opening a book. If a fracture occurs in the pelvic area, the potential is there for major bleeding, organ and nerve damage, so to repeat what I mentioned at the start of this section, any injury to the pelvis must be treated with the greatest of care until a fracture is ruled out and even then, if there is any shadow of doubt, treat the injury as a fracture.

Major fractures of the pelvis can occur as a result of high-speed motor vehicle accidents or falls from a height. If you are treating an elderly person with brittle bone disease such as osteoporosis who has taken even a minor fall, you should always suspect a fracture. It's worth noting that where the elderly are concerned, the fracture may occur spontaneously and the fall may be secondary, so a history of what and how it happened and what they were doing before and when it happened will be very important.

People with pelvic fractures will have severe pain in the groin, hip, or lower back. There may be difficulty urinating, and the patient may have numbing or tingling in the groin or legs. There may also be bleeding from either orifice. A visual examination can tell you a lot if you take those few extra seconds to look at the MOI. If, for example, you come upon a high-impact injury such as a motorcycle accident, not only the damage to the motorcycle will be obvious, but the injury to the driver may also be obvious. If your patient is lying on the ground with the toes of both feet pointing away from each other, it is almost a sure bet that they have an open book fracture. The normal position for feet would be toes pointing upwards or at best, a few degrees away from each other. That's why it's called an open book fracture as the feet resemble an open book.

It can be difficult in the pre-hospital setting to make a definitive diagnosis unless you can actually see the problem; therefore, our diagnosis when dealing with anything internal is often based solely on signs, symptoms, and suspicions. It is worth noting that depending on the nature of the accident, the patient may also have a spinal injury. In this case, someone must take C-spine control and maintain it while reassuring the patient until help arrives.

Previously, checking for a fracture was carried out by placing a hand on both sides of the pelvis and gently compressing to feel for movement or a grating sensation of the end of the broken bone (crepitus). This is now discouraged as new guidelines suggest that compressing or springing the pelvis not only created more pain and discomfort for the patient but in some cases led to secondary and possibly more serious injuries.

The new guidelines for pelvic assessment are far safer and easy to remember. First, study the MOI and the position of the patient to help you form part of your general impression. If the patient is conscious, ask them if they feel pain in the pelvic area or with their consent, *lightly* (and I stress the word lightly) feel for tenderness. If the patient is unconscious, and you are suspicious due to the MOI, then treat as a fracture. Under no circumstances should you check for give or movement. It's far better to assume there is a fracture and be told afterwards you were wrong. There's no shame in being wrong for all the right reasons!

The best treatment that any first-aider or responder can give to a patient with a pelvic fracture is to prevent too much movement. Moving your patient may make the situation worse. Call the ambulance (999/112) and tell them what you suspect. You may be asked a few simple but relevant questions from the call taker at ambulance control. This will help the crew en-route to prepare for treatment. It's worth knowing how long the ambulance will take to get to you and it's a question you should ask whenever you call EMS. Remember, you are the one dealing with the patient, so it important to know how long you or your co-responder will be on your own.

The treatment this patient really needs is for the pelvis to be immobilised properly using a pelvic sling. This device is not authorised for use by anyone other than practitioners, but the first-aider can certainly assist the ambulance crew under direction as it can take at least two and sometimes up to four people to stabilise a pelvic fracture. However, a first-aider can immobilise such a fracture using triangular bandages and padding. First, place soft padding such as a small towel between the knees and ankles as this will keep the legs slightly apart as they would be normally. This will also prevent the knees and ankles from rubbing together and create a little comfort space between the legs. Bring the feet and toes slowly together and secure them using a narrow-fold bandage in a figure of eight. Always tie the feet first. If there are any issues in relation to the patient's pain tolerance, it will show at this point. If the patient is still comfortable, continue by tying the knees together using a broad-fold bandage and placing a pillow or equivalent under the knees for support. Your patient is now immobilised at first-aid level. *A word of caution:* if the patient complains of pain when you attempt to immobilise them, do not continue. Place a small pillow, cushion, or folded blanket under the knees as this will fill the void between the back of the knees and the ground and be more comfortable for the patient, and then support the injured area by surrounding it with padding.

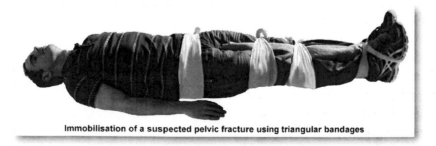

Immobilisation of a suspected pelvic fracture using triangular bandages

If the patient is lying in the same place too long, they will become restless, anxious, and cold, especially if they are on a surface such as a sidewalk. Cover the patient with a blanket or two in order to prevent hypothermia. You may be able to slide a light blanket or even a space blanket (foil blanket) under the arch of the back without moving the hips. If this can be done safely, then do so. This is a two-person operation as it entails sliding the blanket from the arch (slightly above where you would wear a belt on jeans) upwards toward the shoulders as far as you can go without too much movement. This will help to keep out the cold and form insulation between the patient and the ground. Do not give your patient anything to eat or drink, and above all, do not give any unprescribed pain relief. Stay with the patient and monitor their vital signs until help arrives. All patients with pelvic injury are treated for shock. However, *do not* raise the patient's feet until they are secured on a spinal board.

8.2. Spinal Injury

The spine consists of thirty-three vertebrae held together by ligaments. The vertebrae are separated by discs of cartilage which act as shock absorbers. These discs have a soft jelly-like centre covered by a tough fibrous outer layer. Each vertebra has a hollow centre that allows a mass of nerves known as the spinal cord to pass through to where it is connected to the brain. This cord is a two-way communication system which carries information to and from the brain. If any part of this cord is cut, the information cannot be transferred beyond that point,

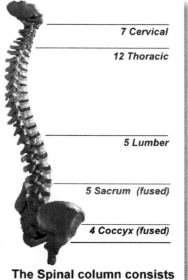

7 Cervical

12 Thoracic

5 Lumber

5 Sacrum (fused)

4 Coccyx (fused)

The Spinal column consists of 33 bones called vertebrae.

resulting in the patient being paralysed below the injured area. If the spinal cord is severed high up in the neck, the diaphragm is paralysed resulting in death. Spinal cord trauma can be caused by a number of injuries to the spine, including, falls, assault, gunshot wounds, industrial accidents, motor vehicle accidents, sports injuries, and diving into shallow water. Spinal cord injury is not the same as back injury, which may result from pinched nerves or ruptured disks.

Injuries to the spine can result in temporary or permanent paralysis. For example, a blunt injury that jars the cord but doesn't sever it may cause temporary paralysis which may last for days, weeks, or even months. The extent of an incomplete injury is generally determined after spinal shock has subsided which could take around six to eight weeks after the injury. In the majority of cases, where we suspect that a spinal injury has occurred, it turns out to be a false alarm but until that is confirmed by X-Ray, we must assume that the injury exists and that is why emergency services will always fully immobilise the patient at an accident scene.

Assessment and treatment of a spinal injury

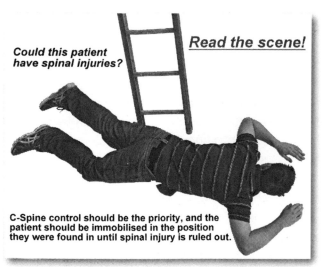

Could this patient have spinal injuries?

Read the scene!

C-Spine control should be the priority, and the patient should be immobilised in the position they were found in until spinal injury is ruled out.

A spinal injury is a life-threatening injury and must be treated quickly and carefully. After you have checked that the scene is safe for you to approach, as you glove up, read the scene and see what it tells you. Apart from looking at the casualty, what part of the scene stands out that helps to identify the possibility of spinal injury? If you are alone, call EMS as soon as you have established patient contact and carried out a quick assessment. If you have help, get them to call while you examine the casualty. If your patient is conscious, try to approach them from the front so they can see you. As you approach, introduce yourself and ask the patient not to move and especially not to turn their head.

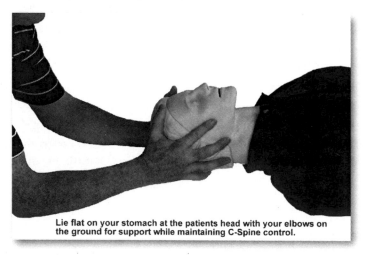

Lie flat on your stomach at the patients head with your elbows on the ground for support while maintaining C-Spine control.

If a vertebra is cracked or broken in the neck, it may be displaced and have sharp edges, and any sudden movement could sever the spinal cord and the patient may die. After you have conducted a primary survey, refer to your appropriate guidelines for guidance (Ref: CPG's Secondary Survey Trauma—Adult, and Spinal Immobilisation—Adult). If necessary, control any major external haemorrhage before moving on to your assessment. Take control of their head as soon as possible but explain to the patient what you are doing and why. If the patient appears to be unconscious, kneel at the patient's head, place a hand either side of their head, and hold it in the position you found it in. This is known as C-Spine Control (Cervical Spine Control) Then check for a response by asking in a reasonably loud voice, 'Hello. Hello, can you hear me?' If the patient was only semi-conscious, and you tapped his or her shoulder without supporting the head, the sound of your voice may startle them and they would move their head in reaction creating a serious problem. More often than not, when dealing with spinal injuries, although a part of the spine may be fractured, the cord remains intact. It's the inexperienced or careless handling that leaves the patient paralysed.

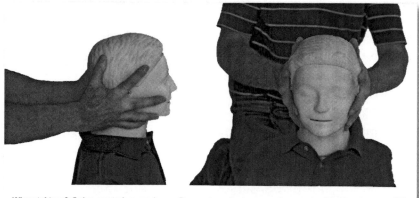

When taking C-Spine control, spread your fingers in order to support as much of the head as possible.

If you have help, have them lie down flat on their stomach at the patient's head and take C-Spine control. Lying down flat at the patient's head is the only safe way to maintain C-Spine control as you are completely wrested and your elbows can rest on the ground allowing you full control. This allows you to continue your assessment. If you are alone, you will have to control and maintain C-Spine until help arrives, but assuming you have help, if the patient is conscious, talk to them and reassure them. Complete a full patient assessment starting with a primary survey (Airway, C-spine breathing, circulation [AcBC]). The primary survey is a crucial element in the 'initial assessment' of a seriously injured patient. While assessing and managing the patient's airway, great care should be taken to prevent excessive movement of the cervical spine. The patient's head and neck should not be hyperextended, hyperflexed, or rotated to establish and maintain the airway. However, in order to immobilise the head properly for transportation, the head is usually returned to the neutral position. This is only possible if on movement, there is no increase in pain or no resistance during movement. In any event where the LOC was altered by blunt trauma above the shoulder line, you should assume that a C-Spine injury is present until ruled out. If the airway is patent and breathing is adequate and there is good circulation (pulse), move on to establish the LOC (AVPU Scale). Once you have established their LOC, if the patient has any life-threatening injuries such as open wounds, this is the time to deal with them.

If the patient's injuries are serious and life-threatening and you feel out of your depth, call EMS. They will update you on their arrival time and help you to deal with the patient over the phone. You could put your phone on speaker and put it on the ground near to you so you can both listen to instructions and have both your hands free to help the patient. If the injuries are not serious, move on to your secondary survey. This is where you examine for any obvious injuries and check the patient's vital signs. Make notes!

Take a SAMPLE history. Make more notes! Now you can do a complete head-to-toe survey to rule out any other injuries using your DCAP-BTLS acronym as a guide. Check the patient for medical alert bracelets or medication they may be carrying. Remember, your partner *must not* let go of the head at any time while you are doing your assessment until EMS arrives. When the ambulance service arrives, one of them will take over C-Spine control, while the other will bring the necessary equipment to fully immobilise and move the patient. This equipment will consist of a scoop-stretcher, spinal board (aka longboard), head blocks to place at either side of the patient's head, a blanket to cover them, and straps known as spider straps to secure them to the board. Alternatively, they may choose to place the patient in a vacuum mattress which also fully immobilises the patient. The crew will also do a full survey and compare their findings with your notes.

When we summarise what treatment you as a first-aider can give to a very serious injury, you can do quite a lot. By maintaining C-Spine control, you are stabilising the head and preventing a serious injury from becoming a life-threatening or at the very least a life-changing injury. By talking to the patient and explaining your actions, they get reassurance. By placing a blanket on them, you keep them warm. By making that phone call, you bring advanced care. And all that treatment is possible with only a pair of hands, a borrowed blanket, and the knowledge you acquire by doing a first-aid course.

8.3. Facial Injuries

Facial injuries can vary from a simple black eye to fractures of one or more bones. Injuries to facial areas that include the upper or lower jaw, nose, cheek or forehead are often caused by blunt or penetrating trauma associated with road traffic accidents, falls, sports, and assault, to name but a few. When dealing with facial injuries, there is also the possibility that a head injury may be involved at the same time.

Serious facial fractures can be life-threatening as blood, saliva, bone fragments, or swelling may cause breathing problems. It must be remembered that the face is a very complicated structure that carries out so many functions. The facial skeleton serves to protect the brain; (see musculoskeletal system). It houses and protects the sense organs of smell, sight, and taste and provides a frame on which the soft tissues of the face can act to facilitate eating, facial expression, breathing, and speech. The primary bones of the face are the mandible (lower jaw bone), maxillae (upper jaw bones), frontal bone (forehead), nasal bones (bony roof of the nasal cavity), and zygomatic (cheek).

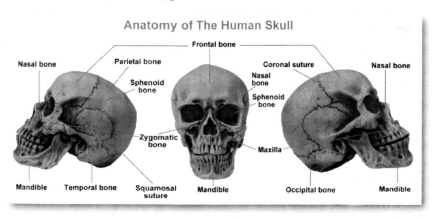
Anatomy of The Human Skull

When assessing the injury or injuries, take into account the MOI as there may also be cervical spinal issues. Your initial focus in your primary survey must be on the patient's ABCs as the throat can become compromised quite easily as a result of bone fragments or a foreign body becoming lodged. Vomiting caused by swallowing blood or as a result of gag reflex can also compromise the airway. Swelling is also a consideration. The nasal passage can also become compromised if the bridge of the nose is damaged, broken, or blocked due to swelling, blood clots, or the presence of a foreign body. Once the patient's ABCs are intact, perform a quick visual assessment as you carry out your secondary survey. Look for a symmetrical face. Always compare one side with the other. Look for any sign of deformity. Look for missing teeth or swelling around the eyes, nose, or cheeks. Impact injuries around the eye area may cause swelling and visual problems such as blurred or double vision or even blindness. Check eye movement and assess the pupils. Check also that there is no change in sensation or sensitivity in or around the injured area. Check for bleeding in the nose or mouth. If there is bleeding, ensure that your patient doesn't swallow it as it will eventually cause them to vomit and this will lead to other problems such as aspiration (breathing in a foreign object) into the respiratory tract. Palpate (examine by touch) the whole face gently for deformities or crepitus. Has the patient any trouble with their hearing such as ringing in the ears (tinnitus)? Is there blood or CSF coming from the ears? Is the patient's ability to bite down compromised in any way?

Get a history of the event. If the patient is conscious, get them to tell you in their own words what happened. If they are unconscious, examine the MOI for clues and try to get information from witnesses (if any). Was the patient involved in an argument? Have they been drinking or taking drugs? Has the patient been mugged? Has the assailant left the scene? Is it a crime scene? If it is a crime scene, have you notified the police? And most important question of all, are you safe? You should try to get as much information as possible before you decide on what treatment to give. Do a SAMPLE history

Treatment for facial injuries

Although facial injuries can look serious and bleed considerably, they are rarely life-threatening unless the airway is compromised. Your first step when treating the patient is scene safety and gloves on. Take C-Spine control and ensure ABCs are intact. If the patient is lying down, gently open the airway and clear away any vomitus, blood, or other debris that could obstruct the airway. If the mandible (jaw) is broken or dislocated, the patient will have difficulty swallowing, and this must be addressed as saliva or blood will trickle into the airway causing the patient to aspirate, or if blood enters the stomach, it will cause the patient to vomit and in turn, aspirate. If the patient is on the ground, you will require help to logroll the patient on their side to allow fluids to drain from the mouth while still maintaining C-Spine control.

If the patient is sitting and there are no indicators of spinal injuries, have the patient lean well forward in about the same position as you would if dealing with a nosebleed. This will allow the mouth to drain also. If the patient has false teeth, they should be removed. Bleeding should be controlled by placing a dry sterile padded dressing directly on the wound and applying firm but gentle pressure. If the damage is around the eye area, be sure not to put direct pressure on the eye itself. Use a ring bandage or donut bandage, as it is sometimes referred to, to protect the eye before bandaging. Applying an icepack or cold compress will help to keep swelling under control. Treat any other injuries that may be present. Treat the patient for shock by covering them with a blanket. Call EMS as soon as possible as stable patients can suddenly deteriorate on realisation of their injuries. Revisit the primary and secondary survey with the emphasis on ABCs and AVPU scale. Document as much information for your handover as possible as it will save time when the ambulance arrives. Be prepared to provide rescue breathing or even CPR, if necessary.

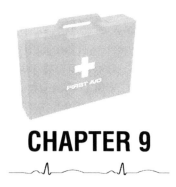

CHAPTER 9

9.1. Altered Levels of Consciousness

Altered level of consciousness (ALOC) also referred to as altered mental status (AMS) is characteristic of nervous system dysfunction and warrants thorough examination to rule out all possible causes. It can be due to number of causes involving both trauma and medical conditions. It can also be characteristic of psychiatric or emotional conditions. Casualties can be disoriented, confused, or unconscious. ALOC is an indication that a person is experiencing a sudden illness that may or may not be life-threatening.

As a tool for remembering some of the more common causes of ALOC, we use the acronym FISH SHAPED: F—Fainting, I—Infantile convulsion, S—Shock, H—Head injury, S—Stroke, H—Heart attack, A—Asphyxia, P—Poison, E—Epileptic seizure, D—Diabetes. Other causes include infection (sepsis), drug overdose, alcohol, and psychiatric disorders.

Signs and symptoms

This topic is included to provide clarity so as not to get confused between what a sign is and what a symptom is. A sign is something that we can literally see such as a nosebleed which can tell us that there is a problem with a blood vessel within the nasal cavity, whereas a symptom is something that is experienced by the affected individual that only they can describe, such as pain or tiredness or dizziness.

Some signs can be that of aggression, memory loss, disruptions in psychomotor skills, and even paranoia. There are so many conditions that alter a person's LOC either directly or indirectly that it's difficult not alone to name them all but even to remember them all. From a simple faint or urinary tract infection to a stroke, from a head injury to asphyxia, they all contribute to the patient's LOC to a lesser or greater degree depending on the severity of the ailment.

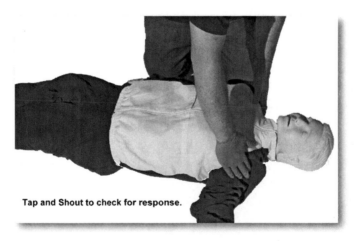

Tap and Shout to check for response.

The AVPU scale is the simplest method of ascertaining a patient's response level. If they are sitting up talking to you normally and quite alert, then you have no problem. They would be classed as A on the scale. If you have to raise your voice to get their attention, (assuming they don't have a hearing problem), they would be mildly unresponsive, so they would be V on the scale. If the patient didn't respond to voice and you had to resort to applying pain by tapping their shoulder, pressing a biro or pencil flat on their fingernail, rubbing their sternum hard with your knuckles, or pinching the earlobe (which is frowned upon!) to get their attention, then they are P on the scale. If you can't get any response no matter what you do, then they are U on the scale. The rule of AVPU is simple. Any letter other than A warrants a trip to hospital. The exception to that rule, of course, is if you enter a room where someone is having an afternoon nap. Obviously, if the person is in a deep sleep, they may not hear you the first time you call out. We don't want to fill the hospitals with tired people just because they catnapped in the afternoon!

AVPU Scale		
A	Alert	Patient is fully alert and responsive.
V	Responsive to voice.	Patient unable to respond spontaneously but responds to voice.
P	Responsive to pain.	Patient is not alert and only responds to pain stimulus.
U	Unresponsive.	Patient unconscious and unresponsive, it's time to call 999 / 112.
When the patient is V, P or U on the AVPU scale, they must be transported to a hospital.		

Take an easily recognisable sign such as confusion. The patient appears dopey as if staring into space or abnormally drowsy (lethargic) and will tend to ask the same questions more than once. To the untrained eye, the patient may appear to be inebriated, or in the case of the elderly, one might assume that the person is becoming forgetful and perhaps suffering from some form of dementia, but compare your observations (signs) with what the patient tells you (symptoms), then add the history of the event into the equation, and you should be able to form a general impression as to what is going on with your patient. However, it isn't always as simple as that. Sometimes getting a reliable history can be difficult if not impossible. This is where a more thoughtful and comprehensive approach is called for.

Assessment and treatment of patient with ALOC

The primary concern must be the patient's ABCs. Their breathing status requires constant monitoring as the patient's ability to manage their own airway adequately diminishes as they become less responsive. It is quite 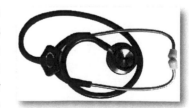 possible that you may not be able to move on to do anything else for your patient other than maintaining their ABCs until the emergency services arrive. If that's the case, then so be it; you are doing all you can do under the circumstances and no more should be expected of you.

It is essential to obtain as much information as possible if you are to accurately diagnose and treat your patient. I emphasise the phrase 'your patient' quite a lot, mainly to make the point that you are the person who has stepped up to the mark and taken control of a situation. Therefore, you have taken responsibility for the welfare and treatment of the sick or injured person making them your patient until they are handed over to a higher level of care.

Treatment should always start with your own safety foremost in your mind. Glove up if possible before you touch the patient. Read the scene. If the cause is due to trauma, the MOI will tell you a lot if you take a minute to study it carefully. The injuries that the patient has sustained as a result of trauma may also be obvious, so you can form an initial impression and plan your treatment faster.

Assuming you have established an adequate airway and the patient's breathing is acceptable, you should try to get a history of what led to the event. You may have to rely on third party information if your patient isn't coherent. If there are relatives or a spouse present, they should be able to give you a history and perhaps clarify what brought about the event. If the condition is medical, you will want to know what their ailment is, what medication they are on, did they take it, and when they last took it. If they collapsed, have they sustained any injuries as a result? Have you enough information to form an initial impression?

On your AVPU assessment, where does your patient fit in? If they are V, P, or U on the scale, you must, as is standard procedure, request immediate medical assistance. Call 999/112. If C-Spine injury is not indicated, place the patient in the recovery position (aka Safe Airway Position) and maintain a patent (clear) airway. Keep the patient warm. If ALOC was brought about as a result of trauma, try to locate the injury. If there is a bleed, apply direct pressure on the wound and apply a pad and bandage. The less blood lost, the better the chance of stabilising the patient. If the wound is to a limb, elevate it if it is safe to do so. Knowing the history and MOI will tell you if C-Spine is indicated or not. Remember, it's important to make notes! (Ref: CPGs Primary Survey—Adult.)

9.2. SAMPLE History

At this stage, you should obtain a SAMPLE History. You have already studied the signs and symptoms, so you must now establish if the patient has any allergies. Perhaps an allergy is at the core of the problem? Are they on any medications, and if so, have they taken it? What kind of medication are they on? Perhaps they are diabetic and haven't taken their insulin for a few days and may be slipping or have slipped into a coma as a result? Have you noticed a sweet smell from the patient's breath? Will their past medical history give you an insight? If they have to undergo surgery, you need to know how long it has been since the patient had anything to eat or drink. Finally, what was the patient doing before they became unwell? If you can get all the answers to these questions, it will be of great benefit for the management and treatment of the patient. Make notes!

Having acquired the SAMPLE history, you should move on to assess the patient's skin colour and temperature. Assess the temperature by pulling away the glove and placing the back of the hand on the patient's forehead. Check the pupils. Are they equal and reacting to light? Are they sluggish? Are they bloodshot? What size are they (dilated or pinpoint)? Check the skin for any form of rash. Does the patient have any medical alert bracelet or pendant? If the patient is talking to you, a diagnosis is easy, but if they are unconscious, obviously it's more difficult. If the patient is conscious, check a radial pulse. If unconscious, check a carotid pulse. Reassess the patient's breathing. Provide reassurance and keep them calm until help arrives. (Ref: CPG's Secondary Survey Trauma or Medical—Adult.)

Taking a few examples of illness and injuries that can lead to ALOC, we can see case by case just how much or how little of the overall assessment is realistically required to make a diagnosis.

Take for example stroke. As we have previously discussed, a stroke is a CVA that occurs when blood flow to the brain is interrupted by a blocked or burst blood vessel. It is one of the leading causes of death and long-term disability throughout the world. Stroke is also referred to as a brain attack. We use the FAST assessment as a means to quickly access the patient in order to correctly diagnose the problem. As we have already discussed the signs and symptoms in great detail, we will only touch on a few here in order to set the scene.

You are called by a neighbour to give assistance to her sixty-year-old husband who is acting strange and appears drunk or confused. His wife tells you that he usually has a few drinks after work on a Friday evening with his work colleagues, but on this occasion, when he arrived home, he complained of a splitting headache and insisted that he came directly home from work. In her own words, she describes how after he sat down on the couch, he started to act very strange and she couldn't make sense of the situation and that is when you were called.

He isn't in a position to give you much help in the line of information, but he does appear to understand what you are saying to him. As part of your procedure, you introduce yourself and even though you know him, as part of your assessment, you ask him his name. He only mumbles, but you notice there is no smell of alcohol or sweetness on his breath which leads you for some reason to suspect he may be having a stroke. As you study the patient in greater detail, you notice that his face isn't symmetrical and he's dribbling from the corner of his mouth. You reassure him and tell him you are going to help him, and he acknowledges by attempting to smile. This is the giveaway as you can clearly see facial muscles droop to one side. Just to be 100% sure, you help the patient to hold out both hands, and after asking him to keep them outstretched, when you let go, one hand slumps onto his lap. You have just completed the FAST assessment, apart from calling ALS which you will now do because you know the patient is having a stroke and that time is brain.

F.A.S.T. Assessment		
F	Facial weakness.	Can the patient smile? Have the eyes or face drooped?
A	Arm weakness.	Can the patient raise both arms and hold the position?
S	Speech problems.	Can the patient speak clearly and understand what you say?
T	Time.	If any of these symptoms are present, it's time to call 999 / 112.

As the name suggests, this is a fast assessment and generally takes only a few minutes to carry out. It is an easy assessment to do, and if the patient is indeed having a stroke, and you know what to look for, the signs are right there in front of you. It is also worth pointing out that at the onset of stroke, the patient may not show all the signs right away; in fact, in some cases, the symptoms are so subtle and transient they can be difficult to recognise. The point here is if you suspect the patient is having a stroke and you're not sure, don't wait too long to find out. Call for help. They may be having a TIA or mini stroke which is a warning that the big one could happen anytime.

So how complex is a stroke assessment? We looked for facial droop (F), we got the patient to hold out their arms to assess weakness on one side (A), we identified that his speech was slurred (S), and we called EMS as quickly as possible (T). That is the full assessment. (Ref: CPG's Stroke)

What else can we do while waiting for the ambulance? The main concern should be the patient's airway. There may be paralysis of the muscles of the tongue, face, or throat which could impair or obstruct the airway, so positioning is vital. If it is appropriate, put your patient in to the recovery position as this will help to drain spittle from their mouth and prevent it from being inhaled into the lungs. Be sure to monitor them constantly, and be prepared to provide rescue breaths if their breathing becomes inadequate. If you have oxygen and you are trained to administrate it, do so. Try to get a SAMPLE history and write everything down, especially the time of onset if it is known. Cover the patient with a blanket and reassess and reassure. What we learn from this example is that for such a serious event, the assessment and treatment is quiet straight forward and uncomplicated and easily remembered and that is really what first aid should be about. The other thing to remember is that you are dealing with another human being, and you should treat them with respect and without bias. Show concern for what they are going through and empathise with them. In the medical world, it is considered a privilege to be allowed help someone.

9.3. Fainting (Syncope)

Another event that happens regularly is fainting (syncope). There are people who will faint if a room is stuffy or suddenly exposed to an unpleasant sight or experience, such as the sight of blood or a sudden intense episode of stress, emotional upset, fear, or anxiety. Dehydration can also cause a person to faint. The list is endless. So what causes it? Fainting (syncope) is caused by a temporary reduction in blood flow to the brain.

There are different types of fainting, because blood flow to the brain can be interrupted for different reasons.

The most common type of fainting is caused by a temporary malfunction in the autonomic nervous system. This type of fainting is called neurally mediated syncope. The autonomic nervous system is made of the brain, nerves, and spinal cord and regulates a number of automatic bodily functions, including heart beat and maintenance of blood pressure.

Fainting can occur when your blood pressure falls suddenly as you stand up. This drop in blood pressure as you stand up is called orthostatic hypotension. It is more common in older people and is the reason for fainting in 1 in 10 persons aged sixty years or above who faint. It is a common cause of falls in elderly people.

Fainting can also occur when the blood supply to the brain is interrupted due to an underlying problem with the heart. This type of fainting is called cardiac syncope. Cardiac syncope becomes more common as people get older. For example, it is estimated that a third of people aged sixty years or above who have fainted may have fainted as a result of a heart problem.

Treatment for Fainting

First, if you see someone about to faint, help them down onto the floor and raise their legs. Ideally, you should kneel down, and putting both ankles together, support them on one of your shoulders as this will improve the blood flow to the brain. If you don't want to or are not able to put their feet on your shoulder, use a chair, footstool, or several pillows or cushions. If you are dealing with an elderly person, be careful when lifting their legs as you may cause problems with their joints. In reality, you only need to raise the legs higher than the heart as you would when treating for shock. About 18 inches (45 cm) is adequate. Leading up to a faint, the patient may feel weak and dizzy and possibly complain of blurred vision. They may also feel nauseated. A faint can happen quite quickly, so don't delay in reacting; otherwise, they may fall and injure themselves.

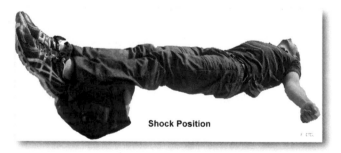

Shock Position

Loosen any tight clothing such as a necktie or shirt button or anything that may be tight around the neck and ensure a good supply of fresh air by opening a door or window. As they recover, allow them to sit up slowly and offer them a few sips of water. Always reassure the patient during their recovery as they may feel a certain amount of embarrassment. Another option where a person is feeling light-headed is to sit the patient down on a chair and place their head between their legs until the episode passes. This is all fine if you are dealing with a small or petit person whereby you can easily control them if they do faint and severe weight issues don't arise when having to get them onto the floor, whereas if it is a large person and they do faint, you may not be able to control them and they may slump from the chair to the floor hurting themselves along the way. You could also strain yourself in the process while trying to break their fall. The better option is help the patient on to the floor from the beginning while they are still conscious because from a health and safety point of view, it's safer both for the patient and for you the responder. If the patient doesn't regain consciousness quickly, open their airway and check their breathing. If there are family members present, ask them if the patient was on any medication or has any medical problems that may have contributed to the event.

Let's recap and see how we assessed and diagnosed this issue and just how much work went into the treatment and handling of this patient. Because a faint happens so suddenly, your reaction is almost immediate. If the patient felt faint while sitting at the dinner table, for example, you would support them with their head between their legs or preferably put them on the floor and raise the legs and ensure a supply of fresh air in the hope that the episode would subside. If your actions worked and the patient responded, you would get them to rest for a while. If the patient is alert and talking, offer them a small amount of water. *Do not* give water to anyone who isn't fully alert as they may aspirate. A fainting episode passes quickly and the patient should be back to normal within minutes. As you can see, dealing with a fainting episode is very straight forward and uncomplicated. In essence, you have diagnosed and treated the problem and all within two or three minutes without any need for equipment apart from know-how.

9.4. Concussion

Concussion is a common enough injury brought about as a result of falls, traffic accidents, or sports injuries. It happens when the brain is shaken within the skull as a result of the head hitting or being hit by an object. The blow then sends shockwaves that temporarily disrupt the brain's function. The severity of the concussion is determined by the severity of the force sustained and can vary from a momentary loss of function that the person may not even be aware of to severe bruising or bleeding of the brain. A major complication of bleeding into the brain is increased intracranial pressure (ICP) which requires urgent advanced care and transport to hospital. Mild concussion as a rule leaves no lasting damage apart from impaired consciousness, short-term confusion, and a headache. The patient may describe seeing stars or images like being in a whiteout or blackness as if in a dark room and in mild cases, may be able to recall the events that led up to and after the event. Children are more likely to experience nausea, vomiting, and drowsiness even after a minor event and should be checked by their doctor as a precaution.

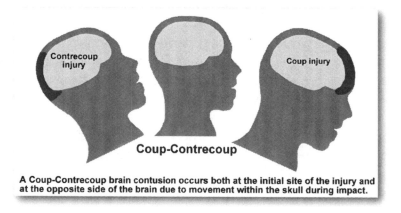

A Coup-Contrecoup brain contusion occurs both at the initial site of the injury and at the opposite side of the brain due to movement within the skull during impact.

People involved in RTC can suffer ALOC as a result of their head being slammed into an object. An injury known as coup-contrecoup injury occurs when the brain bounces back and forth inside the skull. The coup injury happens when the head stops abruptly because of an impact and the brain then crashes into the skull. The contrecoup injury occurs when the brain then bounces and impacts the opposite side of the skull. This type of injury can also be as a result of assault and shaken baby syndrome.

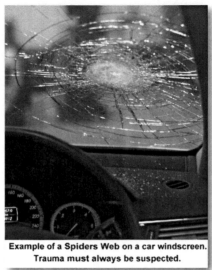

Example of a Spiders Web on a car windscreen.
Trauma must always be suspected.

If the concussion produces swelling, the brain will not function properly, and depending on the location of the bruise, it may contribute to loss of motor ability to part or all of one side of the body or cause visual impairment. If a bleed occurs as a result of the injury, it can result in ICP. This is referred to as a secondary complication. When this happens, the patient's LOC will deteriorate. You will find it difficult to rouse the patient as they may only respond to painful stimuli or not respond at all. Other conditions that cause ICP are meningitis, ruptured aneurysms, haemorrhagic stroke, and hydrocephalus (increased fluid around the brain), but knowing the history of the event and the MOI can help you to rule out such conditions, so you can focus on getting advanced treatment to the patient and doing what you can for them until help arrives.

The general signs and symptoms of concussion are a brief period of impaired consciousness following a blow to the head, dizziness, nausea, and mild to severe headache depending on the severity of the blow. There may be confusion and loss of memory in relation to the events at the time of the injury or immediately after. Blurred vision can also develop. In severe cases, the patient's LOC may deteriorate from being conscious to semiconscious to unconscious.

Treatment for concussion

ALOC is a medical emergency. As there is usually nothing an onlooker can do to treat the cause, the best advice for the untrained person is to call EMS right away. However, as a first-aider or responder, there is a lot you can do to prevent or slow down the deterioration of the patient.

As with all assessments and treatments, once you have protected yourself by gloving up and ensuring that you are working in a safe environment, you should read the scene to establish the MOI. As you approach the patient, if there are bystanders or witnesses, try to get a history of the event.

If the patient is conscious but groggy, introduce yourself and establish that there is a clear airway and that they are breathing adequately and have a good pulse (primary survey). Ask them if they can to describe in their own words how they feel. *Do not put words in their mouth.* Explain to the patient what you are doing or about to do, and always ask their permission before you touch them. If the patient has no apparent injuries, there has to be a reason for their condition. If they fell and hit their head on the sidewalk, for example, was it a helpless fall, or did they put their hands out to break the fall? As part of your secondary survey, examine the hands for graze marks, especially the palms. A conscious person who trips or falls will instinctively try to break their fall, whereas someone who suddenly loses consciousness will simply slump to the ground. If the palms are cut or grazed, you should also examine both limbs to rule out a fracture. If you have ruled out fainting, and on the AVPU scale the patient is V, P, or U, you should call an ambulance. (Ref: CPG's ALOC—Adult) Stay with the patient, and try to keep them conscious. Be aware that they may deteriorate and you may have to resort to doing CPR. Try to get as clear a picture as possible on what happened. If the patient is able to speak to you, or if there is someone there who knows them such as a relative, friend, or neighbour, try to get a SAMPLE history. When speaking to a patient or a bystander, use simple language that everyone can understand. Don't use medical jargon.

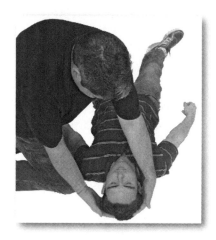

If the patient is unconscious, you are totally dependent on witness information, visible injuries, and MOI. First, confirm that the patient is unresponsive. If so, call for help, 999/112. If C-Spine injury is indicated, you or your partner should take C-Spine control immediately before continuing. If you are satisfied that the MOI doesn't warrant C-Spine immobilisation, start your primary survey and ensure ABCs are intact, and do a secondary survey to rule out life-threatening injuries. Examine the head for any swelling, cuts, deformities, or crepitus (DCAP-BTLS) (Ref: CPG's Secondary Survey Trauma or Medical—Adult).

Check the ears and nose for fluids and in particular, CSF which is a straw-coloured almost clear fluid. If blood is present, there may be CSF mixed with it and you may miss it. A simple test if you aren't sure is to roll out a few inches of roller bandage, dip the end into the blood and hold it up to the light. If there is CSF present, you should see a separation that resembles a rainbow effect on the bandage. The effect is similar to that of oil on water. If there is CSF or blood leaking from the ear or nose, place a loose sterile dressing over it to prevent contamination from dirt or debris but do not obstruct or block the flow. If there is bleeding from any other part of the head, use direct pressure to control it. Take care if the bleed is at a fracture site as applying too much pressure may push a skull fragment into the brain. Check for Battle's sign . . . named after Dr William Henry Battle, an English surgeon, a Battle's Sign, in medical terminology, is called a mastoid ecchymosis (bruising behind the ears) that indicates a posterior basal or base of skull fracture and potential brain injury.

Although not visible right away, another sign of basal fracture is raccoon or panda eye. This is another form of ecchymosis or bruising around the eyes and worth knowing about for future reference. This is a dark purple discolouration which forms around the eyes, giving an appearance similar to that of a raccoon or panda. While the phrase aptly describes the patient's appearance, it should not be confused with an ordinary black eye. Raccoon or Panda eyes develop two to three days after a closed head injury that results in a basilar skull fracture.

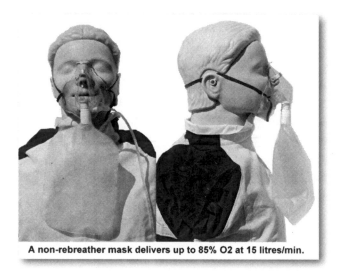

A non-rebreather mask delivers up to 85% O2 at 15 litres/min.

If you are trained in oxygen administration, give the patient 15 litres per minute (100%) using a non-re-breather mask. If the patient is conscious but cannot tolerate a mask, use nasal prongs and give no more than 4-6 litres per minute. If appropriate, put the patient in the safe airway or recovery position and cover them with a blanket. Reassess the patient regularly in accordance with your allowed protocols.

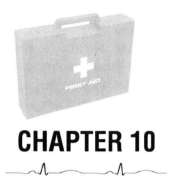

CHAPTER 10

10.1. Burns, Scalds, and Electric Shock

Burns are injuries to the body tissues caused by heat, electric Shock, chemicals, or radiation. Scalds, on the other hand, are caused by wet heat such as steam or hot liquids. As we have discussed earlier, the skin has three layers: the epidermis (outer layer), the dermis (middle layer), and the subcutaneous, which is the inner layer, and these layers play a big part in this section. Other examples of types of burns are friction burns, caused by coming into contact with fast moving belts on machinery, and cold burns, caused by bare skin contacting ice.

Because the skin is one of the biggest organs in our body and represents approximately 16% of the total body weight, it plays a major role in protecting us from infection and injury. It also maintains our body at a constant temperature. When we receive a burn, the skin becomes damaged and infection can set in, but the location, size, and depth of a burn can determine the difference between a superficial burn and a serious and life-threatening burn. Burns are categorised according to their depth, and as we examine the different types of burn, you will be able to understand what we mean by the three degrees of burn and be able to treat each one accordingly.

The seriousness of a burn is determined by the percentage of the body burned, the type and severity of the burn, the location of the burn, and the age of the person. Burns can be a devastating injury emotionally as well as physically and can affect the entire family. The legacy of a bad burn can be serious disfigurement and scarring. Nightmares and flashbacks are common, and the victim can suffer from depression. All burns are serious if they involve the face, head, hands, and feet, flexion joints, and groin area.

Superficial or first-degree burns

Superficial burns are the most common of all burns. Sunburn is probably the best example as nearly everyone at some time in their life has been caught off guard and burnt by the sun to some degree or another. Working in the kitchen will also on occasion contribute to someone getting a superficial burn. This can happen by coming into contact with steam while taking a lid off a saucepan or boiling a kettle or glancing off a hot pot for a split second. The signs and symptoms of a superficial burn are redness of the skin and warm and dry to the touch. It involves the outer layer (epidermis) of the skin and can vary from tingling to being quiet painful. These types of burns generally heal well without complications following a descaling of the affected epidermis. This is part of the normal healing process.

Partial-thickness or second-degree burns

Partial-thickness burns are more serious as they involve both the epidermis and dermis. These types of burns are caused by scalds from hot liquids and flash injuries where heat is more intense. The danger with this type of burn is if the burn has surrounded a limb, swelling caused by fluid retention (oedema) can restrict blood flow. The signs and symptoms are pink, red, or dark blotchy skin (depending on depth of burn), or swelling and blistering caused by damage to tissue and the accumulation of plasma from injured capillaries. Pain following a partial-thickness burn is intense. Blisters should never be burst intentionally as they provide a barrier to infection. With partial-thickness burns, the sensitivity at the burn sight may vary depending on the depth. If the burn is deep into the dermis, nerve damage may occur resulting in decreased sensation. If some of the skin structures such as hair follicles and sweat glands remain intact, the injury will eventually heal itself, but progress will take a while and there may be scarring. Pain management may be necessary for the first few days or weeks.

Full-thickness or third-degree burns

Full-thickness burns are the most serious of all. Not only are both the epidermis and dermis involved, but also the hypodermis or subcutaneous tissue as it is mostly referred to in first-aid circles is involved. Any full-thickness burn has lasting consequences because there are no cells left in the area of the dermis affected that can reproduce or generate new skin tissue. Because of the severity of such a burn, healing will only occur at the margins of the wound; therefore, skin grafts from an unaffected area of the body will have to be transplanted to the affected area. The grafts (called autografts) will ideally come from locations that are not ordinarily visible, such as the buttocks or upper thighs, because the donor sites will not be normal in appearance after they heal.

This type of burn is normally associated with prolonged exposure to flames, extreme heat or radiation, or emersion scalds. The skin will appear charred, dark red, brown, or yellow. It can also appear waxy or translucent with a leathery texture. Unlike superficial and partial-thickness burns, a victim of a full-thickness burn will have no sensation or pain due to the destruction of nerves. In some cases, the burn may extend to the muscle and bone. This is sometimes referred to as the fourth-degree burn. Because the skin is charred and leather-like, its flexibility is lost, and in the case, for example, of a person whose chest is badly burned, the skin's inability to move will also restrict lung expansion. Similarly, as with partial-thickness burns, if the burn has surrounded a limb, the swelling caused by fluid retention (oedema) can continue to swell over time and greatly restrict blood flow to the unaffected distal area.

Electrical burns

Electrical burns are one of the most dangerous injuries for a first aider to respond to. This is where scene safety and heightened awareness are paramount for the responder's safety, simply because electricity may still be flowing through the casualty. As an electric shock travels through a victim as a result of catching a live cable, the heat it generates burns any tissues in its way as it follows the path of least resistance on its way to the ground. This pathway is generally blood vessels and nerves. Slightly stronger resistance would be muscle, with bone and skin offering the most.

Wet skin is easier to penetrate than dry skin, and whether you come into contact with an overhead power line or a faulty household appliance, if your skin is wet, the contact is more positive and the shock can cause cardiac arrest. It is indeed a true saying that water and electricity do not mix! Electricity causes serious internal injuries that aren't immediately noticeable, but be aware that a strong current travelling through the body can cook internal organs, blood vessels, muscles, and nerves. What is noticeable, however, is the burn where the current entered the body. This is referred to as an entrance wound and can resemble a small-to-medium charred burn mark. The exit wound, however, is much more extensive and deep. It has been compared to a miniature explosive charge being detonated inside the limb blasting the flesh outwards. The exit wound can vary from a hole the size of a small coin to several inches of flesh being blown out. These types of wounds are generally associated with contact with high voltage.

It's worth clarifying the difference between getting an electric shock and being electrocuted. When we hear that a person has had an electric shock, they are generally likely to be alive but injured to a greater or lesser degree and in need of emergency treatment. Electrocution, however, is death caused by electric shock, either accidental or deliberate, so if you hear that someone has been electrocuted, and it's from a reliable source, the person is already dead.

Respiratory burns

Respiratory burns, also known as inhalation burns, are always treated as serious. This injury is one of the most common causes of death in house fires. Smoke inhalation in a lot of cases kills long before fire comes in contact with a victim, and in some cases where the victim is asleep in bed, they asphyxiate and die totally unaware of events.

Breathing in extremely hot air, smoke, or other hot gasses causes airway oedema or bronchospasm resembling an asthmatic attack which can lead to acute respiratory distress syndrome (ARDS), which is often lethal. Inhaling steam can overwhelm the airway quickly as it carries more heat than air and will scald the respiratory tract which may cause acute swelling and could completely occlude the airway. The clinical presentation of an inhalation injury may be subtle and often does not appear in the first twenty-four hours. Inhalation injuries

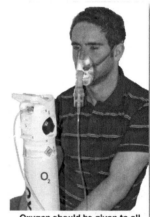

Oxygen should be given to all smoke inhalation victims. Consider humidified Oxygen.

are frequently accompanied by carbon monoxide poisoning. Other substances in smoke that can cause breathing problems include benzenes, ammonia, acrolein, nitrogen oxide, and hydrogen cyanide produced by burning wool and plastics.

Look for signs such as burns to the nose, mouth, and face, singed nostril hairs or irritated sinuses, hoarseness, and difficulty breathing. Sooty sputum (burned saliva) or soot around the nose and mouth are also signs of smoke inhalation injury. Symptoms range from coughing and vomiting to nausea and confusion. Treatment depends on the severity of the smoke inhalation, and humidified oxygen plays an important role in the cooling down process. Oxygen should be administered to all victims of smoke inhalation as the presence of carbon monoxide (CO) must always be a consideration. Asthmatics in particular should be monitored if they have inhaled smoke due to the existing weakness and sensitivity that exists in their lungs.

Chemical burns

Burns from chemicals are similar to thermal burns with one exception, chemicals continue to burn until they are removed. We also have to take into consideration the type of chemical, how corrosive it is, how concentrated it is, and how long the patient has been exposed to it, and if water is poured on the chemical, will it exacerbate the problem. Chemical burns to the eyes are extremely painful and serious and even the mildest form of chemical can be quite irritating. It's very important to locate the container and read the label before you attempt to treat the patient. Don't touch anything without wearing gloves, and if you aren't sure of what to do, tell the emergency operator what type of chemical you are dealing with and he or she will help you as they have a list of every known chemical at their disposal.

10.2. Rule of Nines

The rule of nines is known worldwide as the recognised method for assessment for burns. Being able to determine the percentage of the body burnt is vital in order to report accurately and arrange for the appropriate treatment. The percentage of burn and the depth of burn determine the severity of burn injury. Usually, burns covering more than 20% of the body surface are considered as life-threatening. Burns covering more than 30% of the body surface are usually fatal to adults without immediate treatment.

To approximate the percentage of the burnt surface area, the body has been divided into eleven sections:

1—Head. 2—Right arm. 3—Left arm.

4—Chest. 5—Abdomen. 6—Upper back.

7—Lower back. 8—Right thigh. 9—Left thigh.

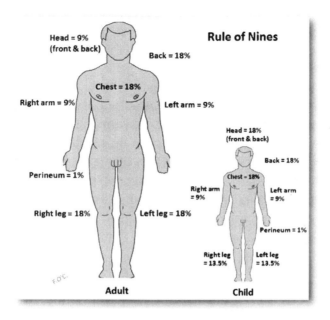

Adult

Child

10—Right leg (below the knee).

11—Left leg (Below the knee).

Each of the above sections takes about 9% of the body's skin to cover it. Added all together, these sections account for 99%. The genitals make up the last 1%.

10.3. Treatment for Burns and Scalds

In the majority of cases, most minor burns are treated in the home or workplace successfully without any complications; however, if a burn is serious, it's important to know how to apply the correct treatment.

Treatment for burns and scalds starts by removing the casualty from the source or the source from the casualty and stopping the burning process. Remember that your own safety is your first priority. In a case where there is an active fire in progress, call 999/112 and wait for the fire service and other associated agencies. Never enter a burning building. Fire and Rescue personnel wear helmets and special fire resistant clothing and use breathing apparatus (BA) for protection, whereas you could be overcome by smoke and normal clothing that contains certain synthetic materials that may melt or ignite.

If it's a minor burn or scald that doesn't cause blistering, run cool (not cold) water over it for fifteen to twenty minutes. Ice packs are acceptable also, but initially, they may be just that bit too cold. The problem with ice packs is that after a few minutes due to the heat radiating from the burn area they become ineffective and need to be replaced often in order to continue the cooling process.

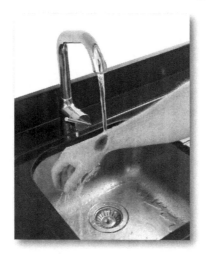

As with any use of ice packs, wrap the ice pack in a tea towel or triangular bandage to prevent direct contact with the skin. If it's more practical to immerse the burnt area such as a hand or foot in cool water, do so. Cooling will reduce swelling as heat is conducted away from the skin. Do not use burn sprays as these can freeze the area and cause even more damage if sprayed too close to the skin. Never use butter on a burn (believe it or not people will use it!) as it will hold in the thermal energy and the burn site will continue to burn for longer. The old rule for first-aiders was no lotions or potions and it's a very safe rule to adhere to. If the burn is to the hand, remove any rings, watches, or bracelets as soon as possible as the area may swell and the jewellery may restrict or cut off circulation (see hand and finger injuries on how to remove a ring from a swollen finger). As with any treatment given to a patient; he or she should be advised to have the burn looked at by a doctor as there is always the danger of infection. Equally the patient may feel the need for pain relief, and this is something that may be outside the scope of practice of a first-aider or responder. For more serious burns, it is important as with the minor ones to remove the patient from the source and cool the burn as quickly as possible. Call for help as soon as it is realistically possible or ask a bystander or colleague to do so. The quicker you cool the burn, the better the chances you have of reducing the degree and depth of the burn. You may have to use whatever resources are available such as the garden hose, the kitchen sink, or even the shower. It is also important to point out that a burn will continue to burn causing more damage even after the source has been removed so rapid cooling is important.

If the clothing is smouldering, saturate the area with water first before attempting to remove but never attempt to remove clothing that is stuck to a burn site as you will only cause further injury. With any level of burn, it is very important that you don't over cool the patient. This applies particularly to young children and elderly people as they are always considered an increased risk. Never use cold water over a large area for too long as you will only promote hypothermia. Cool or lukewarm water is best. The idea is to bring the affected area back to a normal body temperature. As long as the burnt area feels warmer to the touch than the surrounding skin area, treatment should be continued. Burns to the perineum are extremely serious. This is the region of the body between and including the anus and the genital organs, including some of the underlying structures. Burns to this area require urgent treatment and transportation to hospital.

Water-Jel products are also very effective for any level of burn and have the advantage of not contributing to hypothermia and are an approved emergency first-aid treatment in a pre-hospital setting. They can be used on both wet and dry burns and are designed to draw the heat out of the burn, spreading it over the whole gel surface and releasing it at the outer surface.

Apply the rule of nines. This will give you an approximate measurement of the burnt area that you can pass on to EMS. The rule of palm is another way to estimate a burn area. The size of the victim's own palm (not including fingers or wrist) is about 1% of their body. If you aren't sure, simply describe the size of the affected area. If there is an inhalation or facial injury, check that there is a patent airway, and if your protocols or CPGs allow you, humidified oxygen should be considered as airway oedema or bronchospasm may occur. With an inhalation injury, you should also suspect that the patient has inhaled carbon monoxide (CO) of which high-concentration oxygen is the main treatment. In some rural areas where organised First Responder groups are set up where there is a medical director in place, the responder can administer oxygen among other medications under the medical director's instruction.

Pouring water directly over the face can be dangerous as the patient may aspirate (inhale) causing more problems. A wet towel or cloth is ideal to cover the face which should be immersed in cool water often. Don't rub the face; you may pull the skin or burst a blister. Just lay the cool, wet cloth or water-gel mask gently over the burn site. Remember to monitor any cool compresses that you place on a patient and remove them when normal body temperature returns. Check for circumferential burns especially around the neck. If the neck is burned, treat this as a priority and start your cooling there and work your way downwards. If there is a necklace or chain, remove it quickly as it may still be hot and will continue to burn. Treat the patient for shock and cover any parts of the body (within reason) that aren't burnt with a blanket to prevent hypothermia. Do not give anything to drink as the patient may not be capable of swallowing. Cover any burned areas with clean dressings, but do not use cotton wool of any

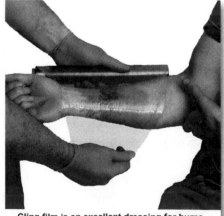

Cling film is an excellent dressing for burns.

material that may stick. Cling film is an excellent dressing as it allows you to see through and monitor the wound. Be especially careful when dressing burns as the affected area may continue to swell and tight dressings will restrict blood flow. Always check CSMs before and after you bandage a wound.

When treating electrical burns, treat as you would a thermal burn, but check that there is no danger of electrocution to you and that all associated dangers are removed before you attempt to touch the patient. Be particularly aware if the victim was near high-tension overhead power lines (pylons) as you may still be in danger from arcing. High-voltage electricity may jump (arc) up to 18 m (60 feet). Although we generally treat electrical burns on scene as you would thermal burns, we do so cautiously as these type of burns may be far worse than what you can see. If the shock was severe, there may be damage to internal organs in the form of cooking. This patient needs rapid transport to hospital, and calling EMS at the onset would be prudent. With electric shock, the patient may go in to respiratory or full cardiac arrest, so be prepared to resuscitate. Remember also that most victims that get serious burns may eventually go into shock and you should be prepared to treat them.

If there is a chemical burn, it's worth remembering that chemicals will continue to burn until removed. The responder should use maximum protection to protect their eyes, hands, and body as splashes while treating are inevitable. Because you may have a lot of physical contact with the patient, caution should be exercised. Wear two pairs of surgical gloves as an added precaution or use rubber kitchen gloves, and keep an eye on them for cuts or tears. If you are dealing with dry or powdered chemicals, be sure to wear protective glasses and a mask as there is a danger of both inhalation through the nose or mouth and absorption through the tear ducts. Be advised that if dealing with this type of chemical outdoors, the

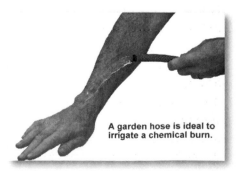

A garden hose is ideal to irrigate a chemical burn.

slightest breeze may blow it into your face. Powder can also accumulate in folds in your clothing or get inside your shoes, so check yourself out before you leave the scene. Spare a thought for family pets that may be attracted to the water on the ground as they may drink it. Be sure it's well diluted and washed away in a safe manner. Any contaminated clothing including the responders used materials should be bagged and sealed for disposal in clearly marked bags.

The treatment here is to irrigate using large amounts of water for at least twenty minutes. Be aware that a lot of chemically contaminated water will run off the patient; therefore, positioning of the patient is important. If they are lying down, for example, and the contamination is to their chest, position yourself at the back of the patient while irrigating. A shower or garden hose with a sprinkler with medium pressure is ideal for washing down the patient as the flow is controllable and constant. When dealing with powdered chemicals, brush off as much as possible before irrigating. Lime, for example, is a widely available product sold as hydrated Lime in 25 kg bags and is used extensively in the building and farming industry. It was a much-used product in some countries as a whitewash. Farm outhouses and rural cottages were painted with it every year as it produced a blinding white finish. It is so taken for granted that people don't realise that it's a chemical that can give quite a burn if it gets in the eye or makes contact with the skin. If only a speck gets into the eye, the tears will activate it, and it will burn until it's washed out. The problem with lime is that because water activates it, it takes constant irrigation of about twenty minutes to dilute and wash it away. If only a small amount such as a half-litre of commercially bottled drinking water was available, it may only activate the powder and not wash it away. If a chemical gets into the eye, you should advise the victim to place their head sideways, affected eye down, and irrigate it for at least twenty minutes. Some chemicals may also give off toxic fumes. If you are in any doubt when dealing with chemicals, call EMS, and they will give you the proper information about the chemical and how to treat it.

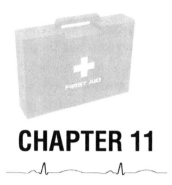

CHAPTER 11

11.1. Recognition of Poisons or Toxins

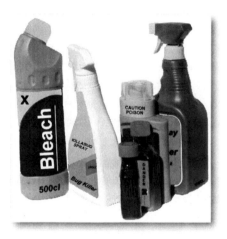

A poison or toxin is a substance that when taken into the body in sufficient quantity can cause temporary or permanent damage or even death. Poisoning should be suspected if a person is sick for an unknown reason. Many conditions mimic the signs and symptoms of poisoning, including seizures, intoxication from alcohol, strokes, and insulin reactions.

Poisons enter the body in four different ways:

1. Absorption: Poisons or toxins can be absorbed through the eyes and through the skin itself or through cuts or abrasions. These

poisons can be anything from cleaning products to garden sprays, weed killers, insecticides, DIY products, and industrial poisons. Drugs such as cocaine can be absorbed through the nasopharynx having been snorted through the nose.

2. Inhalation: Poisons or toxins such as fumes from cleaning and DIY products are easily inhaled as can industrial poisons. Plant poisons that are sprayed using pressurised vessels that deliver a fine spray can be carried in the breeze and inhaled at a distance from the source. Aerosols, carbon monoxide (CO), paint thinners and glue are other examples.

3. Ingestion: Ingestion (swallowing) is probably the more common route for taking poisons or toxins into the system either accidently or intentionally. The list in this instance is rather large and varied. For a start, there are a vast amount of cleaning and DIY products that are poisonous and toxic to a lesser or greater degree depending on how concentrated the product is. Some, such as paint stripper or thinners, will burn while others may only make you feel ill and cause you to vomit. Antifreeze and windscreen wash are other substances that are commonly found in the home. Chemicals such as pesticides, plant sprays, and weed killers that we use on the farm, on the lawn, or on the flower beds are also varied and easily accessible. Alcohol and drug overdoses are probably dealt with in hospitals more frequently than any other form of poison.

Storing poisonous or toxic fluids in plastic mineral or fruit juice bottles is a sure way to kill or seriously harm a child. The child will think they have found dad's secret stash of orange or cola or whatever in the shed, and because they recognise the bottle, they won't give it a second thought. Every product of a dangerous nature should be kept in its own original container, clearly labelled and put out of harm's way. One we should always be mindful of is food poisoning. There are more than 200 known types of bacteria, viruses, and parasites that can cause food-borne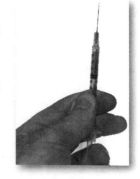

disease, and reactions to these germs can range from mild gastric discomfort to death.

4. Injection: Both prescription and illicit drug overdoses are another form of poisoning although a lot of prescription drug overdoses can be accidental. Venom from bites and insect stings can also cause problems, but in the majority of cases, pain followed by swelling is the main concern.

Signs, symptoms, and treatment

If you are called to help someone who has taken poison, you should be extremely careful about how you approach the situation. (See assessment and treatment of an ALOC patient) If it's a drug overdose for instance, was it accidental?

If the patient is a diabetic, for example, were they confused and injected too much insulin because they had difficulty reading the syringes or vials or were unfamiliar with a new product, or simply forgot they had taken it earlier?

Too much insulin released into the bloodstream causes low blood sugar levels, (hypoglycaemia). Symptoms of hypoglycaemia include anxiety, confusion, extreme hunger, fatigue, irritability, sweating or clammy skin, and trembling hands. If sugar levels continue to fall during an insulin overdose, serious complications such as seizures can occur. The patient may go unconsciousness or go into diabetic shock. Worst case scenario, the patient could die.

If the patient is conscious, give them a sugary drink (not diet drinks) or apply Glucose gel to the inside of the cheek (buccal), if available. Glucose gel is a non-prescription treatment which contains 10 g per tube of fast-acting glucose. This should help to restore their sugar to a reasonable level. Don't worry about pushing their sugar too high if it's only for a short time. One high level won't hurt, but a very low sugar level can. If the patient goes unconscious, call EMS as the patient needs a glucagon injection to prevent further deterioration. This injection is given intramuscular into the deltoid muscle in the upper arm to treat episodes of severe hypoglycaemia where a patient is either unable to treat themselves or treatment by mouth has not been successful.

That would be an example of a relatively safe call, as most diabetics are by nature glad of assistance and don't pose a threat to responders. It's generally the users of narcotics and the hallucinogens that pose the threat to the responder. The important thing to be aware of when being called to any drug-related incident is the possibility of needle stick. *Never* put your hands in the patient's pockets or anywhere you can't see clearly. You may be dealing with an addict who has Hepatitis C or Aids. You may even be entering a crime scene. Scene safety is paramount in this environment. As with any dangers, if the scene looks unsafe and you feel threatened, leave immediately and wait for the police to arrive.

11.2. Medical Safety Data Sheet

It is also worth mentioning that every medication both prescription and non-prescription carries what is known as a Medical Safety Data Sheet (MSDS). This leaflet or sheet is usually found inside the box or packet and gives all relevant information relating to that particular drug. It will tell you what the drug is, what it contains, what it's used for, how it's taken, and the correct dosage and side effects. It will also advise on the contraindications.

A contraindication is a specific situation in which a drug, procedure, or surgery should not be used because it may be harmful to the patient. There are two types of contraindications: relative and absolute. Relative contraindication means that caution should be used when two drugs or procedures are used together. (It is acceptable to do so if the benefits outweigh the risk.) For instance, a person who takes warfarin to thin the blood should not take aspirin, which is also a blood thinner. An absolute contraindication means that that event or substance could cause a life-threatening situation. A procedure or medication that falls under this category should be avoided.

11.3. How to Recognise Some of the Effects of Drug Poisoning

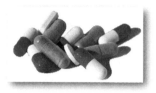

The main part of your diagnosis here is the history. If a person having taken a drug is not yet showing symptoms, don't wait to see if symptoms develop. If the container is nearby or you know what the person has taken, call the ambulance service and give them as much information as possible. They may be able to give you direction on what or what not to do over the phone. If the patient stops breathing, be aware that the poison they ingested may be corrosive, so mouth to mouth may not be an option. Always use a barrier device such as a pocket mask or a BVM if you have to give breaths. Protect yourself at all costs. The following section gives you an idea of some of the type of drugs associated with overdoses both accidental and deliberate that the ambulance service has to deal with on a regular basis. Even knowing a little about the effects of different types of drugs on the human body helps you to understand the reason the patient is reacting the way they are.

Aspirin

Aspirin is a trade name for acetylsalicylic acid (a·ce·tyl·sal·i·cyl·ic acid) which is an over-the-counter painkiller. Aspirin belongs to a group of medicines known as non-steroidal anti-inflammatory drugs (NSAIDs) and works to relieve pain and inflammation. It comes in both regular tablet form and soluble and is taken orally.

The effects of aspirin poisoning vary from nausea and vomiting to ringing in the ears, confusion, dizziness, delirium, and upper abdominal pain.

Paracetamol

Paracetamol is an over-the-counter medicine that is used to ease mild to moderate pain such as sprains, toothache, or the symptoms of a cold. It is also used to control fever (high temperature, also known as pyrexia) when someone has the flu (influenza). Paracetamol is taken orally in tablet form. Calpol is a liquid form for small children. Paracetamol works as a painkiller by affecting chemicals in the body called prostaglandins which are substances released in response to illness or injury. It is important to remember that, when used at therapeutic levels, paracetamol is usually safe and effective; however, taking 4 g per day (or slightly more) for more than a few days has been known to result in hepatotoxicity (chemical-driven liver damage). A single overdose of twenty to thirty standard tablets can result in serious liver damage or death if not treated promptly. The threshold may be lower in a person who is an alcoholic, seriously undernourished, or takes certain medicines. Symptoms may not show within the first twenty-four hours after the overdose, although in some cases, there may be mild nausea and vomiting. If the overdose is large, then liver function may start deteriorating leading to either jaundice, confusion, or loss of consciousness. Death due to overdose of Paracetamol is rare, but when it occurs, in the majority of cases, it's due to liver failure; therefore, immediate treatment is essential in case of paracetamol overdose.

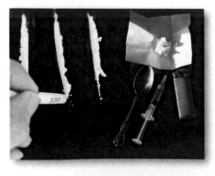

Narcotics

The word narcotic comes from the Greek word 'narkos', meaning sleep. Therefore, 'narcotics' are drugs that induce sleep. Opiates such as heroin and morphine fall under the narcotics category. Morphine, which is one of about twenty alkaloid substances extracted from the opium poppy, is one of the most powerful analgesics known. Heroin, on the other hand, is a derivative of morphine. For this reason, heroin is known as a semi-synthetic opiate. The three basic acute (immediate) effects of heroin are sedation (inducement of a relaxed state), euphoria (intoxication), and analgesia (pain relief). When heroin is injected, it crosses the blood-brain barrier which exists between circulating blood and the brain preventing certain substances from reaching brain tissue. In order for drugs to be intoxicating, they must be capable of crossing this barrier. In the brain, heroin is converted to morphine and binds (attaches) rapidly to opioid receptors on the surface of certain brain cells into which opiate substances fit. The reason that heroin is so addictive is that it can enter the brain so quickly.

Morphine causes slow breathing, lowered heart rate, dopiness, constipation, euphoria, and itchiness. A large overdose can cause asphyxia and death by respiratory depression if the person does not get medical attention or an antidote (Naloxone) immediately. Although heroin is slightly more potent, the symptoms of overdose of both opiates are almost the same. Pinpoint or small pupils (black part of the eye) are a giveaway as far as signs are concerned, and of course, track marks or needle marks will also be visible, but they aren't always where you expect to find them. Addicts stick needles wherever they can find a vein, so unless track marks are visible, don't go looking for them. EMS use sheers to cut away clothing when examining this type of patient. This limits the dangers of needle sticks, and furthermore, most addicts are known both in their community and by the ambulance crews who look after them on a regular basis.

Solvents

Teenagers can obtain an intoxicating high similar to alcohol simply by inhaling products found in their homes. Traditionally referred to as 'glue sniffing', the vast majority of solvent abusers are between the ages of eleven to sixteen and usually male. Things such as lighter fluid, deodorant, gasoline, paint thinners, cleaning products, and furniture glues are examples of commonly used items. A feeling of strong intoxication kicks in almost immediately with some users experiencing hallucinations. The effects are short-lived, resulting in the prospect of repeated abuse. While some users inhale the product through the mouth from the can or whatever, others pour the substance into paper or plastic bags sealing the bag over their mouth and nose and inhaling the fumes without taking in fresh air at the same time. Small doses of *volatile substances* produce effects similar to alcohol, but with greater exposure and higher doses, solvents can have severe effects such as central nervous system (CNS) depression, respiratory distress, convulsions, pulmonary oedema (fluid in the lung), coma, and in rare occasions, cardiac arrest. The signs are hallucinations, fixed stare, blurred or double vision, appearance of being drunk, erratic behaviour, running nose and eyes, persistent cough, tiredness and lack of energy, abdominal cramps, respiratory distress, and abnormal heart beat. There may be a smell of solvent from clothing or from the person's breath. Finding the container will give vital information that you can pass on to the ambulance crew.

11.4. Stimulants and Hallucinogens

Stimulants

Stimulants are drugs that stimulate the brain and CNS, speeding up communication between the two. Coffee, for example, is a stimulant to which many people form an addiction to and can suffer withdrawal symptoms when they stop drinking it. Stimulants usually increase alertness and physical activity. They include amphetamines, cocaine, crack, ice, speed, Ecstasy, crystal meth, and some inhalants like amyl or butyl nitrites. Originally produced as a treatment for angina, amyl nitrite is a vasodilator which means it dilates blood vessels. It is classified as an inhalant and evaporates at room temperature. When inhaled, the vapour released from amyl or butyl nitrites causes your veins and arteries to dilate resulting in the blood flowing faster through the heart and the brain. Short-term effects may include warm sensations, light-headedness and dizziness, euphoria, increased sensual awareness, increased libido, removal of inhibitions, skin sensitivity, nauseous, rash, headache, sinusitis, nosebleeds, allergic reactions accompanied by wheezing and breathing difficulty, and loss of consciousness.

Hallucinogens

Hallucinations interfere with the brain and CNS in a way that results in radical distortions of a user's perception of reality. Profound images, sounds, and sensations will be experienced, but they will not actually exist. These are vivid hallucinations. Common hallucinogens would be LSD, magic mushrooms (psilocybin), PCP (phencyclidine) often referred to as Angel dust, ozone, wack or rocket fuel, ketamine, and mescaline. Ketamine, Special K or K, is a fast-acting 'dissociative anaesthetic'. Rather than blocking pain like traditional painkillers, it shuts off the brain from the body. With the brain no longer processing information from nerve pathways, awareness expands, resulting in a hallucinogenic state. An overdose can slow down a person's breathing and cause them to lose consciousness.

Mescaline is a dark-brown powder ground from 'buttons' of the Mexican cactus peyote, one of the psychotropic plants. Mescaline is generally taken orally. But like LSD, it may be injected. The average dose is 350-500 mg. This yields a 'high' lasting anywhere from five to twelve hours. Because of its bitter taste, mescaline is often taken with tea, coffee, milk, orange juice, soda, or soft drink.

The general side effects of mescaline are what are termed creative closed-eye visuals, dream-like scenarios, euphoria, mystical experience, fear of not being able to return to normal consciousness, dizziness, vomiting, a fast heart rate, headaches, anxiety, feeling of dying or annihilation, hallucinogen persisting perception disorder (HPPD), and irrationality of the thought-process.

11.5. Alcohol and Tobacco (For information purposes only)

It's difficult to give examples of drug addiction and drug abuse without mentioning the two most common drugs of all, alcohol and tobacco.

Alcohol

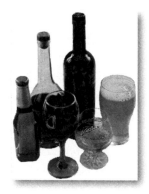

Alcohol comes in many different forms such as beer, spirits, and wine. Initially, it gives the person a high and appears to cure all worries and increase sexual desire, but excessive consumption can cause vomiting, mood swings, dehydration, hangovers, and loss of consciousness. The majority of us who take a drink do so in a sensible and responsible manner and know our limits. However, there are occasions such as weddings, Christmas parties, and other various social gatherings where one may end up having a few too many. When the party atmosphere kicks in, the extra one or two drinks can be tempting and we wouldn't be truthful to ourselves if we didn't admit to letting the hair down once in a while. I would never set out to promote alcohol, but we must also find a balance between the person who takes the occasional drink and the person who can't get through the day without one. Having spent time on the streets with the ambulance service, it becomes very clear that alcohol abuse is a big problem and is not going away anytime soon.

In the cities, the homeless drug addicts and drunks are so well known that they are referred to by some in the ambulance service as frequent fliers because they end up in the back of an ambulance so often. The teenage population has its problems also with cheap drink available in abundance in supermarkets and off-licences. Some of these teenagers as young as thirteen and fourteen are already hardened drinkers and party animals as they often refer to themselves as! The amount of teenage drunks (both women and men) that get involved in late-night fights among themselves or with nightclub staff or just fall and hurt themselves as a result of over-intoxication is incredible. Big concert events also put a strain on EMS resources. It's horrible to see young well-dressed educated people having spent hours getting ready to have a night out, end up lying unconscious in their own vomit, and boast about how much they had to drink the next day. This type of drinking is referred to as alcohol abuse. Calls like this make up over 60% of calls received annually by the ambulance service and can be frustrating to paramedics who have to respond to these party-goers while genuine emergencies stack up while they spend half the night decontaminating and cleaning the vomit both off themselves and the ambulance floor.

So how do we know when there's a problem?

Do you spend long hours at the bar counter on a regular basis? Do you pay more than the occasional visit to the off-licence? Are you missing days at work because of a hangover? Are you getting arrested for offences under the influence? Are you regularly taking the chance driving under the influence? Do you have a secret stash somewhere in the house? Apart from the regular verbal abuse, do you physically hurt family members? Despite all the advice and help from family and friends, do you still continue to drink? When the doctor tells you to stop because your liver is damaged, do you ignore him?

This list is endless, and apart from the domestic, social, and financial chaos, there is also the health issue which if not addressed in time will kill you. Alcohol-related problems are highest among the eighteen to thirty age groups. Alcohol dependence is a chronic disease and affects both genders although men seem to be higher on the list than women. The thing to bear in mind with alcoholism is first, it is a disease that is influenced by generic factors and pressure from society, and second, an alcoholic is an alcoholic for life. Even when a person gets help and attends Alcoholics Anonymous (AA) meetings and has the love and support of family and friends, they are always only one drink away from a relapse. It is a great symbol of strength and courage when someone in this situation finally decides to get help. It is without doubt, the biggest and most important step they will ever take and deserve every support available.

For the responder being asked to help someone who has injured themselves as a result of over-intoxication, there isn't a lot you can do apart from treat any obvious injuries and ensure they are taken care of either by EMS if they are injured, or looked after by family or friends if not. Remember, you can only treat the physical injury; getting treatment for the addiction is up to them. The main thing to remember is that the person may become violent and assault you if the mood takes them. Do not be judgemental, and if permitted, treat that person as you would treat any other.

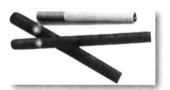

Tobacco

When we talk about tobacco, we automatically think of cigarettes, cigars, and the pipe. We also have snuff and chewing tobacco. Nicotine addiction is the second leading cause of death worldwide, and people don't realise that when we inhale tobacco smoke, along with nicotine, we inhale over 7,000 other chemicals.

According to Medscape, in their article on nicotine addiction, there are in the region of 1.3 billion smokers worldwide with the majority of these (approx. 84%) in the developing countries. It is estimated that if the current smoking trend continues, by the year 2020, around 10 million people per year will die from tobacco-related illnesses. At present, studies show that the average age of first-time smokers is fourteen to fourteen and a half years, while the average age of those who smoke on a daily basis is seventeen to eighteen years of age.

Tobacco accounts for more than 85% of all deaths due to lung cancer. In 1988, laryngeal cancer accounted for 1.1% of cancer-related deaths in men and 0.3% of cancer-related deaths in women. Oral cancer accounted for approximately 2.1% of male cancer-related deaths and 1.2% of female cancer-related deaths. Cigarette smoking and tobacco chewing are major causes of this disease. Oesophageal cancer accounted for 2.6% of male cancer-related deaths and 1% of female cancer-related deaths. Approximately, 50% of overall oesophageal cancer mortality is due to cigarette smoking.

Non-smokers who inhale passive smoke have a significantly higher risk of developing cancers and pulmonary diseases because the concentrations of toxins and carcinogens are higher in sidestream smoke. Children exposed to passive or second-hand smoke develop a variety of respiratory disorders and morbidity.

Getting help

Smoking cessation therapy has been around since the mid-1980s and started off as a prescription-only medication in the form of nicotine gum. Although it worked for some, there were people who couldn't tolerate the taste of the chewing process. In the early 1990s, Nicotine Replacement Treatments (NRTs) were becoming the way forward, and the Food and Drug Administration (FDA) approved four transdermal nicotine patches of which two were made available in 1996 as over-the-counter products. Apart from patches and gum, nasal sprays and inhalers are now available and all work equally well, so there is something to suit everyone who wants to give up smoking.

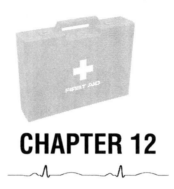

CHAPTER 12

12.1. Respiratory Emergencies

Anything that prevents or restricts a person from breathing such as choking, strangulation, allergic reactions, or severe asthma or other conditions that cause inadequate breathing are classed as respiratory emergencies.

Signs of adequate breathing include a breathing rate and rhythm within the normal limits for the patient's age. Normal breathing should be effortless, regular, and gentle with only slightly visible but equal rise and fall of the chest.

Signs of inadequate breathing include a rate outside the normal range for the patient's age, irregular breathing and rhythm with diminished breath sounds, the use of accessory muscles as the patient makes an increased effort to breathe, inadequate depth of respirations, and unequal chest rise. The patient may be pale or even cyanosed (blue from lack of oxygen), and their skin may be cool and clammy. Patients with advanced lung disease such as COPD will often assume a tripod position (leaning forward, hands on knees). This provides a position that optimises respiratory ability. Intercostal retractions due to reduced air pressure inside the chest can happen if the upper airway (trachea) or small airways of the lungs (bronchioles) become partially blocked. As a result, the intercostal muscles are sucked inward, between the ribs, when the patient breathes. This happens particularly in children. Nasal flaring and seesaw breathing may be seen in infants. (See also Respiratory Arrest and Respiratory Distress). In this section, we shall deal with some of the common respiratory emergencies.

12.2. Respiratory Failure

Respiratory failure is a condition in which not enough oxygen passes from your lungs into your blood. Your body's organs, such as your heart and brain, need oxygen-rich blood to work well. Respiratory failure can also occur if your lungs can't properly remove carbon dioxide (a waste gas) from your blood. Too much carbon dioxide in your blood can harm your body's organs. Both a low oxygen level and a high carbon dioxide level in the blood can occur at the same time.

Diseases and conditions that affect your breathing can cause respiratory failure. Examples include chronic obstructive pulmonary disease (COPD) and spinal cord injuries. COPD prevents enough air from flowing in and out of the airways. Spinal cord injuries can damage the nerves that control breathing.

In respiratory failure, gas exchange is impaired. Respiratory failure can be acute (short-term) or chronic (on-going). Acute respiratory failure can develop quickly and may require emergency treatment. Chronic respiratory failure develops more slowly and lasts longer. Signs and symptoms of respiratory failure may include shortness of breath, rapid breathing, and air hunger (feeling like you can't breathe in enough air). In severe cases, signs and symptoms may include a bluish colour (cyanosis) on your skin, lips, and fingernails; confusion; and sleepiness. One of the main goals of treating respiratory failure is to get oxygen to your lungs and other organs and remove carbon dioxide from your body. Another goal is to treat the underlying cause of the condition. Acute respiratory failure usually is treated in an intensive care unit. Chronic respiratory failure can be treated at home or at a long-term care centre.

The outlook for respiratory failure depends on the severity of its underlying cause, how quickly treatment begins, and your overall health. People who have severe lung diseases may need long-term or on-going breathing support, such as oxygen therapy or the help of a ventilator. When respiratory failure causes a low level of oxygen in the blood, it's called hypoxemic respiratory failure. When respiratory failure causes a high level of carbon dioxide in the blood, it's called hypercapnic respiratory failure.

12.3. Causes of Respiratory Failure

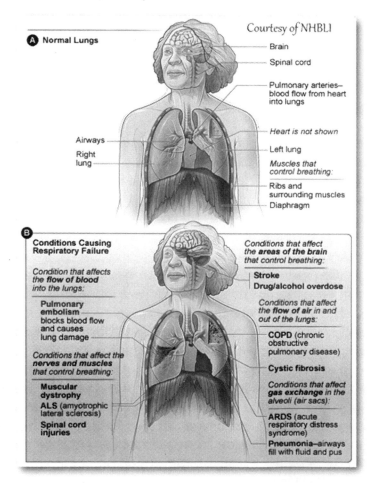

Diseases and conditions that impair breathing can cause respiratory failure. These disorders may affect the muscles, nerves, bones, or tissues that support breathing, or they may affect the lungs directly. When breathing is impaired, your lungs can't easily move oxygen into your blood and remove carbon dioxide from your blood (gas exchange). This can cause a low oxygen level or high carbon dioxide level, or both, in your blood. Respiratory failure can occur as a result of conditions that affect the nerves and muscles that control breathing. Examples include muscular dystrophy which is a group of genetic diseases characterised by progressive weakness and degeneration of the skeletal or voluntary muscles which control movement, amyotrophic lateral sclerosis, or ALS for short, which is a nervous system disease that attacks nerve cells called neurons in your brain and spinal cord. Other examples are spinal cord injuries, stroke, and damage to the tissues and ribs around the lungs. Problems with the spine, such as scoliosis (a curve in the spine), can affect the bones and muscles used for breathing. Drug or alcohol overdose affects the area of the brain that controls breathing. During an overdose, breathing becomes slow and shallow. Lung diseases and conditions, such as COPD, pneumonia, ARDS, pulmonary embolism, and cystic fibrosis (CF), are diseases and conditions that can also affect the flow of air and blood into and out of your lungs. ARDS and pneumonia affect gas exchange in the air sacs. Acute lung injuries, for example, inhaling harmful fumes or smoke can also injure your lungs.

COPD

COPD is a progressive disease that makes it hard to breathe. 'Progressive' means the disease gets worse over time. COPD can cause coughing that produces large amounts of mucus (a slimy substance), wheezing, shortness of breath, chest tightness, and other symptoms. Cigarette smoking is the leading cause and people who have this disease smoke or used to smoke. Long-term exposure to other lung irritants—such as air pollution, chemical fumes, or dust—also may contribute to COPD.

Overview

To understand COPD, it helps to understand how the lungs work. The air that you breathe goes down your windpipe into tubes in your lungs called bronchial tubes or airways. Within the lungs, your bronchial tubes branch into thousands of smaller, thinner tubes called bronchioles. These tubes end in bunches of tiny round air sacs called alveoli. Small blood vessels called capillaries run through the walls of the air sacs. When air reaches the air sacs, oxygen passes through the air sac walls into the blood in the capillaries. At the same time, carbon dioxide (a waste gas) moves from the capillaries into the air sacs. This process is called gas exchange. The airways and air sacs are elastic (stretchy). When you breathe in, each air sac fills up with air like a small balloon. When you breathe out, the air sacs deflate and the air goes out. In COPD, less air flows in and out of the airways because of one or more of the following: The airways and air sacs lose their elastic quality; the walls between many of the air sacs are destroyed, the walls of the airways become thick and inflamed, or the airways make more mucus than usual, which can clog them.

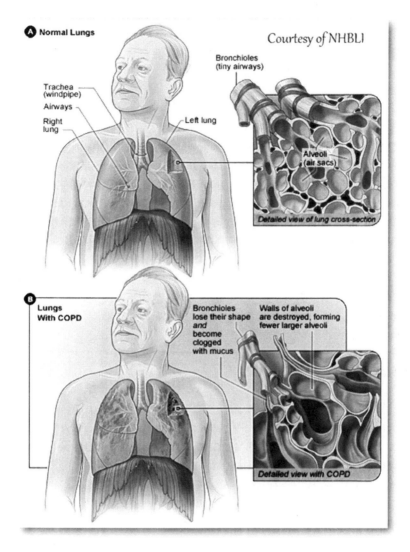

The term 'COPD' includes two main conditions—emphysema and chronic bronchitis. In emphysema, the walls between many of the air sacs are damaged. As a result, the air sacs lose their shape and become floppy. This damage can also destroy the walls of the air sacs, leading to fewer and larger air sacs instead of many tiny ones. If this happens, the amount of gas exchange in the lungs is reduced.

In chronic bronchitis, the lining of the airways is constantly irritated and inflamed. This causes the lining to thicken. Lots of thick mucus forms in the airways, making it hard to breathe. Most people who have COPD have both emphysema and chronic bronchitis. Thus, the general term 'COPD' is more accurate.

Outlook

COPD is a major cause of disability, and people may have the disease and not even know it. COPD develops slowly. Symptoms often worsen over time and can limit your ability to do routine activities. Severe COPD may prevent you from doing even basic activities like walking, cooking, or taking care of yourself. Most of the time, COPD is diagnosed in middle-aged or older adults. The disease isn't passed from person to person—you can't catch it from someone else. COPD has no cure yet, and doctors don't know how to reverse the damage to the airways and lungs. However, treatments and lifestyle changes can help you feel better, stay more active, and slow the progress of the disease.

Bronchitis

Bronchitis is a condition in which the bronchial tubes which carry air to the lungs become inflamed. People who have bronchitis often have a cough that brings up mucus. Mucus is a slimy substance made by the lining of the bronchial tubes. Bronchitis also may cause wheezing, chest pain or discomfort, a low fever, and shortness of breath. The two main types of bronchitis are acute (short-term) and chronic (ongoing).

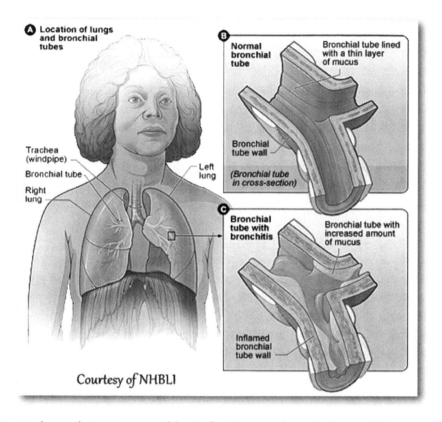

A Location of lungs and bronchial tubes

Trachea (windpipe)

Bronchial tube

Right lung

Left lung

B Normal bronchial tube

Bronchial tube lined with a thin layer of mucus

Bronchial tube wall

(Bronchial tube in cross-section)

C Bronchial tube with bronchitis

Bronchial tube with increased amount of mucus

Inflamed bronchial tube wall

Courtesy of NHBLI

Acute bronchitis is caused by infections or lung irritants. The same viruses that cause colds and the flu are the most common cause of acute bronchitis. These viruses are spread through the air when people cough. They are also spread through physical contact (e.g., on hands that have not been washed). Sometimes, bacteria cause acute bronchitis. Acute bronchitis lasts from two or three days up to as long as eight or ten days. However, coughing may last for several weeks after the infection is gone. Several factors increase your risk for acute bronchitis. Examples include exposure to tobacco smoke (including second-hand smoke), dust, fumes, vapours, and air pollution. Avoiding these lung irritants as much as possible can help lower your risk for acute bronchitis. Most cases of acute bronchitis go away within a few days. If you think you have acute bronchitis, see your doctor. He or she will want to rule out other, more serious health conditions that require medical care.

Chronic bronchitis is an ongoing, serious condition. It occurs if the lining of the bronchial tubes is constantly irritated and inflamed, causing a long-term cough with mucus. Smoking is the main cause of chronic bronchitis. Viruses or bacteria can easily infect the irritated bronchial tubes. If this happens, the condition worsens and lasts longer. As a result, people who have chronic bronchitis have periods when symptoms get far worse than usual. Chronic bronchitis is a serious, long-term medical condition. Early diagnosis and treatment, combined with quitting smoking and avoiding second-hand smoke, can improve quality of life. The chance of complete recovery is low for people who have severe chronic bronchitis.

Elderly people, infants, and young children are at higher risk for acute bronchitis than people in other age groups. People of all ages can develop chronic bronchitis, but it occurs more often in people who are older than forty-five. Also, many adults who develop chronic bronchitis are smokers. Women are more than twice as likely as men to be diagnosed with chronic bronchitis.

Acute bronchitis caused by an infection usually develops after you have been affected with a cold or the flu. Symptoms of a cold or the flu include sore throat, fatigue (tiredness), fever, body aches, stuffy or runny nose, vomiting, and diarrhoea.

The main symptom of acute bronchitis is a persistent cough, which may last two to three weeks. The cough may produce clear mucus (a slimy substance). If the mucus is yellow or green, you may have a bacterial infection as well. Even after the infection clears up, you may still have a dry cough for days or weeks. Other symptoms of acute bronchitis include wheezing (a whistling or squeaky sound when you breathe), low fever, and chest tightness or pain. If your acute bronchitis is severe, you also may have shortness of breath, especially with physical activity.

The signs and symptoms of chronic bronchitis include coughing, wheezing, and chest discomfort. The coughing may produce large amounts of mucus. This type of cough often is called a smoker's cough.

12.4. Asthma

Asthma is a chronic (long-term) lung disease that inflames and narrows the airways. Asthma causes recurring periods of wheezing, chest tightness, shortness of breath, and coughing. The coughing often occurs at night or early in the morning. To understand asthma, it helps to know how the airways work (See Anatomy and Physiology). People who have asthma have inflamed or swollen airways which make them very sensitive. They tend to react strongly to certain inhaled substances. When the airways react, the muscles around them tighten. This narrows the airways, causing less air to flow into the lungs. The swelling can worsen, making the airways even narrower. Cells in the airways can make more mucus than usual which is a thick sticky liquid that can further narrow the airways. Patients can die from asthma if the attack is severe enough and goes untreated as it can get to the stage where no effective air exchange occurs due to the severity of the attack. The patient can also die from exhaustion caused by trying to breathe.

Triggers can include allergens from dust, animal fur, cockroaches, mould, and pollens from trees, grass, and flowers. Irritants such as cigarette smoke, air pollution, chemicals or dust in the workplace, compounds in home DIY products, and sprays such as hairspray can also trigger an attack. Medicines such as aspirin or other non-steroidal anti-inflammatory drugs and non-selective beta-blockers or even Sulphites in foods and drinks will also bring on an attack. Viral upper respiratory tract infections, such as colds and even physical activity, including exercise, can also trigger an attack.

Common signs and symptoms of asthma include coughing which can worsen at night or early in the morning, making it hard to sleep. Wheezing from narrowing of the airway occurs when you breathe accompanied by chest tightness. This may feel like something is squeezing or sitting on your chest. Shortness of breath is obvious. Some people who have asthma say they can't catch their breath or they feel out of breath. You may feel like you can't get air out of your lungs.

Asthma is a long-term disease that has no cure. The goal of asthma treatment is to control the disease. Good asthma control will prevent chronic and troublesome symptoms, such as coughing and shortness of breath, and reduce the need for quick-relief medicines and help to maintain good lung function allowing the patient to maintain a normal activity level and sleep through the night.

Treatment for asthma

Treatment for asthma although it can appear stressful is reasonably straight forward. The first thing is to get the patient to relax. If you are dealing with a child, you may have to work a little harder to get them to relax. Good eye contact and bringing yourself down to the patient's level is a good start. Eye contact gets their attention and gives them a sense that you genuinely care, while kneeling down to be at their level does 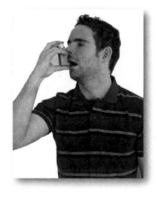 away with that sense of intimidation they would feel if you were otherwise standing up and looking down on them. You should adopt this procedure as standard regardless of the age of your patient. Speak in a soft compassionate voice and reassure them that everything will be OK, and do likewise to the parents because it can be very stressful for them also to see their child suffering such an attack. Get them to sit in a position that is comfortable for them that gives them relief. Generally, sitting the patient forward with their hands resting on their lap gives some relief as the lungs more or less hang free, allowing them to work better. This is known as the tripod position. Alternatively, when a patient is in a standing position leaning forward with their hands resting on a table for support, they are also able to breathe somewhat easier. This is also referred to as tripoding.

If the patient has medication, get them to take it. The fact that they are regularly using this medication means it has been prescribed for them and there are no worries about contraindications. The usual medication would be Ventolin. The active ingredient salbutamol works by acting on receptors in the lungs called beta 2 receptors. When salbutamol stimulates these receptors, it causes the muscles in the airways to relax. This allows the airways to open. Salbutamol is most commonly taken using an inhaler device. Inhaling the medicine allows it to act directly in the lungs where it is needed most. It also reduces the potential for side effects occurring in other parts of the body, as the amount absorbed into the blood through the lungs is lower than if it is taken by mouth. Don't get confused if the patient has two different colour inhalers as the one that the patient inhales during an attack will normally be blue which is also known as a 'reliever' inhaler. The other type you are likely to see will be a brown or red inhaler. This is known as a preventer inhaler, and as the name suggests, it is given to prevent asthma attacks and should not be used to treat an attack.

A new device on the market is *the turbohaler*. This is administered by unscrewing and lifting off the cover, turning the grip fully in one direction then turning it all the way back until you hear a click. Once you hear that click, the device is loaded and ready to use. The patient then simply breathes out (not through the inhaler) and places the inhaler between their lips and breathes in as deeply and as hard as they can. The mouthpiece should be cleaned often with a dry tissue but never washed.

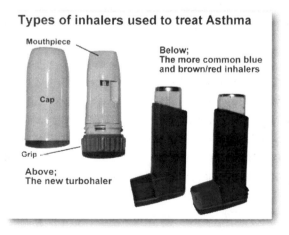

Types of inhalers used to treat Asthma

Mouthpiece

Below;
The more common blue
and brown/red inhalers

Cap

Grip

Above;
The new turbohaler

If it's a mild attack, one puff from the inhaler should see results within a few minutes. The patient may sometimes use a spacer or extension tube that attaches to the inhaler which allows more medication to be deposited into the lungs instead of the throat and airways, which makes a single dose more efficient. When using a spacer, you do not need to match an inhale with the medication release, allowing an easier inhalation. If the first puff appears not to be making a difference after five minutes, get them to take a second puff. If the patient isn't making signs of recovery within five minutes of taking the second dose, you should call the emergency services. Get the patient to purse their lips as if they were blowing out a candle and blow forcibly as it helps to relieve some of the internal lung pressures that are responsible for the attack.

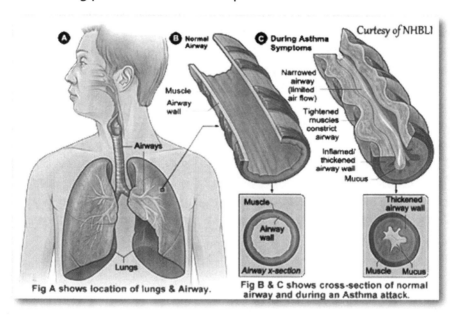

Fig A shows location of lungs & Airway.

Fig B & C shows cross-section of normal airway and during an Asthma attack.

Legal note: It's safe to advise or hand the patient their medication allowing them to self-administer as they know the correct dosage, but unless you are qualified to administer these drugs, you should never attempt to do so. Your priority when dealing with inadequate breathing should be to assess and maintain the airway, and if your protocols or CPGs allow, you should apply oxygen and monitor the patient until EMS arrives. (Ref: CPG's Inadequate Respirations—Adult) If it's a first ever attack, you should call EMS immediately as it may not be asthma. You should assess and maintain the airway, and if trained to do so, apply oxygen. Keep in mind that oxygen will dry out the throat if administered over too long a period. Humidified oxygen is preferred if possible. Keep the patient calm and get them to concentrate on their breathing. If they are in an open area, keep them warm. Find out what lead up to the event as this may help with your diagnosis. It may even be an allergic reaction to a sting of food item. Get a SAMPLE History. *Do not* attempt to give or assist with medication if it's not theirs or hasn't been prescribed specifically for that patient. On arrival, if it is asthma, EMS may administer salbutamol through a nebuliser mask. This mask is similar to a regular non-rebreather mask except that it has a medication bowl attached where they will put the medication in liquid form and attach it to low-flow oxygen which converts the medication into a fine mist allowing the patient to breathe it in a humidified fashion.

12.5. Croup

Croup is an infection of the upper airway that occurs in children from around six months to four years. It is caused by inflammation in the trachea (windpipe), the vocal cords (larynx), and the bronchial tubes (bronchi), which results in hoarse whooping noise during inhalation, unlike asthma, where the patient will wheeze on exhalation. Sometimes croup can be more distressing for the parents than the child, and for that reason, the parent dealing with it must try to be calm and reassuring because if the child sees that you are distressed, the child will also become distressed and the attack may get worse. These attacks usually occur during the night. Children aren't dumb; they can read and sense panic and emotion from the parent. Croup generally passes without causing any lasting problems and can be treated at home.

When an attack occurs, it is essential to keep calm. This attitude will in turn help to prevent the child from being panicked. The home cure generally means steam. Sit the child on your lap in the bathroom and run the hot tap in the bath or shower keeping the door and window closed to allow the bathroom to fill with steam. Alternatively boil a kettle or saucepan of water to create steam but always use caution with hot liquids. This helps to relax the vocal cords lessoning the croupy noise. If the steam isn't helping, wrap a blanket over the child and call EMS. Continue the steam treatment until they arrive as it's possible that the child could be suffering from epiglottitis.

12.6. Epiglottitis

Epiglottitis is a severe inflammation of the epiglottis caused by bacterial infection. This is a potentially life-threatening condition that occurs when the epiglottis, a small flap that covers your windpipe, swells, blocking the flow of air into the lungs. When a child has this condition, they will want to sit upright and will not want to lie down. Drooling is a good indicator as the child will have difficulty or be totally unable to swallow. They will be extremely anxious, and the treatment you can give is very limited. The number one priority in this case is to call the EMS. Keep the child calm and allow them to find their own comfortable breathing position. They will most likely want to sit up leaning forward which allows their mouth to drain. If they are old enough, give them a facecloth or something of that nature so that they can wipe their mouth. If for no other reason, this will give them something to do. If you are trained in the administration of oxygen, give it to them. Monitor them and keep reassuring them until help arrives.

Note: It is sometimes worth bearing in mind that things aren't always what they appear to be. If the child is distressed and can't breathe or has difficulty breathing, consider looking in the mouth first. They may have swallowed something that got lodged in the throat and may be choking. With any condition concerning children, if you have any doubt as to what is wrong with them, call EMS. They don't mind if it was a false alarm provided your intentions were good. Better sure than sorry.

12.7. Choking

(Adult and Child/Adult and Child CPR)

For the purposes of categorising and determining age, a child is someone that is aged between one and eight, while an adult is someone aged from eight and above.

Choking or FBAO as it is referred to in the medical world is a common life-threatening occurrence among all ages, particularly in young children and the elderly which can be as a result of food or other foreign bodies becoming lodged in the throat and blocking the airway. When something gets stuck in the throat, the muscles contract and go into spasm which adds to the problem of clearing it. However, when the patient goes unconscious, the muscles relax, but you don't ever want the episode to get to that stage if it can be helped. If someone is choking, they may be grasping their neck with both hands. (This is known as the universal sign of choking.) They need help right away. If you see someone who appears to be choking, ask them, 'Are you choking?' If they nod, reassure them and tell them you are going to help.

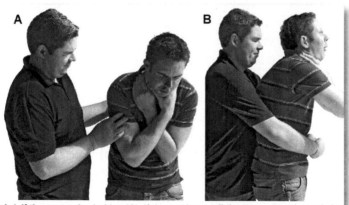

Ask if the person is choking (A). If they nod yes, tell them you are going to help. Stand behind the victim and give abdominal thrusts until the airway is clear (B).

In some cases, the airway may only be partially blocked, and the best person to clear this is the person themselves. If this is the case, encourage the victim to cough hard and keep doing it until they cough the object out. If the airway is fully compromised, you need to perform abdominal thrusts (aka the Heimlich manoeuvre). To perform abdominal thrusts, you need to stand behind the victim. Get them to spread their legs about 12 inches or so (30 cm) apart so that you can place your foot between them (as if you were taking a step forward). This will give you a stance or solid platform to work from. If the victim's legs are together and they go unconscious while your hand is wrapped around their waist, they will either fall back on top of you or pull you forward on top of them as they hit the ground. Having a good stance gives you a chance to help the unconscious victim to the ground in reasonable safety because you can slide them down along your leg. If you are dealing with a child, you may have to kneel down to be at the appropriate level.

Once in position, place one hand around their waist making a fist as you go. Place the second hand around the waist also and locate the bellybutton. Place the fisted hand on the stomach about an inch (25 mm) above the bellybutton (do not go any higher) turning the thumb side in as if you were looking at your watch. Grab the fist with your other hand and pull inwards and upwards toward you. This needs to be done with force. Do this for as long as it takes to remove the object. If this works and the object is expelled, let the victim rest for a few minutes to get their breath back. It is advisable for the victim to see their doctor as soon as possible as bruising will have occurred internally.

If the victim is large or in the late stages of pregnancy, stand behind them, and rather than performing abdominal thrusts, place your hands under the victim's armpits and put the fist of one hand slightly above the nipple line in the centre of the chest (thumb side in toward the chest) and grab your fist with your other hand and pull straight back toward you with force. Keep doing it until the object is expelled or the victim goes unconscious. If your hands aren't long enough, the alternative is to back the victim against a wall and place one hand on top of the other and push on the centre of the chest, slightly above the nipple line hard and fast (a bit like doing CPR standing up).

Another issue that could arise in that you may be a small or slightly built person and not have the physical ability to help. If you know how to relieve an FBAO, and there are other people nearby, get one of them to assist the victim while you explain to them what to do step by step. It's amazing what you can do if you put your mind to it!

If you fail to expel the object and the victim goes unconscious, lower them onto the ground. Establish that they are unconscious, and if so, call for help (999/112) and ask someone to get an AED. If no one comes, make the call yourself and get the AED (if available). Return to the victim and begin the steps of CPR with one exception, every time you go to give a breath, look in the mouth for the object. If you can see it, fish it out. If you can't see it, don't go looking for it by blind finger-sweeping as you may push the object further down. Start with thirty compressions (hard and fast, at a rate of at least 100 per minute) followed by two breaths using the head tilt, chin lift method looking in the mouth first (see also CPR/AED). Continue rotating thirty compressions followed be two breaths, remembering to look in the mouth first before giving a breath until help arrives.

An alternative means of reliving a FBAO is taught to CFRs. This is a method whereby five abdominal thrusts and five back slaps or blows between the shoulder blades are used in continuous rotation. When it is established that a person is choking, the responder gives five abdominal thrusts in the same way as previously discussed. If the object isn't expelled, the responder then moves to the victim's side placing one hand across their abdomen to support the victim from falling. They will then ask the victim to lean or bend slightly forward (anywhere between 40° and 60°) so that the victim is basically looking at the ground, and then with the heel of the other hand; give five hard slaps between the shoulder blades. Keep rotating abdominal thrusts and backslaps until the object is expelled or the victim goes unconscious. If this happens, continue the steps of CPR as discussed in the previous paragraph.

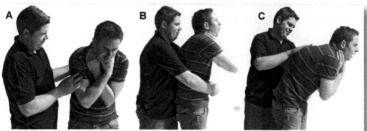

Helping a choking victim using a combination of abdominal thrusts and backslaps.
Ask the person if they are choking (A)?   If they nod yes, tell them you will help.
Do 5 abdominal thrusts (B) followed by 5 backslaps (C).   Repeat as required.

While these steps are used both in adults and children, there is a slight difference as to when you call for help when dealing with a child or infant. It is important to note that cardiac arrest in children is rarely the primary event unless the child or infant was born with a heart defect or condition. Cardiac arrest is almost always secondary to respiratory inadequacies due to suffocation or trauma. Therefore, it is recommended that for children and infants, if you are on your own, you do five cycles of CPR first before you call for help. Remember, the rate, ratio, and depth of compressions are the same for both adults and children.

12.8. Choking

(Infant/Infant CPR)

For the purposes of categorising and determining age, an infant is someone who is between zero and one year old. When an infant is choking, it seems far more traumatic than if it was an older person because they are so helpless. If an infant is lying on their back after a bottle or semisolid feed for instance and they get sick, the vomit may be aspirated into the lungs or become stuck in the airway. Unlike children and adults, infants aren't able to alert you to the fact that they are choking, and for that reason, they need to be monitored regularly, especially after feeding. If the infant can cough or make sounds, the blockage is mild. Stand by and let them cough.

If the infant cannot make a sound or has a cough with no sound, or cannot breathe, then the blockage is severe and you need to act fast. When an infant has severe choking, use a combination of back slaps followed by chest thrusts to help relieve the blockage.

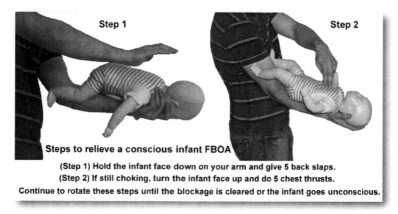

Steps to relieve a conscious infant FBOA

(Step 1) Hold the infant face down on your arm and give 5 back slaps.
(Step 2) If still choking, turn the infant face up and do 5 chest thrusts.
Continue to rotate these steps until the blockage is cleared or the infant goes unconscious.

To relieve an infant airway obstruction, do the following steps:

1. Hold the infant face down on your forearm, supporting the head and jaw with your hand. Try to keep the baby's head in a neutral position to get the maximum effect.

2. Give up to five back slaps with the heel of your other hand between the infant's shoulder blades. Do this quickly taking no more than one second between blows.

3. If the object does not come out, turn the infant on its back, and supporting the head in the neutral position, give up to five chest thrusts using two fingers of your other hand to push straight down on the chest in the same place you push during CPR (slightly below the nipple line). Do these compressions over one second each to a depth of at least one-third the depth of the infant's chest which would be approximately 1½ inches (4 cm).

4. Repeat giving five back slaps followed by five chest thrusts until the infant can breathe or cough or cry or until they stop breathing.

5. If they stop breathing, put them on a hard flat surface such as a table and continue the steps of CPR with one exception. Look in the mouth before you give breaths.

One important note: When doing backslaps and chest thrusts on an infant you always keep their head supported in the neutral position and keep the head lower than the body. You can also use your knee to support your hand. Remember also that an infant's head is heavy in proportion to the rest of the body. If it isn't supported and allowed to flop around, you could also cause injuries to the neck or head.

12.9. Paediatric Chain of Survival

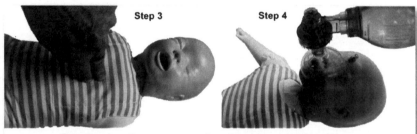

Step 3 **Step 4**

The steps to relieve an unconscious infant airway obstruction

When an infant goes unconscious or stops breathing, call for help, then place them on a hard surface and do 30 compressions (Step 3) followed by 2 breaths (Step 4). If dealing with a FBOA, always check the mouth before giving breaths. Continue giving compressions & breaths until the infant responds or help arrives.

There is a difference when it comes to the Paediatric Chain of Survival because the first link of the chain here is prevention of cardiac arrest. With the exception of being born with a heart defect, children in general have healthy hearts. Usually a child's heart stops because they can't breathe or are having trouble breathing. If the rescuer leaves a child with respiratory arrest to call EMS, the child may progress to cardiac arrest and the chance of survival will be much lower. For this reason, if a lone rescuer finds an unresponsive child who is not breathing or gasping, the rescuer should provide 5 cycles (about 2 minutes) of CPR before calling for help (999/112). This is why early high quality CPR becomes the second link in the chain followed link three which is rapid activation of EMS. The fourth link is effective advanced life support followed finally by integrated post-cardiac care.

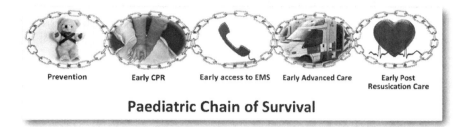

Prevention   Early CPR   Early access to EMS   Early Advanced Care   Early Post Resusication Care

Paediatric Chain of Survival

When an infant becomes unresponsive and stops breathing, you need to act fast and follow the steps of infant CPR.

1. Tap and shout for response. This is generally done by tapping the sole of the infant's foot and calling their name out loud. If there is no response, *call for help.* Check for breathing, and if they are not breathing, start compressions.

2. After thirty compressions, open the airway by tilting the head no more than slightly beyond the neutral position. Look in the mouth. If you can see the object, remove it; if not, cover the infant's mouth and nose with your mouth and give two breaths. Remember that infants' lungs are small, so you only want to see slight chest rise. Your breaths for an infant should be no more powerful than a small puff. If the chest doesn't rise, reposition the head and try again. If you fail a second time, go back to compressions.

3. After two minutes (five cycles) of CPR, if help hasn't arrived, you may carry the infant with you to phone for help.

4. After calling for help, return to giving CPR until help arrives.

Remember: After doing chest trusts on an infant, have them examined by a doctor as there will be bruising which in turn leads to swelling that may cause problems later.

12.10. Hanging and Strangulation

This is quite a heavy topic, but because it can happen in every city, town, and village either accidently or intentionally, it's important to know what to do.

Hanging is a form of strangulation that involves suspension by the neck. Hangings are categorised into two types. Hanging where the body is freely suspended is known as complete hanging, while hanging with incomplete suspension whereby part of the body such as the tips of the toes are resting on a solid surface partially supporting the victim's weight is known as an incomplete or partial hanging. Where a fall involves a distance greater than the height of the victim, significant cervical spinal cord (C-Spine) injuries are most common with poor outcomes due to fractures of the upper cervical spine and transection of the spinal cord with loss of all sensation below the level of lesion resulting in almost instant death. Incomplete suspension, however, can result in the person dying mainly due to strangulation. This would involve severe or complete obstruction of all blood vessels of which the latter is sometimes referred to as global cerebral ischemia which leads to cerebral hypoxia (when the brain is completely deprived of oxygen). The victim will be rendered unconscious followed in turn by loss of muscle tone and final arterial and airway obstruction. It is well documented that a large amount of suicides by hanging are in reality suicides by strangulation.

Blocking of the carotid artery by applying external pressure deprives the brain of oxygen and likewise, blocking the jugular vein prevents deoxygenated blood from exiting the brain thereby leading to unconsciousness. If the pressure is maintained long enough, a person will die! In some cases of domestic violence, for instance, women die at the hands of their partners from being strangled or choked to death.

It only takes an applied pressure of 10-12 lbs for approximately ten seconds on both carotid arteries to render someone unconscious. It takes about three times that pressure to close off the trachea. However, not all incidents involving strangulation are premeditated.

Accidents occasionally happen in the workplace whereby loose clothing gets caught up in machinery resulting in the victim being pulled into the machine, or typically that last minute look under the bonnet of the car while the engine is running where a person wearing a necktie gets it caught in the pulley-wheel or fan-belt. The victim will be powerless to help themselves, and unless, help is at hand, the victim will be strangled.

Children and toddlers are also at risk. Young children die every year as a result of being strangled by pull cords on window and door blinds. Or in the case of babies whereby they manage to get their heads stuck between the bars of their cot and strangle themselves trying to get free. Risk assessment is a good foundation for a safe working environment. This also applies to the home where there are young children. Simply by looking around the house, you should be able to identify and remove any potential hazards or dangers.

What can a responder do?

If you are called to help someone who has hanged or attempted to hang themselves, you should take a second or two to mentally prepare yourself. What you witness may not be pleasant and could have a lasting effect on you. In small communities there is a very good chance that the victim will be someone known to the responder which makes dealing with the event even harder. You may even have to get help to deal with it afterwards.

Getting help is not a sign of weakness. People working for years in emergency services occasionally look for help to deal with stressful situations and talking about it openly to someone will help. Sometimes talking things out with a colleague or family member who is prepared to listen and not judge helps a lot. Usually, when a serious incident has occurred, a debriefing for the crew involved is held before the end of shift and any potential problems and other related issues are talked through. When everyone gets together and discusses the incident, people feel that the load is shared and any ideas that your actions in your own mind were questionable are nearly always answered. What if, is a big question, and we all ask it from time to time, but you as a responder must take on board that we can't always save someone who doesn't want to be saved, and often we're not able to save those that do. We also witness things we wish we didn't have to.

Dealing with a suspension (hanging)

When you are called to an incident involving hanging or strangulation, the person may still be alive. They may have in the case of a hanging or attempted hanging been already cut down, or in the case of a strangulation attempt, the perpetrator may have fled the scene, or if it was accidental say, for example, a child, whereby whatever was causing the problem such as a blind cord was already removed by the parent.

The first thing you should do knowing the circumstances is ensure whether the scene is safe for you to enter. Once you have established a few facts, call an ambulance and have the police involved as well. If an AED is available, have someone get it or get it yourself.

Let's address both issues separately dealing first with hanging.

If the victim is still hanging, always assume that they are still alive until proven otherwise. In most cases, the victim is only hanging a few feet from the ground, so it's possible to deal with this with the help of one or two others. First, someone has to support the body while another relieves the constriction or cuts them down. Once that's achieved, lay the victim gently onto the floor, remove the ligature from around the neck, and try to establish a clear airway. Remember, where a fall involves a distance greater than the height of the victim, there may be C-Spine issues; therefore, a trauma jaw thrust is advised, but if, for example, the victim jumped off a chair, and the fall distance was only 1-2 feet (30-60 cm), you should proceed with caution when opening the airway and gently do a head tilt, chin lift as you are more likely to be dealing with strangulation. Either way, if you are not sure and the victim is not breathing, you must apply the life over limb rule and do a head tilt, chin lift.

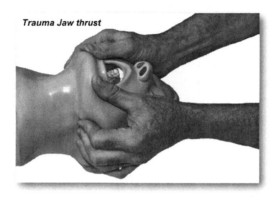

Trauma Jaw thrust

Sometimes there is visible evidence of strangulation. When, for example, the victim realises he or she is slowly choking to death rather than the swift death they planned, they struggle to remove the rope or belt or whatever without success. You may see scratches on the throat around the ligature from their fingernails where they attempted to free themselves before going unconscious.

Once you have established a patent (clear) airway, check for breathing. Place your ear close to the victim's mouth and listen for any breath sounds or gurgling while looking down the chest for any rise and fall. At the same time, check for a carotid pulse. If you can't find a pulse or are not sure of a pulse, start CPR beginning with compressions and continue until help arrives. If there was an AED available, use it in the same way as you would when dealing with a cardiac arrest. If the victim started to cough or breathe and if C-Spine damage wasn't indicated, put them into the recovery position and cover them with a blanket. If oxygen is available and you are trained to use it, give them 100% O2 (15 litres per minute) using a non-rebreather mask.

If the victim was found several feet off the ground, say for example, they climbed onto a high branch of a tree, or they were suspended from a high rafter in a shed and you are unable to reach them, unless there is a ladder nearby, and two or three people to help you, there isn't really a lot you can do until help arrives. However, if with help, you were able to release or cut the victim down, there is a definite possibility of C-Spine damage. Position yourself at the victim's head. Open the airway using a trauma jaw thrust and listen for sounds of breathing and maintain in-line immobilisation. If need be, ask everyone to stop talking and remain silent until you have established whether the victim is breathing or not. If breathing is absent and a pulse isn't detectable, your co-responder should apply the AED and start compressions. It is possible to give breaths through a pocket mask when using a trauma jaw thrust, but practice on a manikin is advised as it is a difficult manoeuvre. If you are using a BVM, it becomes a three-person operation. One person should hold the mask over the face and maintain the open airway, while another rescuer squeezes the bag, and the third person does compressions. If you were the only trained person there, you should ask a bystander to do compression only CPR until help arrives while you maintain the airway.

If the victim shows signs of life after removing the ligature, it is worth knowing that if the blood supply was cut off to the brain for several minutes, the victim may well suffer a reperfusion injury. This is the tissue damage caused when blood supply returns to the tissue after a period of ischemia (blockage) or lack of oxygen, so the level of recovery for the victim both physically and neurologically is time critical.

Strangulation

Strangulation can be accidental or deliberate. In some cases of domestic violence, for instance, women die at the hands of their partners from being strangled or choked. Children and infants also die from strangulation as discussed at the start of this section.

If you were called to an incident where an attempted strangulation was involved, there are a number of things you should do before you commit yourself to giving help. First, you may be entering a crime scene where an act of violence has taken place. And second, you shouldn't respond until you are sure that the scene is safe and help such as the police are already on scene as the perpetrator may still be there. Under no circumstances should you put yourself in harm's way. If in your opinion, the scene looks suspicious, don't disturb or move anything. In these situations you only move something if it is preventing you from treating your patient. If you must move something, make a mental note of where it was. In the event that it is a crime scene, the more preserved the scene is the better the outcome of the investigation.

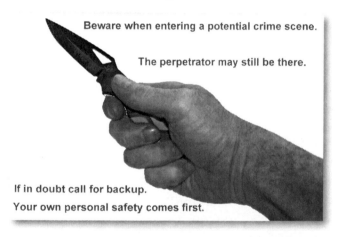

Beware when entering a potential crime scene.

The perpetrator may still be there.

If in doubt call for backup.
Your own personal safety comes first.

If you find someone that appears lifeless, check for response as you would with any unconscious patient. If there is no response, you should ensure that help is on the way and an AED is available. Put the victim on the floor. Open the airway using the head tilt, chin lift method, and check for signs of breathing while at the same time checking for a pulse. Take into account that the trachea may be damaged and it may be difficult for the victim to breathe. Listen for any gurgling or wheezing or any other noise that might indicate breathing. If there is no breathing and you can't find a pulse, start CPR beginning with compressions and attach the AED as soon as it arrives. Keep doing cycles of five sets of thirty compressions followed by two breaths and switch roles every two minutes, or if the AED is in use, switch every time it analyses to avoid fatigue.

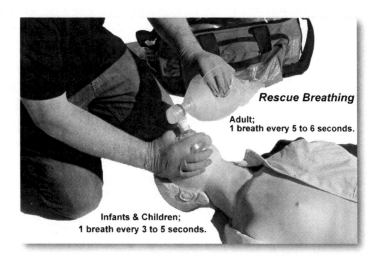

If there is a pulse but their breathing is shallow or inadequate, you should perform rescue breathing. For an adult, you should give one breath every five to six seconds (about 10-12 BPM). When giving rescue breaths for infants and children, you should give one breath every three to five seconds (about 12-20 BPM). Give each breath over one second and look for reasonable chest rise. You should also check the pulse every two minutes. Bear in mind that when dealing with infants and children that although you are providing adequate ventilations and oxygenation, if their pulse is less than 60 beats per minute, you should start CPR. If the victim recovers, put them into the recovery position and keep them warm. If you are trained to administer oxygen, give 100% (15 litres per minute) using a non-rebreather mask.

If the adult victim is able to communicate with you, you should introduce yourself and reassure them that they are safe as they will be extremely anxious. Check their ABCs. They may not want to talk about the incident to you, so don't push for information. The only concern for you is that your patient is stable and hopefully will remain so until the ambulance arrives. The circumstances of the incident are a police matter. Try to obtain a medical history, and if you are trained to administer oxygen, give 100% (15 litres per minute) using a non-rebreather mask. Do a secondary survey and make notes of any changes.

When dealing with children or infants, it's better to have a parent or guardian present as strangers may only frighten them and cause further distress. If you are called to a strangulation involving a child, you need to act fast as children can deteriorate quite quickly. If, for example, the child was caught in a window blind cord, you should quickly take the weight of the child and release the cord from around their neck. If the child is unresponsive, check their ABCs as already discussed in this section. The trachea or windpipe of a young child won't be as strong as that of an adult, so care must be taken as it may have been damaged during the event. If there are no signs of life, begin the steps of CPR; do five cycles (two minutes) before calling EMS. If others are present, have them call EMS while you start CPR. If an AED is present, attach it and follow the prompts.

If the child is responsive and able to breathe but with difficulty, have the parent calm the child as best they can. Remember, this event is just as traumatic for the parent as it is for the child; this means you are actually dealing with two casualties. The parent will need as much reassurance as the child, but you need to get the message quickly to the parent that they must remain calm in order to reassure the child as the child will sense fear and anxiety and may take longer to relax. It's important not to give anything to eat or drink until they are checked out in a hospital setting.

The same applies to infants and toddlers (a toddler is aged between one and three years), and although there are a lot of hazards that a grown-up may be aware of, there are always surprises. It may happen that the infant could put their head through the bars of their cot or crib, and in the process of trying to get out of the situation, their neck gets squeezed resulting in them being rendered unconscious. The problem here is they can't call for help or bang on things to attract attention. The word infant after all comes from the Latin word infans meaning unable to speak or speechless. Dealing with this scenario can be emotionally as well as physically challenging. First, because of the age, the trachea hasn't yet developed and can kink easily. Getting the head out from between the bars may be just a matter of manoeuvring the infant into the right position, but if you are struggling, don't waste time, bend or break one of the bars away from their head. Cots can be replaced! Place the infant on a solid surface such as a table and check for signs of life (ABCs). When tilting an infant's head to open the airway, *don't* do a head tilt, chin lift as you would an adult or child as this will block an infant's airway. You only want to tilt the head back just slightly more than the neutral position. Any more may kink the airway. If there are no signs of life, begin the steps of infant CPR, then call EMS after doing five cycles or two minutes of CPR and continue until help arrives. As mentioned earlier, if there are others present, have one of them call EMS while you get to work on the victim. If the infant is conscious, place them with the mother and let her comfort it. Infants respond better to the familiar voice of a parent than that of a stranger. If they are struggling to breathe, you may have to assist by giving one breath every three to five seconds (about 12-20 BPM). If oxygen is available and your CPGs or protocols allow you to give it, do so. However, infants won't tolerate a mask, but you can put it close to their nose and mouth and they will still get some benefit.

Evidence of strangulation

Evidence of strangulation is quite varied and may include any of the following. Swallowing may be painful and difficult and feel as if there's a lump in the throat. The victim may have a hoarse, raspy, or total loss of voice. Breathing may be laboured, or they may not be able to breathe at all. The victim may witness near or total loss of consciousness. Memory loss is also possible as is confusion, agitation, and restlessness. The victim may be nauseous and have the inclination to vomit. In the event that the victim was attacked, they may have defensive wounds such as scratches, scrapes, or bruises. Vision and hearing can be affected. There may be ligature marks and also fractured bones in the back of the neck. Blood may be visible in the eyes. There may be involuntary incontinence.

Prevention of strangulation

While we can't always know what adults get up to, we do have a certain role to play in keeping our children safe. The key to keeping our children from harm is prevention. Most accidents involving children happen in their own familiar environment, the home. There is so much we can do to prevent tragedies such as strangulation and entrapment happening in our homes. Prevention is also the first link in the paediatric chain of survival.

Anything you can put around your child's neck has the potential to strangle them! Bibs should be removed during sleep as there is potential for the tie strings to cut off circulation or be swallowed. Necklaces or any form of jewellery or toy that can dangle or hang around the neck can get caught in something. When choosing a cot or crib, check that the bars or slats are close enough (less than 3 inches or 75 mm apart) so that the infant can't get their head through, or talk to the shop owner for advice and recommendation. Clothing with draw strings can be a hazard for toddlers as they could get snagged in all sorts of places. Doors that are left ajar are lethal as the toddler may get their head or fingers trapped between the door and frame. Mobiles on cots or cribs can be a danger especially for a four- or five-month-old as they may be able to reach it and get tangled in the cords that the shapes are suspended with. Pull cords in window blinds and curtains are well up there when it comes to hazards. Toy boxes with lids can also pose a danger.

The more common accidents are where infants and toddlers pick up small objects and put them in their mouth or get into the kitchen cupboards where detergents and cleaning agents are or stick things in electrical power sockets. Child locks and catches can be bought at any hardware shop, as can doorstops, blank caps for power sockets and even baby listening devices and monitors.

You could literally write a book on hazards, and I have only touched the tip if the iceberg, but common sense works wonders. You don't have to empty every room to keep your child safe; remember you live there too! Child safety is just about common sense, compromise, and having a watchful eye. There are great websites and books dedicated to child safety where you will pick up great tips.

12.11. Drowning

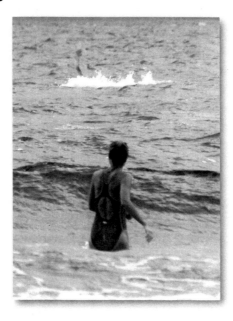

Drowning is defined as a process resulting in primary respiratory impairment as a result of submersion or immersion in a liquid. Drowning itself is quick and silent, although it may be preceded by distress which is more visible. Submerging the face in water colder than about 21°C (70°F) triggers what is known as the mammalian diving reflex. This reflex protects the body by putting it into energy-saving mode to maximise the time it can stay under water. The strength of this reflex is greater in colder water and has three principal effects: first, the heart rate can slow down by as much as 50% (bradycardia) followed by peripheral vasoconstriction whereby blood flow to the extremities is restricted in order to increase blood supply and oxygen to the brain and other vital organs. Finally, blood is redirected into the thoracic cavity which is the region of the chest between the diaphragm and the neck. This is known as blood shift. This protects the lungs from collapsing should the victim be in deeper water. Generally, when a person realises they are in difficulty, the first thing they try to do is hold their breath while splashing around to try to keep their head above water. Panic then sets in, and they use up more oxygen forcing them to gasp for more air. This is the critical point as they may be unable due to fatigue to get their head above water in order to take a breath resulting in water entering the mouth. At this stage, the victim may try to cough it out or swallow resulting in involuntary inhalation which leads to laryngospasm whereby the larynx (voice box) constricts to seal the airway. While laryngospasm prevents water entering the lungs, it can also prevent air which will cause the victim to go unconscious due to hypoxia. When the victim becomes unconscious, the laryngospasm relaxes allowing water to enter the lungs. This is known as wet drowning. About 8%-10% of victims have been known to maintain laryngospasm until they go into cardiac arrest, and in this instance, no water enters the lungs. This is known as dry drowning.

Secondary drowning is a condition that can be difficult to recognise. A person who was involved in a near-drowning incident that may have aspirated a small amount of water can look and feel OK, and yet they can die within anything up to forty-eight hours after the event. In most cases of secondary drowning, there is very little water found in the lungs but yet enough to prevent enough oxygen entering the bloodstream resulting in death by hypoxemia, or low blood oxygen as a result of pulmonary oedema (fluid in the lungs).

For this reason, anyone who has ingested water or has been involved in a near-drowning incident should, as a cautionary measure, be taken to a medical centre or hospital to rule out the likelihood of secondary drowning.

Attempting a rescue and providing treatment

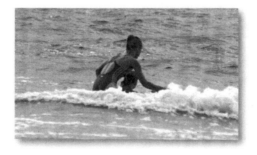

Drowning isn't something we come across every day, but it does happen, and for someone who witnesses it, it can be very traumatic and frightening and can make that witness do the most brave or stupid things. No one wants to see someone drowned, and we all would like to help, but unfortunately, and it is well documented, rescuers can also become victims.

Giving advice to someone who has never witnessed a person in difficulty in the water is a hard thing to do and even more difficult for the learner to imagine how they would react. However, on any given day, you could be the one person to witness such an event while strolling along the beach or the riverbank. It could be that you are by a lake or even by a swimming pool. People on occasion (especially young children) have even drowned in their own bathtub. All these places have the potential for accidents to happen and it takes very little water to drown in.

If you see someone in difficulty in the water, the first thing you should do is call for help. If there are lifeguards on duty, describe the location and what you witnessed and let them handle it. You can offer them assistance if you feel you can help. Lifeguards only work beaches and swimming pools at set working hours, so there is a possibility of no one hearing you or coming to help. You could also be in an isolated area such as by a river or lake. If there are no lifeguards in the area, look around and see if there are life buoys or rings with a rope attached that you can throw to the victim and haul them to safety.

There are dozens of reasons why you shouldn't attempt a rescue, but there are a few why you should. It's never like in the movies where the hero swims out and casually grabs the victim and brings them to shore safely and smiles for the camera, quite the contrary. There is an old saying 'clutching at straws' which is what happens when you swim into deep water to rescue someone. The minute you make contact with a drowning victim, they will grab you anywhere they can to get above water and will push you under. If you can't react or haven't been trained to do so, you will drown along with the victim.

If the victim is in shallow water that may be chest level to you and you can reach them in safety, then, there is a level of safety for you to provide rescue because you can stand on the bottom, but remove any heavy clothing that may weigh you down before entering the water. You will need something dry to wear afterwards to prevent you from getting cold. The main thing before you do anything is to call 999/112 and ask for marine or water rescue and ambulance. Give a location and directions, if possible. It often happens that someone thinks they see someone drowning, but when the rescue services arrive, it turns out to be a false alarm. This is never a problem because that person, who called, genuinely thought someone was in trouble and the coastguard or inshore rescue units understand this and it gets logged as a false alarm with good intent. Rescue units prefer that you call if you think someone is in trouble rather than thinking you might be wasting their time. It could be that one time someone hesitates to call that a real emergency occurs and instead of making a rescue, the rescue services spend days or weeks looking for the body as a result.

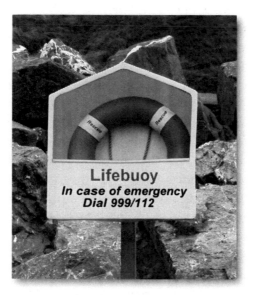

If you witness someone in difficulty in a swimming pool, river or beach, first call for help. If there is a life buoy with a rope attached near you, grab it, hold the end of the rope, and throw the buoy to the victim and pull them to safety. When throwing a life buoy, you should if possible throw it beyond the victim and pull it towards them rather than throwing it directly at them. This way the victim may swim into it or they may be able to grab the rope. If you throw it directly to them, they may only have a split second to grab it and may be too tired or in too much of a panic to grab it and it will float away out of reach. If there isn't a life buoy in the area, use a branch or pole or anything they might be able to grab. A towel or even a jumper would do if they were near enough. However, if you witness someone face down or floating lifeless, in the water, only you know if you are confident enough to perform the rescue. If you can't swim, wait for help. If there is someone with you and there is a life buoy nearby, ask them to hold one end of the rope while you take the buoy and wade into the water to retrieve the victim but never attempt a rescue if the water is higher than your waist unless you are a strong swimmer and trained in lifesaving techniques. A person who is alone will rarely enter water without having support ashore.

Before you enter the water, remember scene safety! Beaches by nature slope gradually, so depth of water is also gradual and currents depend on tide. Rivers because they flow all the time are more flooded in winter and may also be tidal. They can have deep and shallow pools, so every foot you travel is different and currents can be rapid in times of flood, usually after heavy rain. Certain times of the year, a good runner wouldn't be able to keep up with the speed of a river in flood. Lakes are extremely dangerous. A foot or two from shore and you may only be in several inches of water, but 5 or 10 feet from shore, you could be in 50 feet of water or more. Lakes can go to depths of hundreds of feet plus the fact that it is fresh water from the mountains means it will have less buoyancy than sea water, so the victim will sink faster also. You should never attempt a rescue if you can't swim, as lakes in particular tend to be ice cold because of their depth and surroundings. The cold could cause you to cramp in a very short time or even the shock of a warm person hitting the cold water could bring about a cardiac arrest.

Let's say, for example, the victim is in a position whereby you can get to them to shore safety. If they are face down, turn them face upwards and quickly drag them ashore or out of the swimming pool. In the majority of cases, C-Spine isn't an issue unless the victim was seen falling from a height into shallow water or hitting the floor of the pool. If C-Spine is an issue, ideally, the victim should be rolled in the water as a unit, keeping the head straight in the neutral position and in line with the body. However, this procedure requires three or four people and that might not be possible.

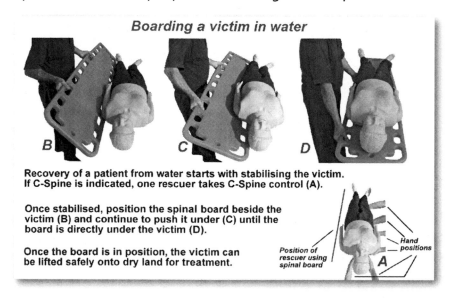

Boarding a victim in water

B   C   D

Recovery of a patient from water starts with stabilising the victim. If C-Spine is indicated, one rescuer takes C-Spine control (A).

Once stabilised, position the spinal board beside the victim (B) and continue to push it under (C) until the board is directly under the victim (D).

Once the board is in position, the victim can be lifted safely onto dry land for treatment.

Position of rescuer using spinal board

Hand positions

A

Ideally, a spinal board should then be floated under the victim and the victim secured before being lifted on the board to safety. However, if you are alone or with a partner or there is a bystander willing to help you, and there isn't the luxury of a spinal board or any equipment until EMS arrives, rather than struggling and injuring yourself or anyone else, if it means pulling the victim outruns the risk of spinal damage or leaving them in the water to die, you should apply the life over limb rule and remove the victim from the water as best you can.

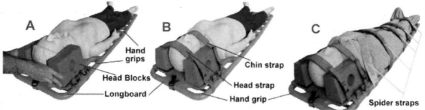

Spinal immobilisation without the use of a cervical collar

A — Hand grips / Head Blocks / Longboard

B — Chin strap / Head strap / Hand grip

C — Spider straps

Position the patient correctly on the longboard and place a head block at either side of the head (A) insuring snug contact for support.

Secure the head in place by fixing a head strap over the forehead and a chin strap across the chin (B) insuring that both straps are snug tight to minimise movement.

Cover the patient with a blanket and secure the entire body and legs using spider straps, insuring the straps are appropriately positioned (C).

Maximum weight capability for a longboard is 500lbs (approx 226KG's).

It is very important that the victim is removed horizontally to prevent shock. (Ref: CPG Submersion Incident CFR, OFA, EFR.) Try to shelter the victim from the elements to prevent their temperature from dropping any further as they may already be in the mild to moderate stages of hypothermia (see Hypothermia Causes and Treatment). Do a complete primary survey, quickly checking the mouth for debris as part of your ABCs.

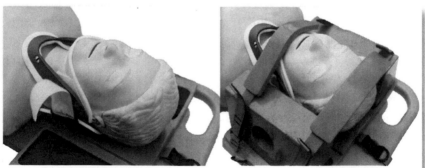

This is an example of full Cervical Spine immobilisation

Spinal immobilisation using a cervical collar should only be carried out if the rescuer or responder is competent and fully trained in C-Spine immobilisation.

Untrained persons attempting this manoeuvre may cause further damage and possible permanent paralysis to their patient.

Check for a pulse and breathing for thirty to forty-five seconds. Unlike the normal primary survey we have been discussing throughout this book, when dealing with a submersion incident where hypothermia is an issue, we check for a pulse for much longer because of the mammalian diving reflex. If there is a pulse but undetectable breathing, start rescue breathing straight away. For an adult, you should initially give two breaths in quick succession, and then give one breath every five to six seconds (about 10-12 BPM). When giving rescue breaths for infants and children, you should also give two quick breaths in succession followed by one breath every three to five seconds (about 12-20 BPM). Giving those two initial breaths helps to oxygenate the blood faster and can benefit the outcome. Give each breath over one second and look for adequate chest rise. You may have to give stronger than normal breaths to achieve chest rise because of poor compliance due to pulmonary oedema (fluid in the lungs). You should also check the pulse every two minutes. Rescue breaths can be given while in the water, if necessary, by supporting the back of the head with one hand and pinching the nose with the other hand. If C-Spine is indicated, keep the head in the neutral position while giving breaths, otherwise, tilt the head back, but the victim will have to be brought on to solid ground before compressions can be done.

Beware, there's a strong possibility that the victim may vomit as a result of ingesting water as they regain consciousness and the gag reflex returns. If this happens, and if there is no indication of C-Spine injury, turn the head sideways to allow the mouth drain and finger sweep any remaining debris to prevent it being aspirated into the lungs. If spinal injury is indicated, logroll them onto their side to allow drainage, and finger sweep any remaining debris ensuring that the head is kept in a straight line with the body to prevent further damage.

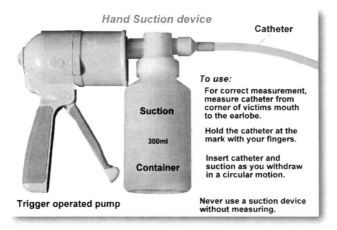

Hand Suction device

Catheter

Suction

300ml

Container

To use:

For correct measurement, measure catheter from corner of victims mouth to the earlobe.

Hold the catheter at the mark with your fingers.

Insert catheter and suction as you withdraw in a circular motion.

Trigger operated pump

Never use a suction device without measuring.

Alternatively, suction can be used if available. If you are at EFR level and trained in using a handheld or mechanical suction device, remember to measure the catheter (rigid suction tip) from the corner of the victim's mouth to the earlobe as this gives you the correct depth for insertion into the mouth. If you do not measure the catheter, you may not go deep enough which will leave debris behind or you will go too deep and stimulate their gag reflex or damage the back of the throat. Once you have sized it, if it's mechanical, turn it on and test it for suction and likewise with a handheld device by touching the tip against your gloved hand. Open the mouth and remove any large debris before inserting the catheter to the measured depth and suction as you slowly withdraw. You should suction for no longer than fifteen seconds. If the victim is to the stage whereby they are breathing adequately and there is no suspected spinal injury, remove any wet clothing and wrap the victim in warm blankets or whatever is at hand and put them into the recovery or safe airway position. If trained, you should administer oxygen (warmed if possible), give 100% (15 litres per minute) using a non-rebreather mask. Monitor the patient until EMS arrives.

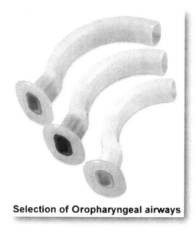

Selection of Oropharyngeal airways

If there is no breathing and you can't find a pulse, ensure that EMS has been called and that an AED is available and then start CPR right away. If you are at EFR level or upwards, you should insert an appropriate-sized OPA as this will help to maintain a patent airway and prevent the tongue from falling back in the throat. If the patient is on a longboard or spinal board, lift the end about 9 or 10 inches (about 25 cm) off the ground and support it well (especially midway to prevent bounce when performing compressions) as this will assist drainage and help to prevent water or vomit entering the lungs. Alternatively, if you are on sloped ground such as a riverbank, position the victim whereby their head is at the lower point of the slope.

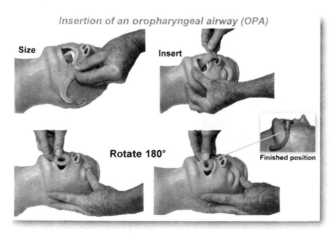

Insertion of an oropharyngeal airway (OPA)

Size

Insert

Rotate 180°

Finished position

Remove wet clothing as soon as possible and continue CPR and attach the AED as soon as it arrives. Follow the prompts and change places every time the AED analyses to avoid fatigue. If no AED is available, continue CPR, changing places with your partner after every five cycles (two minutes) to avoid fatigue. When hypothermic, the human body can do without oxygen for a longer period of time than when the body temperature is normal; therefore, you should also continue CPR for an extended period of time until the victim begins to show signs of life or the emergency services arrive.

When EMS arrives, they will ask for information regarding the incident. They may ask how long the person was in the water, for how long, and what treatment was given, or if the victim was witnessed entering the water or not. It is also important to obtain a history either from a witness or whoever was with them or from the victim if conscious. This will give you some idea of the mechanism and type of injury. Was it a diving accident, alcohol-related, a fall from a height? If it was in a pool, did the victim hit the bottom as a result of a high dive and pass out or land awkward from a water slide or perhaps the victim may not have been able to swim in the first place and inhaled water? Just tell them what you know.

Resuscitation of a drowning victim is slightly different to that of someone who has to be resuscitated in the home or workplace, etc. The noticeable difference is in giving compressions. If the victim has swallowed water and also inhaled water into the lungs, there will be a greater resistance in getting depth into your compressions due to the lungs being full or partly full of water, so a greater effort has to be made. When you give a breath, in the worst case scenario, although you achieve chest rise, you will in fact only be filling whatever space the water hasn't taken, so poor oxygen exchange is inevitable. This, however, equates more so to someone that has been submerged for a long period, and in the majority of these situations, the outcome is poor.

Another issue that arises after we take a victim from water is when do we stop all effort? There is an acronym that covers a lot of these questions (U18, CHOPP 15). It is a great reminder and applies to out-of-hospital resuscitation in general. You should continue all efforts of resuscitating a victim if they are *under eighteen* years of age, a victim of *cold water drowning*, suffering from *hypothermia* or drug *overdose*, if they have taken *poison*, if they are *pregnant* and less than *fifteen* minutes from a hospital.

12.12. Decompression Sickness

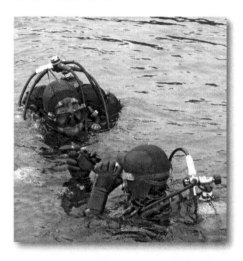

Decompression sickness, also called the bends, is caused by nitrogen bubbles forming in the bloodstream and tissues of the body as a result of rapid decrease in the pressure that surrounds you. When a person dives, they use tanks filled with compressed air which results in the diver taking in more than the normal amount of oxygen and nitrogen. Because the body continually uses oxygen, the extra oxygen molecules breathed in under pressure usually do not accumulate, whereas the extra nitrogen molecules build up in the blood and tissues during the dive until the tissue becomes saturated at the ambient pressure. When the pressure decreases, the excess nitrogen is released.

When ascending from a deep dive, the diver ascends at a slow rate to allow the body to adjust to the decrease in pressure allowing the nitrogen to clear from the blood at an acceptable rate. If for any reason the diver ascends from a deep dive too quickly, the nitrogen that can't be immediately exhaled doesn't have time to clear from the blood, instead it separates and forms bubbles in the blood or the tissues. The effect is similar to opening a can or bottle of fizzy drink too soon after shaking it. If nitrogen bubbles form in your blood, they can damage or block blood vessels in any part of the body and block normal blood flow to various organs causing pain and other symptoms that can show anywhere between one and twenty-four hours after the dive. Statistically, 50% of divers develop symptoms within the first hour after a dive and 90% within six hours. However, 98% of divers can develop symptoms within the first twenty-four hours.

Decompression sickness can be divided into two types. Type one which affects the joints in the arms and legs is not life-threatening but may precede more serious problems. The victim may also be bent over as a result of severe abdominal pain if an air bubble obstructs the blood flow in this area, hence the name 'the bends'.

Type two is far more serious as it involves the nervous system. Symptoms will range from mild numbness to paralysis and even death. At the onset, as the spinal cord is also affected, the symptoms may be mild in the form of tingling or weakness in the arms and legs, but in a matter of hours, it will progress to paralysis which is irreversible. Other symptoms caused when nitrogen bubbles affect the brain are headache, double vision, confusion, and speech difficulties which have similarities to stroke symptoms. Vertigo is another legacy of decompression sickness as the nerves are affected in the inner ear.

During an ascent from a deep dive, the recommendation is that the diver should make a safety stop (aka decompression stop) every 5 m and not ascend at a pace of more than 10 m per minute. Even this doesn't guarantee that one will avoid decompression sickness as other factors such as cold, exertion, current, obesity, age, physical condition, and dehydration can all contribute. Repeated dives as opposed to a single dive during a one-day period are likely to cause compression sickness because excess nitrogen can remain dissolved in the body tissues for at least twelve hours. Flying shortly after a deep dive should be avoided as it can also bring about decompression sickness as that person will be exposed to an even lower atmospheric pressure.

Anyone who is thinking of taking up diving as a pastime should have a medical evaluation done, preferably by a doctor who understands or is involved in the sport in order to rule out certain risk factors. Some of these risk factors include congestion of the nose or sinuses, epilepsy, obesity, asthma, emphysema, type 1 diabetes, history of heart problems, history of pneumothorax, history of syncope (fainting), ear problems, any medications that cause drowsiness, pregnancy, old age, and history of alcohol or drug abuse. Proper training and certification goes without saying as does making sure that the equipment you purchase is of a high standard and quality. Unlike riding a bicycle and getting a puncture where you can pull over and fix it without any danger, the same can't be said about equipment failure at 30 or 40 metres, especially if you are new to the sport. Panic can make you do strange things. Check and service your equipment regularly and above all, never dive alone.

Signs and symptoms

Signs may include; blotchy skin, mild to extreme confusion, personality changes and behaviour outside the norm, staggering as if inebriated, weakness in the arms or legs or both, mild to severe paralysis, problems with speech such as slurring or their words, the patient may be seen to double over with abdominal pain, they may find it difficult to urinate even though the bladder is full, the victim may cough up blood tinged frothy sputum or may be semi or fully unconscious.

Symptoms may include; complaining of pains in the joints or muscles or both, fatigue, tingling, numbness or paralysis, complaining of an unusually high level of tiredness, amnesia, dizziness/vertigo, double vision, itchy skin and shortness of breath (dyspnea). However, joint pain, numbness and tingling, muscle weakness and difficulty urinating appear to be the more common complaints.

Treatment for decompression sickness

Treatment for decompression sickness at the scene is rather limited but still effective enough to make a difference. (Ref: CPG Decompression Illness EFR) Oxygen is the key factor and should be given as soon as possible. Mild forms of decompression sickness can resolve without any treatment although administering 100% (15 litres per minute) oxygen will help enormously to minimise any risk. If you suspect that a diver may have decompression sickness, you should alert the emergency services immediately as the patient may deteriorate over time. A helicopter may be dispatched in order to transport the patient quickly to a hospital that has a hyperbaric (recompression) chamber as 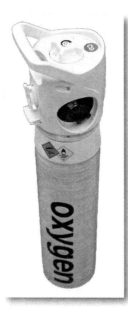 not every hospital has this facility. A history of the dive either from the patient themselves or from their diving buddy should give you a lot of information. For example, how deep was the dive? How long did they stay at that depth? Was it the first dive of that day? How fast did they surface? Did they make a safety stop? Did they go unconscious for any length of time either during or after they surfaced? Did the other diver surface at the same rate? When you are called to a decompression incident, it is possible that the dive buddy may also be suffering from submersion sickness and not be aware of it for the simple reason that symptoms haven't begun to show yet. As a precaution, that diver should also be checked out by a doctor in order to rule it out.

He or she may refuse treatment or advice and they are entitled to do so, but the fact that you showed concern and offered treatment or made a recommendation to seek treatment exonerates you from any liability should anything happen later on. However, in order to substantiate this, you should either get that person to sign the appropriate section in your patient care report (PCR) form to that affect or have a witness sign it alongside your signature.

Early intervention is the key to a successful outcome as delaying treatment may only increase the risk of complications at a later stage. As with any treatment, the patient's airway, breathing, and circulation must be maintained, and it is also essential to ensure that they are at a normal body temperature. When a diver has been in deep water for a while, especially in the winter months, even though they would be suitably dressed, they may still become hypothermic, so it's essential that they are kept warm. Diving in colder than normal conditions is considered a contributing factor to the onset of decompression sickness due to the fact that the body has to work harder to keep warm as it becomes colder. A cold body also loses its efficiency to absorb gas normally. Oxygen should be given at 100% which is 15 litres per minute using a non-rebreather mask. This will help to flush the nitrogen out of the lungs. Monitor the patient's vital signs and make notes on any changes in their condition. Also try to get a medical history. When the patient is being transported, it is essential to transport their diving equipment also so that equipment failure can be ruled out.

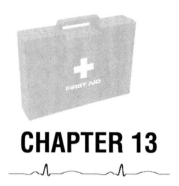

CHAPTER 13

13.1. Causes and Treatment of Hypothermia

Hypothermia occurs when heat is lost faster than the body produces it. It is a potentially life-threatening condition most commonly caused by exposure to cold weather conditions or being immersed in cold water. Paediatrics and the elderly can also suffer the effects as a result of poorly heated accommodation that may only feel mildly cool to others as they have less capacity to self-generate heat. The severity of hypothermia is determined by how low your body temperature drops as a result of exposure. The body has its own built-in temperature regulator or thermostat called the hypothalamus situated at the base of the brain which works constantly to help us to maintain a normal body temperature of around 35.5-37.5°C (95.9-99.5°F).

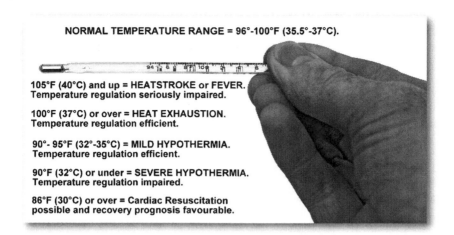

NORMAL TEMPERATURE RANGE = 96°-100°F (35.5°-37°C).

105°F (40°C) and up = HEATSTROKE or FEVER.
Temperature regulation seriously impaired.

100°F (37°C) or over = HEAT EXHAUSTION.
Temperature regulation efficient.

90°- 95°F (32°-35°C) = MILD HYPOTHERMIA.
Temperature regulation efficient.

90°F (32°C) or under = SEVERE HYPOTHERMIA.
Temperature regulation impaired.

86°F (30°C) or over = Cardiac Resuscitation
possible and recovery prognosis favourable.

Medical conditions such as hypoglycaemia, hypothyroidism (aka underactive thyroid), Parkinson's disease, severe arthritis, malnutrition, or fatigue can interfere with the body's ability to combat cold exposure. Alcohol consumption increases the risk of hypothermia through its action as a vasodilator. It increases blood flow to the body's skin and extremities, making a person feel warm, while increasing heat loss. Antidepressants, narcotics, or antipsychotics are only a fraction of drugs that also interfere with the body's ability to generate heat. High humidity, brisk winds, accompanied by rain, sleet, hail, or snow can all magnify the effect of cold exposure on the body by accelerating heat loss from the skin. If a person's body temperature is in the region of 32-35°C (89.6-95°F), they are said to be in mild hypothermia. For simplicity, we will refer to this as stage 1 hypothermia. The symptoms aren't always obvious, but they can include constant shivering, low energy, cold or pale skin, fast breathing (hyperventilation), and the person can appear to be withdrawn.

When a victim reaches stage 2 or moderate hypothermia 27-32°C (80.6-89.6°F), they may shiver uncontrollably in an effort to generate heat, but as the core temperature drops further, shivering may stop altogether. At this stage, you may find that the victim is totally confused, drowsy, and unable to think. They will be unable to make judgments, have difficulty moving, and have little or no co-ordination. Breathing will become slow and shallow, and speech may be slurred. The victims pulse will also slow down. It is not unusual for a victim not to realise they are affected, and in some cases, they will want to remove their clothes. This is known as paradoxical undressing which typically occurs during moderate to severe hypothermia caused either by a malfunction of the hypothalamus or the muscles contracting peripheral blood vessels become exhausted and relax resulting in a surge of blood to the extremities leaving the victim to believe they are overheating.

Severe hypothermia (stage 3) occurs when the body temperature drops to between 27°C and 31°C (80.6-87.8°F). Shivering will have stopped and the victim will be unconscious and appear to look dead. Breathing may be either shallow or undetectable, and pulse will be weak and thready or undetectable and pupils may be dilated. Once the victim's temperature drops below 27°C or 28°C, they may go into cardiac arrest and will have to be resuscitated. It is worth noting that hypothermia can in some cases protect the victim from death.

Understanding heat loss

There are five ways in which we can lose heat from our bodies. Heat loss by conduction occurs when a person comes into direct contact with an object of lower temperature such as cold ground or water. The colder the ground or water, the faster heat will be absorbed. Immersion in water, especially during winter months when there is also a wind chill factor, can bring on severe hypothermia within minutes.

People are surprised when they hear that someone having been rescued from the sea during the hot summer months can also suffer from moderate to severe hypothermia. At the edge of the sea on a beach where the tide flows in and out, because the sand is heated by the sun, when a person stands ankle-high, the water will feel warm. However when we go into much deeper water, the difference in water temperature between the months of winter and summer only varies a few degrees. Therefore when a person gets into difficulty when swimming out of their depth, cramping, tiredness or not being able to swim properly may be the main contributors, but hypothermia will also inter the equation as thermal conductivity of water is over thirty times that of air and the longer the victim is in the water regardless of how warm the surrounding air temperature is, the colder the victim becomes.

Heat is also lost by convection. Our bodies radiate heat that warms the air immediately surrounding our skin. If we do not wear the proper clothing, we can lose this heat by convection to the air outside. In cold weather, windy conditions accelerate the effects of convection as the warm air is literally sucked away from our body. During cold weather conditions, several layers of light clothing are far better than one or two heavy layers.

Radiation is probably the more common way we lose body heat. We are consistently radiating heat from our body into the atmosphere, and the more of our body that is exposed, the more heat we lose. In cold conditions, our head loses heat faster than the rest of our body because we have so many blood vessels close to the surface of the skin. When treating a victim for hypothermia, a simple thing like putting a woollen cap or balaclava on them can make a great difference.

Heat loss by evaporation occurs when water (sweat) evaporates from the skin and as we breathe out during respiration. This is something we cannot control as it is a normal bodily function. We can, however, control it to a certain degree by the use of proper layering of clothes. Respiration is the fifth way we lose body heat as it combines the heat loss mechanisms of evaporation, convection, and radiation when we breathe out as expired air is normally around 36-37°C (96.8-98.6°F) and fully humidified. That hot air is then replaced as we take in the colder air through our mouth and nose. As we continue to breathe, our lungs radiate the colder inspired air over a period of time into our core. Dehydration is always an issue with hypothermia.

Treatment of hypothermia

Mild hypothermia is generally treated aggressively by quickly removing wet clothing and wrapping them in warm dry blankets. Get them into shelter, off the ground away from the elements, and give them warm (not hot) drinks. The victim may complain of thirst as dehydration is always a factor. It's OK to give them water (even cold water) as it won't cause any additional harm to them. Giving a victim a piece of a chocolate bar or small amount of sugar in tea will help to build up their energy level but avoid anything heavily sweetened such as energy drinks. Do not give the victim alcohol. If you have heat packs or warm saline, wrap them in cloth and place them on the neck, under the arms and in the groin area. This will warm the blood that flows through the axillary and iliac arteries. Warm humidified oxygen will help to stabilise the core temperature. Ideally the victim should be heated in the back of a warm ambulance or room.

Treatment of moderate hypothermia is somewhat similar to that of mild hypothermia, although care must be taken to avoid moving the victim suddenly or roughly. The victim may be confused and drowsy and unable to think straight, so reassurance is vital. They will be shivering uncontrollably, and their teeth may chatter leading to a danger that they may bite their tongue accidently. It is important to keep the victim lying down to avoid shock, although, if there is a gradual improvement, and the victim is coherent, allow them to sit up enough to allow them to be able to drink warm fluids. Never allow the victim to attempt to stand up or walk as they are susceptible to hypovolaemia.

If the victim is in cold water and unconscious, they should be removed horizontally to allow the heart to maintain blood flow to the brain. When the body is in water, the water pressure supports it somewhat like a vacuum mattress. When the victim is lifted vertically out of the water, the support is taken away which will cause a dramatic drop in blood pressure causing the victim to go into hypovolemic shock. This happens because the blood that was originally pulled from the peripheries to the core to protect the heart, brain, and other vital organs suddenly drops into the legs and feet, and the heart is too weak to pump it to where it's required most. If, for example, the victim fell from a pier or steep riverbank and there was no other way of removing them from the water other than lifting or dragging them vertically, once you have recovered them, quickly lay them down and raise the legs to allow the blood to flow back to the core. Do not delay in elevating the victims legs.

Severe hypothermia is a priority one medical emergency, and every effort should be made to arrange for ALS to be on scene backed up by rapid transport by an emergency ambulance to a hospital.

At this stage, if shivering has stopped, the victim no longer has the ability to warm up. Although your clinical impression may be such that the victim appears dead, aggressive management may allow successful resuscitation in many instances, and this is the reason for rapid advanced EMS support. Avoid rough handling and keep the victim lying down. Replacing wet clothing with dry blankets will help the warming process, but rapid warming pre-hospital is not advisable as it may prove fatal. Unlike mild hypothermia, with the exception of blankets, heat packs or any form of external heating should be avoided. All that is required is that you prevent the victim from getting any colder.

If the victim has no pulse and isn't breathing, you should start CPR, and if trained to do so, use warm humidified oxygen through a BVM or pocket mask when giving breaths. If oxygen isn't available, the heat from the rescuer's breath (though not as effective) will also help to stabilise the core. It is well documented that severely hypothermic victims who have been apparently dead for several hours have been successfully resuscitated in the hospital setting. In the medical world, if a hypothermic victim is apparently dead, they must be warmed up in order to be officially pronounced dead!

13.2. Frostbite/Frostnip

Frostnip is a mild form of cold injury. Like frostbite, frostnip is associated with ice crystal formation in the tissues. Extreme cold causes the blood vessels of the body to begin to narrow and constrict, reducing blood flow to the extremities, such as ears, the nose, hands and feet. The two conditions are natural survival responses the body makes in order to keep your vital organs from becoming damaged by the cold. With frostnip, little or no damage occurs and rewarming can be done without the need for medical intervention. The person will experience tingling in the affected area until the warming process is initiated. Fingers, for example, can be warmed simply by cupping the hands together and blowing hot air into them or putting them under the armpits. Immersing the hands or feet in warm (not hot) water or applying a warm moist towel to the face is also an effective treatment.

Frostbite is the more serious form of frostnip whereby parts of the body actually freeze. Those that are more commonly affected by this are people who take part in winter sports such as skiing or mountain climbing in snow and icy conditions. The homeless, the elderly who are weakened by age and poor health, and the very young can also be affected. People who have poor circulation or suffer from peripheral vascular disease or vibration-induced white finger can also be affected. Taking certain medications such as beta-blockers also increases the chances of getting frostbite during exposure to severe cold or frosty conditions.

Treatment

First and foremost, as with any other incidents, assess the scene and protect yourself. If you are working in an exposed sub-zero environment, be sure you have the appropriate protection of warm clothing, gloves, and footwear. If a person has been exposed to sub-zero conditions for a long time, first, replace any wet clothing with dry to minimise heat loss and treat them for hypothermia (see Treatment for Hypothermia), and then get them to a warm area. Assess the patient's vital signs (ABC's and AVPU). If they were found to have injuries as a result of trauma, treat those also before addressing frostbite issues. Do not rewarm the skin until you can keep it warm. Warming and then re-exposing the affected area to cold air can cause worse damage. If the patient has been exposed to freezing conditions for an extended period of time, they may have a white waxy appearance and the skin will feel firm to the touch as a result of deep frostbite.

Gently warm the area in warm water or with wet heat until the skin appears pink and warm. *Do not* use direct heat from radiators or fires, and above all, do not rub or massage the skin or break blisters. Give the patient warm drinks, but do not give alcohol as this will have a negative effect. Put gauze or clean cotton balls between fingers or toes to keep them separated and loosely cover them with a roller bandage. Unless it is absolutely necessary, do not allow the patient to walk on frostbitten toes or feet as it may cause further damage. If the patient is suffering from deep frostbite, they should be transported to a hospital where they can be warmed under controlled conditions.

13.3. Heat Exhaustion and Heatstroke

Heat exhaustion is caused by loss of salt and water from the body as a result of excessive sweating which may be due to strenuous physical activity or not being acclimatised to hot humid conditions. Our skin, which is the largest organ in the body, has a big role to play in monitoring temperature control. There are receptors all over the skin that detect any temperature changes and send this information back to the hypothalamus in the brain for processing. The hypothalamus then reacts accordingly by getting rid of excess heat. However, if the system gets overwhelmed, it malfunctions.

Heat exhaustion can occur when exposed to temperatures greater than 26°C (78.8°F), but typically, when the core temperature rises to between 37.5°C (99.5°F) and 40°C (104°F), a person will have already developed visible signs and symptoms of heat exhaustion with excessive diaphoresis (sweating) sometimes being the obvious sign. The victim may feel dizzy and sick and may be inclined to vomit. They may also feel confused and tired. They may develop a weak and rapid pulse and cramping may occur in the legs, arms, or abdomen. Their skin will be pale and clammy. If the victim passes urine, the colour will be much darker than normal, but they may also have little or no inclination to urinate due to peripheral shutdown. As you can see, these signs and symptoms are similar to the early signs of shock; therefore, you should treat the patient in much the same way. The most vulnerable age groups to develop complications from dehydration are young children and the elderly and should receive medical treatment sooner rather than later.

Because of the loss of fluids, the body becomes dehydrated and is unable to sweat; therefore, normal temperature cannot be maintained. As we discussed earlier, when dealing with hypothermia on how easily the body loses heat, we have the opposite problem with heat exhaustion and heatstroke. High ambient temperatures greatly reduce the body's ability to cool itself by radiation, and likewise, high humidity reduces the body's ability to lose heat by evaporation, so the heat is trapped within the body and cannot escape.

Sixty per cent of our bodyweight is made up by water, and the average daily fluid intake that we need to perform properly is around 4 pints (2.5 litres). A little less than half of our fluid intake is obtained from solid foods that we ingest, while the balance is made up of tea or coffee, milk, various juices, water, and other liquids. The body always has a need for fluids, and water should be drunk before, during, and after activities. Never wait until you feel thirsty because once this happens, you are already well on the road to being dehydrated.

Apart from the very young and the elderly, there are other factors that increase the risk of developing heat exhaustion and heatstroke in all ages. These factors include alcohol, pregnancy, obesity, hypertension, respiratory disease, being dehydrated, and anyone that may have a chronic illness or disability. Fair-skinned people are easily burnt by the sun and can easily succumb to heatstroke. In countries such as Ireland and the United Kingdom where our climate can be described as maritime-influenced, mild and humid, with average summer temperatures varying between 14°C and 20°C (57.2-68°F) with 25°C to 27°C or 28°C (77-82.4°F) being exceptional, care must be taken during hot weather to drink plenty fluids and protect the skin. Wearing a hat to protect the head is very important as is not allowing young children's skin become exposed to the hot sun. Sunblock is very important, and although it helps to prevent sunburn, it doesn't prevent heat exhaustion or heatstroke. Certain kinds of medication such as tranquillizers, antihistamines, beta-blockers, and antipsychotics can also interfere with the body's ability to cool itself.

Illicit drugs such as Ecstasy or methylenedioxymethamphetamine (MDMA) to give it its official title can cause heatstroke and occasionally death from the effect it has on the system as it alters the way the body regulates its internal temperature. Combined with the heat of a warm environment and hours of dancing, Ecstasy can cause the body to overheat and suffer severe dehydration in a very short time. While you may think that fluids are the answer, in this case, it can add to the problem as a side-effect of Ecstasy is fluid retention. It is thought that the drug can affect the workings of the kidneys, leading to fluids being retained in the body. If the brain cells absorb too much water, this can lead to respiratory shutdown and death.

For a first-aider or responder who happens upon a person suffering the ill effects of Ecstasy, calling EMS, providing fresh air by moving the victim to cooler safer environment, and attempting to cool the patient until help arrives is as much as you can do.

Heatstroke is defined typically as hyperthermia exceeding 41°C (105.8°F) and is classed as a life-threatening condition. When our body temperature rises above 104°F (40°C), the body systems that regulate the temperature become overwhelmed, and as a result, the body produces more heat than it can release. Heatstroke sometimes referred to as sunstroke occurs when a person is exposed to a hot environment for a long time. If treatment isn't initiated quickly, the body temperature will continue to rise resulting in brain damage or death. The patient's pulse rate will be fast (tachycardia) and up to 130 beats per minute is not uncommon. Symptoms of central nervous system dysfunction will be present and may range from irritability to coma.

The patient may be delirious or go into convulsions or have hallucinations. They may also present with ataxia (lack of muscle coordination). They may also suffer from dysarthria by which the muscles of the mouth, face, and respiratory system become weak resulting in slurred slow speech which may be difficult to understand. Drooling and poor swallowing ability are also an issue. Limited jaw and tongue movement are also part of dysarthria. Although the symptoms of dysarthria are collectively the signs of stroke, they are also a sign of brain damage as a result of heatstroke. The patient may be limp or may show signs of decerebrate posturing, which involves the arms and legs being held straight out, the toes being pointed downward, with the head and neck being arched backwards due to the muscles being tightened and held rigidly. They may also exhibit decorticate posturing in which a person is stiff with bent arms, clenched fists, and legs held straight out. The arms are bent in toward the body, and the wrists and fingers are bent and held on the chest. These collective signs of posturing are also what one might see if the patient was having an epileptic seizure. Pupils can range from pinpoint to normal depending on the extent of cerebellar damage. Muscle tenderness and cramping are common. Acute renal failure (ARF) is a common complication of heatstroke and may be due to hypovolaemia and low cardiac output.

Treatment

Sweating and peripheral vasodilation are major mechanisms of heat loss to maintain proper temperature. Sweat cools the body through evaporation, and peripheral vasodilation provides the blood flow and heat necessary to evaporate the sweat. When this combination fails, the body can't get rid of heat; therefore, it builds up.

As with any patient contact, check that the scene is safe before approaching! Introduce yourself and try to obtain a history of the event. Try to obtain the following information: how long the patient was exposed to the heat? If they are on the beach, where they wearing clothing or sunbathing, were they taking part in physical exercise or sport, were they involved in manual labour, and was any alcohol consumed? Establish that ABCs are intact and take a radial pulse check. While you are doing all this, you should do a visual check at the same time. Getting answers to these questions along with your visual assessment is important in reaching the right diagnosis and helping you to establish what level your victim is at. If the patient is too weak or confused to talk, you may have to depend on bystander information. Get the patient out of the heat and under cover from the sun as soon as possible. A cool room with a draught would be ideal.

Normal temperature taken under the tongue or under the armpit is generally between 36°C and 37.5°C (96.8-99.5°F), and this is a good place to start. People who suffer from heat exhaustion are generally conscious but weak. Generally, when a person in suffering heat exhaustion, one of the more prominent signs is diaphoresis (sweating). However, this may not always be the case as some people have an inability to sweat normally. This is known as Anhidrosis.

Based on the signs and symptoms discussed earlier, once you have established that the person is suffering from heat exhaustion, you can initiate treatment. Lay the patient down on a blanket and elevate their legs (shock position) to allow blood to flow back to the heart and the brain. If they feel better sitting up, that's OK too (patient prerogative). Give them plenty of fluids to drink, but encourage them to drink slowly as it has a better rehydration effect. Isotonic drinks (sports drinks) are excellent for this purpose as they contain similar concentrations of salt and sugar as in the human body. You should continue to monitor the vital signs (ABC's and AVPU) while allowing the patient to recover slowly. Oxygen may be given if breathing is weak, and you are trained to give it, as it will help to clear any trace of hypoxia and help recovery. If the patient recovers within a reasonable time with no ill effects, they will not want and may insist on no further medical intervention. However, it would be advisable for you to suggest that they visit their doctor or medical centre should they feel the need to at a later stage.

Heatstroke, however, requires a more aggressive approach, and EMS must be called as part of your standard operating procedure (SOP). Heatstroke is common in countries with hot climates, but it isn't something we deal with often in countries like Ireland and the UK because of our more moderate weather climate. However, when we do get a sudden burst of heat or a prolonged spell of fine weather, some people can cope better than others, and for those who can't cope for whatever reason and go on to develop heatstroke, it's always good to know what to do.

Reducing the core body temperature is the cornerstone of the treatment because the duration of hyperthermia is the primary determinant of outcome. If temperature reduction treatment is aggressive enough to rapidly reduce the core temperature to an acceptable level within what we call 'the golden hour', there is every chance that complications such as multisystem organ failure can be averted and a more positive outcome can be achieved for the patient. According to the American College of Sports Medicine, the current recommendation is to initiate cooling immediately on scene before transfer to hospital. The goal is to rapidly bring the temperature down to around 38°C or 39°C (100.4-102.2°F). Once this is achieved, further reduction of temperature can be done at a much slower rate and preferably in a hospital setting in order to avoid hypothermia and the patient going into shock.

There are a number of ways in which a responder can cool a victim. First, as with heat exhaustion, get the patient out of the heat and into someplace cool. Remove as much clothing as possible while still preserving their modesty. It is highly unlikely that a first-aider or responder will have enough cold packs or thereafter a continuous backup supply to provide the treatment required, so you will have to improvise. And that's what first aid is all about, thinking outside the box! If there is a garden hose available or indeed if the fire service is involved, the patient should be put lying down and water from the hose should be poured continuously over the patient's torso. If there is a sheet or large towel available, the cooling effect would be even better for the patient because by wrapping them in it and then pouring cold water over them, the fabric will saturate and the cooling process will be more concentrated. If no hose is available, you could continuously pour jugs of water from the kitchen sink or bucket over the sheet or towel. Alternatively, if there is no sheet or towel available, you should ask someone to fan the patient with a newspaper or whatever is available. It is also important to cool the head. This can be done by using a wet sponge or facecloth which can also be used on the body in the absence of sheets or towels. The cooling process will take time, but it is important to monitor their temperature regularly along with their vital signs (ABCs and AVPU). If the patient responds to the treatment and the temperature drops to a near normal level, replace the wet sheet or towel with a dry blanket to avoid them getting cold and continue to monitor until the ambulance arrives. If the temperature rises again, replace the dry blanket with the wet sheet or towel and repeat the process until it drops again.

13.4. Triage Sieve

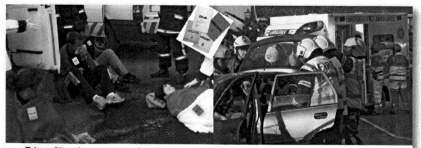

Triage Sieve is a process of sorting casualties according to priority using a colour coded tagging system which gives other agencies on arrival initial information at a glance so that serious and life-threatening injuries are addressed without delay.

Triage is derived from the French word trier, meaning 'to sort or sieve'. In medicine, this refers to the process of sorting patients according to priority and to establish an order for treatment and evacuation. Originally developed for the armed forces for rapid assessment of casualties on the battlefield, the exact same method is used by emergency services throughout the world whenever an incident occurs whereby the number of casualties exceeds the resources available to deal with the event. The aim of triage sieve is to give the right patient the right care at the right time in the right place. Triage is also an ongoing dynamic process as the condition of each patient can change at any time.

Although CPGs say you should be at a practitioner level such as EMT, paramedic, or advanced paramedic in order to understand and execute triage effectively, I believe the responder can play a vital part also, especially if you as a responder happen to be first on the scene of an incident where multiple casualties are involved and help is a while away. Anyone who is at EFR level has acquired a good knowledge of skills and would make a great difference in relation to relaying information to EMS and the treatment skills they could offer casualties. Keeping within their CPGs, the EFR can make the difference between life and death in these situations and can seamlessly integrate and be a great asset to EMS. For this reason, I will try to explain the system so that it is easily understood should the situation ever arise.

Triage is divided into four main categories, and what makes it work is the speed in which triage sieve is carried out. The system that allows us to do this is called the START system. This simply means Simple Triage and Rapid Treatment whereby the maximum time allotted to access each casualty initially is sixty seconds or less. The assessment is based on three primary observations: breathing, circulation, and level of consciousness (BCLOC). Using these three key points, the responder can identify the most serious patient and tag them in order of priority (Ref: CPGs Triage Sieve EMT).

Before you do anything, you must consider a number of things into account as you approach the scene. The first and most important thing is scene safety. Read the scene carefully and rule in or out whatever dangers do or do not exist. This is an out of the ordinary event, and there will be a lot to take in. Things may not be visually pleasant, and there may well be a lot of screaming and calling for help, but under such circumstances, you should try to make a conscious effort to control your emotions and do the best you can.

The information you are looking for in order to bring the appropriate amount of resources should be gathered quickly. For example, was the event caused by a road traffic collision, a collapsed building, a gas explosion, house fire, or whatever? How many casualties are there, and are there children involved? Are there hazards such as oil or fuel spillage, fallen power lines, trees, fire or flooding, or unstable vehicles or buildings? What type of assistance (fire, ambulance, coastguard, or police) is required? And most importantly, give the location of the incident. Ultimately, the number of casualties will determine the level of the emergency. If, for example, there were two cars involved with four or five casualties in total, it would be well within the resources of EMS, but if it was a bus with forty or fifty people on board, it would be classed as a major emergency and extra resources would have to be drafted in from other locations. Make the call (999/112) and try to be calm and deliver your message clearly, and then when the operator asks you to hang up, you can start to triage the casualties.

EMS carry sets of Triage cards which are colour-coded in order of priority. There are only four cards per set which usually have a long elastic string attached so that you can put the appropriate card on each casualty. Priority 1 is a red card. This means the patient's injuries are life-threatening and must be treated and/or transported immediately. Priority 2 would be a yellow card meaning the patient requires urgent treatment but a delay of up to one hour would be acceptable as the injuries would be classed as serious but not life-threatening. Priority 3 would be a green card meaning that the patient has only minor injuries and all vital signs are within normal boundaries. Priority 4 is a white card although in some countries it may be grey or black. This means the patient is dead and requires no treatment.

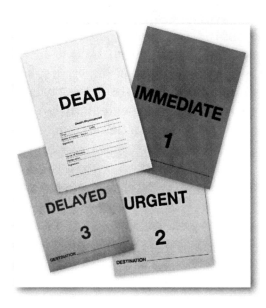

If you don't have triage cards, improvise. Insulation tape that electricians use is very cheap and comes in a variety of colours and takes up very little room in a first-aid kit. You won't have any difficulty getting the four colours you want in any electrical or hardware store. When triaging, simply wrap the appropriate coloured tape loosely around the patient's wrist a few times, preferably not on the skin in case of a reaction to the adhesive, but on the outer sleeve of whatever they are wearing.

Let's say, for example, you are the first to arrive on the scene of a mini-bus with fifteen people on board having overturned after the driver lost control trying to avoid a stray horse on the road. As a result, the bus has ended up on its side near the bottom of a 50-foot embankment after hitting a tree. The bus was doing about 60 mph when it left the road, and there is a lot of material damage. When you get there, you see several people outside the bus, some walking around, some sitting nearby, and others inside the bus. There is a lot of crying and screaming going on and the scene is pretty overwhelming.

This is the point where you take a deep breath and read the scene from a distance for any immediate danger to yourself or any knock-on effects that may occur as a result of the accident before getting involved. At a glance, you see seven people outside the bus and one has come to you asking for you to call for help. You introduce yourself as a first-aider or responder and reassure him you are going to help, but first you want to gather enough information in order to bring the appropriate resources. The man tells you that there are fifteen people including the driver, but some of them are trapped and aren't moving. He also goes on to tell you how the accident happened. Now you have an accurate number of casualties and you have already done a visual examination of the scene. This is when you call for help (999/112). When you get through to the operator, try to be calm, give your name and location and a description of the accident including any dangers or hazards.

The key points to get across are that there are fifteen confirmed casualties, some walking wounded and others trapped inside with possible serious injuries, so multiple ambulances are required. Persons trapped suggest Fire and Rescue are required and police are also required to deal with traffic management and to investigate the incident. It is also important to mention the stray horse as it may be injured and require a vet. If you have a smartphone that you can get GPS coordinates of your location from that would be of great benefit and would insure that resources can find you quickly, especially if it was dark and the incident wasn't immediately visible from the road. Now that help is on the way, you can begin to triage.

The simplest way to start any triage is to ask in a loud voice, 'Can anybody walk?' and if so, get those who can walk to move away from the danger area to a pre-determined safe zone and insist that they stay there. Anyone who is alert and can get up and walk generally isn't considered to have life-threatening injuries and would be classed as walking wounded. They may have a closed fracture to an upper limb or cuts and bruises, but these type of injuries in a triage situation aren't considered life-threatening. Don't force anyone who is having difficulty getting to their feet or complains of pain. They may have injuries to their back or lower limbs. Leave them where they are, but if they tick all the boxes of having no life-threatening injuries, tag them as priority 3 (green tag or tape) and move on. In some instances where triage is necessary, the majority of casualties may only be walking wounded, and once these are out of the equation, your job is made easier. Now you can concentrate on the remaining and more serious casualties. Remember, one minute or less with each one, no more. Another thing to keep in mind is that the casualty who is shouting and screaming is in a far better place than the casualty that is quiet and saying nothing. So a patient shouting can be ticked off as alert, has a patent airway, and is definitely breathing, whereas the silent patient must be taken seriously and given closer examination.

Let's say you have now established that the seven outside the bus are walking wounded and have been moved away from the crash site and given a green tag. Now it remains for you to sieve through the others and prioritise them according to your findings. You have established that the bus is safe to enter and there is no possibility of it moving any further down the bank and there is no fear of fire and the engine isn't running. You are able to gain access through the back window, and starting with the first person you see, check their breathing, circulation and level of consciousness (BCLOC). If their breathing rate is greater than 29 BPM, it is one of the primary signs of shock, so you should tag that individual as priority 1 (red card) and swiftly move on. As you assess the second casualty, you find that their breathing is below 30 BPM. Quickly move on to check LOC and circulation by trying to communicate with them and checking a carotid pulse for five to ten seconds. If the casualty is not breathing, check the mouth for any obstruction. If there is any obstruction such as vomit, quickly clear it away and open the airway with a head tilt, chin lift. If the patient starts to breathe, tag them with a red card and move on. If they make no effort to breathe, tag them as a priority 4 (white card). However, if you are unsure, tag them with a red card but move on quickly to the next casualty. During a triage, there isn't time to check for spinal injuries, so we tend to ignore the guidelines and use the life over limb rule and open the airway in the normal way. If you decide to do a trauma jaw thrust on a victim you suspect has spinal issues during triage, you can't possibly help the others; therefore, never attempt it and move on to your next patient.

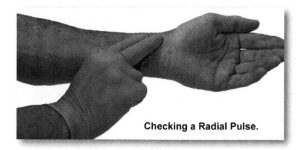
Checking a Radial Pulse.

If the pulse is weak or irregular, elevate their legs to treat for shock and to allow blood to flow back to the heart, lungs, and brain. If the person is bleeding heavily, try to control it. Get the casualty to apply pressure or use one of the walking wounded (green card) to do it. They will be more than willing to help if asked. Tag that casualty priority 1 (red card), and let the green card casualty with them to control the bleeding. Once again to make a point, don't spend time trying to control bleeding yourself because you still have more casualties to evaluate. Again, if there is no pulse, treat them as dead (white card) and move on.

The next casualty is trapped but breathing adequately and has a strong pulse but appears groggy and you know from the grimace on his face that he is in pain. Ask him to open his eyes or ask him his name or day of the week or ask him to squeeze your hand. If he can respond to your voice and understand you without difficulty, it means that on the AVPU scale, he is alert and should be tagged as priority 2 (yellow card). If that patient couldn't understand or follow your commands, give him a red card and move on again. As you move up along the bus, you find three more casualties in similar circumstances, and on quick examination, you tag them as priority 2. Finally, you come to the driver who has sustained obvious fatal injuries due to the impact with the tree. Just to be sure you conduct your BCLOC evaluation and confirm that he is dead. If possible, cover him to avoid causing more stress to the other casualties and then give him a priority 4 tag (white tag).

Now that you have completed your triage sieve, you might find time to focus on the red card casualties, but remember that triage is an ongoing assessment and those who were stable a minute ago may become unstable at any time. Even a walking wounded casualty can deteriorate. It is always advisable to recheck all the red and yellow priorities while keeping an eye of the green priorities as well. Remember, this is something even paramedics don't come across regularly; in fact, it is quite a rare event, but it can and does happen. All you can do is your best until help arrives.

The following is a list to help you understand the triage sieve tag system:

A casualty should be given a red card (priority 1) if

1. The respiratory rate is greater than 29 or less than 10 BPM.
2. The airway was compromised for any period of time due to FBOA.
3. Capillary refill is more than three seconds.
4. The pulse rate is greater than 120.
5. There is any uncontrollable or severe haemorrhage.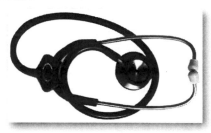
6. There are any abdominal or open chest wounds.
7. There are any severe burns.
8. There are any cardiac or severe medical complications.
9. There are signs of shock.

Yellow cards (priority 2) are given to casualties whose injuries are potentially life-threatening but stable at present due to on-scene treatment or nature of injury; however, to prevent deterioration, they must be transported if possible within an hour of the incident. Other injuries such as multiple fractures, open fractures, head injuries without complications, or mild to moderate burns also fall under this category of serious but not immediately life-threatening. However, patients with these types of injuries have the potential to become unstable if shock sets in and may have to be re-categorised to a red card.

Green cards (priority 3) are given to what we refer to as walking wounded. These casualties are classed as low priority and have no symptomatic or visual life-threatening injuries or ailments. If they can walk and are fully coherent and have only superficial cuts and abrasions, they get a green card. Sometimes, a casualty with multiple minor cuts can look as if they are bleeding heavily after been taken from an accident scene mainly because blood has been smudged (possibly from another casualty) all over their clothes or from rubbing a blooded hand to their face, but if they are walking and talking, tag them green and move on. If a casualty has a fracture to an upper limb, if it's not complicated (open fracture), and if they can walk and talk, sit them down and show them how to support the injured limb with their other hand, tell them someone will attend to them as soon as possible, give them a green tag, and move on.

White or black cards (priority 4) are given to a casualty who has no signs of life or have visual injuries that are not compatible with life such as decapitation, incineration, etc. If a carotid pulse is not palpable or breathing is absent after opening the airway, then that casualty is classed as dead and should, if possible, be covered with whatever is available and given a white card.

Having read all this section, you will see that your approach to a triage sieve situation has to be cold without letting anything distract you. Even if you are dealing with a young frightened person in a lot of pain that you feel you should stay an extra minute to comfort them, that's a minute you could have given to someone else. Triage is about allocating no more than sixty seconds of your time to each casualty regardless of how bad their injuries are. Separating the walking wounded from the more serious only lightens the load, but they also need attention at some stage but not immediately. Once you have taken them away from danger, insist they stay there for their own safety, but also mention that you may need a hand if necessary to help another casualty later on. You will find that some will be more than willing to help, but again, insist they stay away until required. Once everyone is accounted for and tagged, you can then re-triage and concentrate on the worst cases until help arrives.

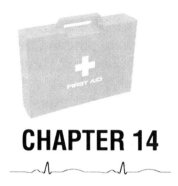

CHAPTER 14

14.1. Oxygen Therapy

(Part I) Administration Guidelines for the Responder

Oxygen (O2) is a colourless, odourless, tasteless gas necessary to sustain life. It is classed as medication and should only be administrated by those who are trained to do so. Although it comes in various sizes, the more popular cylinder for the medical practitioner or emergency medical responder is the CD bottle because it has a built-in regulator, contains 460 litres, and weighs only 3.5 kg (approx. 7.7 lbs). Presently, the clinical levels in the pre-hospital field authorised to administer O2 are cardiac first responder-advanced, (CFR-A), emergency first responder (EFR), emergency medical technician (EMT), and paramedic (P) and advanced paramedic (AP).

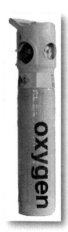

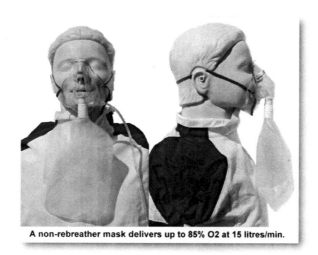

A non-rebreather mask delivers up to 85% O2 at 15 litres/min.

Oxygen is delivered by non-rebreather mask, simple facemask, nasal cannulae (nasal prongs), or venturi mask which is connected by tube to the cylinder. Care must be taken that the tubing doesn't become kinked or ports aren't obstructed and that all delivery systems are fitted correctly so as not to affect the concentrations. A simple facemask when fitted correctly delivers up to 40% O2, and a non-rebreather mask will deliver up to 85% at 15 litres per minute of O2. The venturi mask has six different sized, colour-coded valves to deliver fixed concentrations of between 24% and 60%. The nasal cannula or nasal prongs as they are also known as can deliver concentrations of between 24% and 40% at flow rates of between 1-6 litres per minute. However, with nasal prongs, flow rates in excess of 4 litres per minute may cause discomfort and drying of mucous membranes and should be avoided. Nasal cannulae are often used as a compromise with patients who feel claustrophobic and cannot tolerate a regular mask.

Who gets oxygen?

Oxygen is always given to anyone having difficulty breathing if it's available, and you are trained to give it.

Oxygen should be considered if

1. An adult is breathing fewer than 12 BPM or more than 20 BPM.
2. A child is breathing less than 15 BPM or more than 30 BPM.
3. An infant is breathing less than 25 BPM or more than 50 BPM.

How much oxygen should be given?

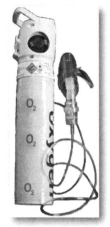

There is nothing to be gained by giving too much oxygen and a huge amount to be lost by not giving enough. You give as much oxygen as is required to return the partial pressure of oxygen (PaO2) in the blood to what is normal for that particular patient. An SPO2 monitor is required to check O2 levels. SPO2 stands for saturation of peripheral oxygen.

You should only administer oxygen if you are trained to give it. The present indications for administrating oxygen (O2) are absent or inadequate ventilations following an acute medical or traumatic event. You should give oxygen if the levels are <94% in adults and <96% in paediatrics. For patients with acute exacerbation of COPD, you should give oxygen if their O2 levels are below 92%. If you have a pulse oximeter, you should use it and titrate O2 to achieve an SpO2 level of between 94% and 98%. For paediatrics, you should titrate between 96% and 98%. For patients with acute exacerbation of COPD, you should titrate to achieve an SpO2 level of 94% or whatever is specified on their COPD Oxygen Alert Card. If a COPD patient has suffered an acute medical or traumatic event, titrate the patient's O2 to achieve SpO2 level of 94-98%. Note:; Prolonged use of O2 on chronic COPD patients may lead to reduction in ventilation stimulus. When the oxygen levels reach their target on your monitor, oxygen should be removed until levels drop again.

For an adult in cardiac or respiratory arrest or other life threats identified during primary survey, give 100% oxygen until a reliable SpO2 measurement is obtained and then titrate the O2 to achieve SpO2 of 94-98%. For paediatric cardiac or respiratory arrest or other life threats identified during primary survey, give 100% oxygen until a reliable SpO2 measurement is obtained and then titrate the O2 to achieve SpO2 of 96-98%. For all other acute medical or traumatic events, O2 should be titrated to achieve SpO2 of 96-98%.

A pulse oximeter is a device intended for the non-invasive measurement of arterial blood oxygen saturation and pulse rate. An oximeter detects hypoxia before the patient becomes clinically cyanosed. When arterial oxyhaemoglobin saturation is measured non-invasively by pulse oximetry, it is called SpO2. Before giving oxygen, it is now advised to use a pulse oximeter to ascertain the O2 level beforehand in order to titrate the amount of oxygen being given to the patient. Pulse Oximeter's may not be 100% accurate. It is recognised that they may register as much as 2% above or below the actual level in the patient. To compensate for this, the practitioner will look for a reading of 98% on the oximeter. This will ensure the patient's O2 level is within an excepted level of between 96% and 100%. Paediatric and COPD patients are also titrated in accordance with their guidelines. Oxygen saturation is affected by breathing rate and depth, lung function, and heart function.

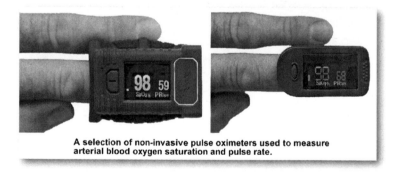

A selection of non-invasive pulse oximeters used to measure arterial blood oxygen saturation and pulse rate.

Note: If you do not have a pulse oximeter, you should give oxygen anyway until one becomes available. Do not deprive the patient.

14.2. Oxygen Therapy (Part II)

for Patients in the Hospital and in the Home

Oxygen therapy is a treatment that provides you with extra oxygen, a gas that your body needs to work well. Normally, your lungs absorb oxygen from the air. However, some diseases and conditions can prevent you from getting enough oxygen. Oxygen therapy may help you function better and be more active. For those in need of oxygen therapy for a chronic (ongoing) disease or condition, this therapy can be carried out in a hospital or any medical facility or even at home.

Oxygen is supplied in metal or carbon fibre hoop-wrapped aluminium cylinders or other containers. It flows through a tube and is delivered to your lungs in one of the following ways;

1. Through a nasal cannula, which consists of two small plastic tubes, or prongs, that are placed in both nostrils.
2. Through a face mask, which fits over your nose and mouth.
3. Through a small tube inserted into your windpipe through the front of your neck. A needle or small incision (cut) is used to place the tube. Oxygen delivered this way is called transtracheal oxygen therapy.

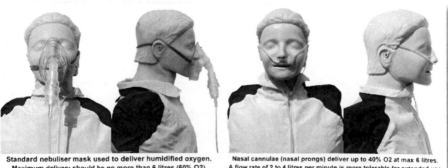

Standard nebuliser mask used to deliver humidified oxygen. Maximum delivery should be no more than 6 litres (60% O2).

Nasal cannulae (nasal prongs) deliver up to 40% O2 at max 6 litres. A flow rate of 2 to 4 litres per minute is more tolerable for extended use.

Overview

To learn how oxygen therapy works, it helps to understand how the respiratory system works. This system is a group of organs and tissues that help you breathe. The respiratory system includes the airways and lungs. The airways carry oxygen-rich air to your lungs and also carry carbon dioxide (a waste gas) out of the lungs.

Air enters your body through your nose or mouth, which moistens and warms the air. The air then travels through your larynx (voice box) and down your trachea (windpipe). The trachea divides into two tubes called bronchi that enter your lungs.

Within your lungs, your bronchi branch into thousands of smaller, thinner tubes called bronchioles. These tubes end in bunches of tiny round air sacs called alveoli. Each of the air sacs is covered in a mesh of tiny blood vessels called capillaries. The capillaries connect to a network of arteries and veins that move blood throughout your body. When air reaches the air sacs, the oxygen in the air passes through the air sac walls into the blood in the capillaries. The oxygen-rich blood then travels to the heart through the pulmonary vein and its branches. The heart then pumps the oxygen-rich blood to your organs. Certain acute (short-term) and chronic (ongoing) diseases and conditions can affect the transfer of oxygen from the alveoli into the blood. Examples include pneumonia and COPD.

A decision is made whether you need oxygen therapy based on the results of tests, such as an arterial blood gas test and a pulse oximetry test. These tests measure how much oxygen is in your blood. A low oxygen level is a sign that you need oxygen therapy. Oxygen is considered a medicine, so your doctor must prescribe it.

Outlook

Oxygen therapy helps many people function better and be more active. It also may help to decrease shortness of breath and fatigue (tiredness), improve sleep in some people who have sleep-related breathing disorders, and increase the lifespan of some people who have COPD.

Although the patient may need oxygen therapy long term, it doesn't have to limit their daily routine. Portable oxygen units can make it easier for a patient to move around and do many daily activities. Oxygen therapy is generally safe, but it can pose a fire hazard. Oxygen supports combustion and must be kept away from any type of naked flame or spark.

Who needs oxygen therapy?

The doctor may recommend oxygen therapy if a patient has a low blood oxygen level. Normally, the lungs absorb oxygen from the air and transfer it into the bloodstream. Some acute (short-term) and chronic (ongoing) diseases and conditions can prevent the patient from getting enough oxygen.

Acute diseases and conditions

A patient may receive oxygen therapy if they are in hospital for a serious condition that prevents them from getting enough oxygen. Once they have recovered from the condition, the oxygen therapy will almost certainly be stopped.

Some diseases and conditions that may require short-term oxygen therapy are;

1. Severe pneumonia. Pneumonia is an infection in one or both of the lungs. If severe, the infection causes the air sacs in the lungs to become very inflamed. This prevents the air sacs from moving enough oxygen into your blood.

2. Severe asthma attack. Asthma is a lung disease that inflames and narrows the airways. Most people who have asthma, including many children, can safely manage their

symptoms. But if you have a severe asthma attack, you may need hospital care that includes oxygen therapy.

3. Respiratory distress syndrome (RDS) or bronchopulmonary dysplasia (BPD) in premature babies. Premature babies may develop one or both of these serious lung conditions. As part of their treatment, they may receive extra oxygen through a nasal continuous positive airway pressure (NCPAP) machine or a ventilator (VEN-til-a-tor) or through a tube in the nose.

Chronic diseases and conditions

Long-term home oxygen therapy might be used to treat some diseases and conditions, such as;

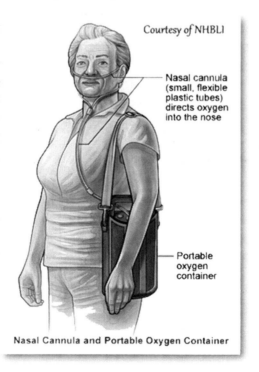

Courtesy of NHBLI

Nasal cannula (small, flexible plastic tubes) directs oxygen into the nose

Portable oxygen container

Nasal Cannula and Portable Oxygen Container

1. COPD. This is a progressive disease in which damage to the air sacs prevents them from moving enough oxygen

into the bloodstream. 'Progressive' means the disease gets worse over time.

2. Late-stage heart failure. This is a condition in which the heart can't pump enough oxygen-rich blood to meet the body's needs.

3. Cystic Fibrosis. CF is an inherited disease of the secretory glands, including the glands that make mucus and sweat. People who have CF have thick, sticky mucus that collects in their airways. The mucus makes it easy for bacteria to grow. This leads to repeated, serious lung infections. Over time, these infections can severely damage the lungs.

4. Sleep-related breathing disorders that lead to low levels of oxygen in the blood during sleep, such as sleep apnea. Sleep apnea (AP-ne-ah) is a common disorder in which you have one or more pauses in breathing or shallow breaths while you sleep. Breathing pauses can last from a few seconds to minutes. They may occur 30 times or more an hour. Typically, normal breathing then starts again, sometimes with a loud snort or choking sound.

How does oxygen therapy work?

Oxygen therapy provides you with extra oxygen, a gas that your body needs to work well. Oxygen comes in different forms and can be delivered to your lungs in several ways. Oxygen therapy can sometimes be referred to as simply oxygen or supplemental oxygen.

Oxygen therapy systems

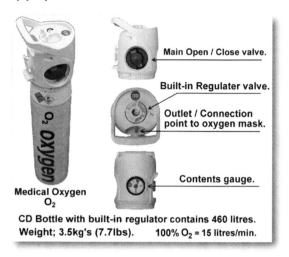

Main Open / Close valve.

Built-in Regulater valve.

Outlet / Connection point to oxygen mask.

Contents gauge.

Medical Oxygen
O₂

CD Bottle with built-in regulator contains 460 litres.
Weight; 3.5kg's (7.7lbs).   100% O₂ = 15 litres/min.

Oxygen is supplied in three forms: as compressed gas, as liquid, or as a concentrated form taken from the air. Compressed oxygen gas is stored under pressure in metal cylinders. The cylinders come in many sizes. Some of the cylinders are small enough to carry around. You can put one on a small wheeled cart or in a shoulder bag or backpack. Liquid oxygen is very cold. When released from its container, the liquid becomes gas. Liquid oxygen is delivered to your home in a large container. From this container, smaller, portable units can be filled. The advantage of liquid oxygen is that the storage units need less space than compressed or concentrated oxygen. However, liquid oxygen costs more than the other forms of oxygen. Also, it evaporates easily, so it doesn't last for a long time.

Oxygen concentrators filter out other gases in the air and store only oxygen. Oxygen concentrators come in several sizes, including portable units. Oxygen concentrators cost less than the other oxygen therapy systems. One reason is that they don't require oxygen refills. However, oxygen concentrators are powered by electricity. Thus, you'll need a backup supply of oxygen in case of a power outage.

Delivery devices

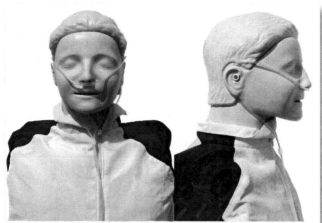

Nasal cannulae (nasal prongs) deliver up to 40% O2 at max 6 litres. A flow rate of 2 to 4 litres per minute is more tolerable for extended use.

Most often, oxygen is given through a nasal cannula. A nasal cannula consists of two small plastic tubes, or prongs, that are placed in both nostrils. To help hold the cannula in place, the patient puts the longer ends of it over their ears. The tubing then comes around the back of the ears and under the chin, where it joins together. From there, it's attached to the tube from the oxygen container. The image shown in the section on chronic diseases and conditions shows how a nasal cannula and portable oxygen container are attached to a patient.

A face mask may be used instead of a nasal cannula. The mask fits over the mouth and nose. This method is mainly used if the patient needs a high flow rate of oxygen or if the nose is clogged from a cold. The face mask is held in place with a strap that goes around your head or with tubes that fit around your ears. The oxygen is delivered through a tube that attaches to the front of the mask.

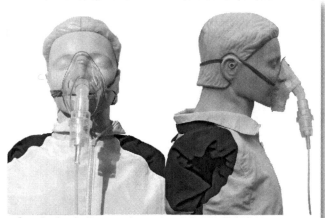

**Standard nebuliser mask used to deliver humidified oxygen.
Maximum delivery should be no more than 6 litres (60% O2).**

Oxygen can also be delivered through a small tube inserted into the windpipe through the front of the neck. A doctor will use a needle or small incision (cut) to place the tube. Oxygen delivered this way is called transtracheal oxygen therapy. If a patient is getting transtracheal oxygen therapy, they will need to have a humidifier attached to the oxygen system. This is because the oxygen doesn't pass through the nose or mouth like it does with the other delivery systems. A humidifier adds moisture to the oxygen and prevents the patient's airways from getting too dry.

Oxygen also can be delivered through machines that support breathing, such as continuous positive airway pressure (CPAP) devices or ventilators. CPAP is a treatment that uses mild air pressure to keep the airways open. CPAP typically is used by people who have breathing problems, such as sleep apnea. CPAP also may be used to treat preterm infants whose lungs have not fully developed. For example, doctors may use CPAP to treat infants who have respiratory distress syndrome or bronchopulmonary dysplasia.

What to expect before oxygen therapy?

During an emergency such as a serious accident, possible heart attack, or other life-threatening event, you might be started on oxygen therapy right away. Otherwise, your doctor will decide whether you need oxygen therapy based on test results. An arterial blood gas test and a pulse oximetry test can measure the amount of oxygen in your blood. For an arterial blood gas test, a small needle is inserted into an artery, usually in your wrist. A sample of blood is taken from the artery. The sample is then sent to a laboratory, where its oxygen level is measured.

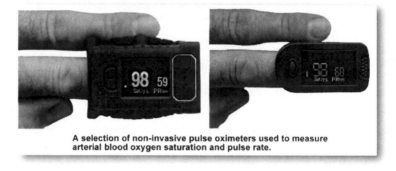

A selection of non-invasive pulse oximeters used to measure arterial blood oxygen saturation and pulse rate.

For a pulse oximetry test, a small sensor is attached to your fingertip or toe. The sensor uses light to estimate how much oxygen is in your blood. If the tests show that your blood oxygen level is low, your doctor may prescribe oxygen therapy. In the prescription, your doctor will include the number of litres of oxygen per minute that you need (oxygen flow rate). He or she also will include how often you need to use the oxygen (frequency of use). Frequency of use includes when and for how long you should use the oxygen. Depending on your condition and blood oxygen level, you may need oxygen only at certain times, such as during sleep or while exercising. If your doctor prescribes home oxygen therapy, he or she can help you find a home equipment provider. The provider will give you the equipment and other supplies you need.

What to expect during oxygen therapy?

Following a medical or traumatic event oxygen therapy is given right away. While you're in the hospital, your doctor will check on you to make sure you're getting the right amount of oxygen. Nurses or respiratory therapists also may assist with the oxygen therapy. If you're having oxygen therapy at home, a home equipment provider will help you set up the oxygen therapy equipment at your house. Trained staff will show you how to use and take care of the equipment. They'll supply the oxygen and teach you how to safely handle it. Because oxygen poses a fire risk, you'll need to take certain safety steps. Oxygen isn't explosive, but it can worsen a fire. In the presence of oxygen, a small fire can quickly get out of control. Also, the cylinder that contains compressed oxygen gas can explode if it's exposed to heat. Your home equipment provider will give you a complete list of safety steps that you'll need to follow at home and in public. For example, while on oxygen, you should never smoke or be around people who are smoking, never use paint thinners, cleaning fluids, gasoline, aerosol sprays, and other flammable materials, and stay at least 5 ft away from gas stoves, candles, and other heat sources.

What are the risks of oxygen therapy?

Oxygen therapy can cause complications and side effects. These problems might include a dry or bloody nose, skin irritation from the nasal cannula or face mask, fatigue (tiredness), and morning headaches. If these problems persist, tell your doctor and home equipment provider. Depending on the problem, your doctor may need to change your oxygen flow rate or the length of time you're using the oxygen. If nose dryness is a problem, your doctor may recommend a nasal spray or have a humidifier added to your oxygen equipment. If you have an uncomfortable nasal cannula or face mask, your home equipment provider can help you find a device that fits better. Your provider also can recommend over-the-counter gels and devices that are designed to lessen skin irritation. Complications from transtracheal oxygen therapy can be more serious. With this type of oxygen therapy, oxygen is delivered through a tube inserted into your windpipe through the front of your neck.

With transtracheal oxygen therapy, mucus balls might develop on the tube inside the windpipe. Mucus balls tend to form as a result of the oxygen drying out the airways. Mucus balls can cause coughing and clog the windpipe or tube. Problems can develop with the tube slipping or breaking. Infection and injury to the lining of the windpipe are also risks associated with transtracheal oxygen therapy. Proper medical care and correct handling of the tube and other supplies may reduce the risk of complications.

Other risks

Oxygen poses a fire risk, so you'll need to take certain safety steps. Oxygen itself isn't explosive, but it can support combustion. In the presence of oxygen, a small fire can quickly get out of control. Also, the cylinder that contains compressed oxygen gas might explode if exposed to heat. Your home equipment provider will give you a complete list of safety steps you'll need to take at home and when out in public. For example, when you're not using the oxygen, keep it in an airy room. Never store compressed oxygen gas cylinders and liquid oxygen containers in small, enclosed places, such as in closets, behind curtains, or under clothes. Oxygen containers let off small amounts of oxygen. These small amounts can build up to harmful levels if they're allowed to escape into small spaces.

Living with oxygen therapy

Portable oxygen units can make it easier for you to travel. If you need oxygen while travelling, plan in advance. If you are travelling on an aircraft, contact the airline company to find out if they can facilitate you. Also, talk with your doctor and home equipment provider if you are planning to travel. They can help you plan for your oxygen needs and fill out any required medical forms.

Ongoing care

To make sure you're getting the full benefits of oxygen therapy, visit your doctor regularly. Your doctor can check your progress and adjust your oxygen therapy as needed. Never change the amount of oxygen you're taking or adjust the flow rate of your oxygen on your own. Discuss any problems or side effects with your doctor first. He or she may recommend adjusting your treatment.

Talk with your doctor about when you should contact him or her in an emergency. Your doctor can advise you about what to do if you have increased shortness of breath, wheezing, or other changes from your usual breathing such as fever, increased mucus production, or other symptoms of an infection. If your lips or fingernails show a blue tint, this is a sign that your body isn't getting enough oxygen. If you become confused, restless, or more anxious than usual, do not hesitate to call your doctor. They are only too happy to help you. During an emergency, you should go to your nearest hospital emergency department or call 999/112. You might want to wear a medical ID bracelet or necklace to alert others to your medical needs.

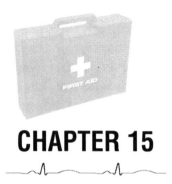

CHAPTER 15

PHECC and CPGs

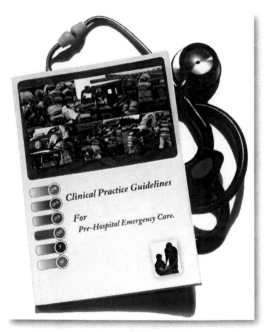

I am sincerely grateful to the Pre-Hospital Emergency Care Council of Ireland for granting me permission to use their Clinical Practice Guidelines (CPGs), and I am sure the algorithms provided will help you to clearly understand the step-by-step actions required in the assessment and treatment of a casualty.

PHECC is an independent statutory body formed in the year 2000. Based in Naas, County Kildare, Ireland, PHECC is responsible for implementing, monitoring, and further developing the standards of care provided by all statutory, private, and voluntary ambulances in Ireland. It is also responsible for conducting examinations at six levels of pre-hospital care and the control of ambulance practitioner registration.

The six levels are divided into two categories which are responder and practitioner level. The responder level consists of CFR, OFA, and EFR. The practitioner levels consist of EMT, paramedic (P), and Advanced Paramedic (AP). PHECC are also responsible for the publication of CPGs.

CPGs are based on the most current scientific research available for the treatment of the sick and injured in the pre-hospital environment. As new evidence becomes available, guidelines are updated and a new edition of CPGs is made available both in the physical book form and pdf format for downloading. The edition used in this book is the third edition version 2 which at the time of going to print is still current. However, the latest version is available on the PHECC website www.phecc.ie. This means that for years to come, as new information on pre-hospital care becomes available, you will be able to keep yourself updated simply by logging in. This is both good for you as a responder as you will always have access to current guidelines, and for the patient as the recipient of good quality care.

To paraphrase a paragraph of the CPG's handbook, the information provided within the CPG's handbook is not intended as a substitute for good clinical judgement. It is merely guidance toward best practice. In frontline emergency response, because of unusual patient presentations, it isn't possible to develop a CPG to match every situation. In this case, common sense should prevail, and only after your patient assessment and clinical impression should you decide what CPG (if any) is appropriate. Remember, you must work within your scope of practice in the best interest of the patient, not forgetting that you can always ask a fellow responder or EMS for advice in unusual circumstances.

The following algorithms explain clearly the role of the responder when other clinical levels are involved and medical interventions have been implemented prior to the arrival of the responder.'

CPGs presume that no medication has been administered or any interventions have been applied prior to the arrival of the responder or first-aider. Should another responder or practitioner administer medication or carry out other interventions during an acute episode, you should be aware of these interventions and act accordingly. When working alongside other responders or practitioners, the duty of care is shared, and each responder or practitioner is responsible for their own actions. It goes without saying that the most experienced or more qualified responder or practitioner takes over the role of clinical leader, and in the interest of the patient and also to avoid confusion, a detailed handover is essential.

15.2. CPG Algorithms

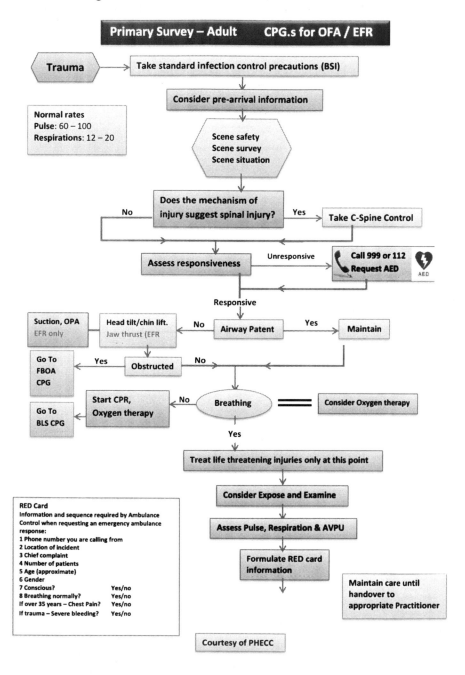

Primary Survey – Adult   CPG.s for OFA / EFR

Trauma → Take standard infection control precautions (BSI)

Consider pre-arrival information

Normal rates
Pulse: 60 – 100
Respirations: 12 – 20

Scene safety
Scene survey
Scene situation

Does the mechanism of injury suggest spinal injury? — No / Yes → Take C-Spine Control

Assess responsiveness — Unresponsive → Call 999 or 112 Request AED (AED)

Responsive

Airway Patent — No / Yes → Maintain

Suction, OPA EFR only

Head tilt/chin lift. Jaw thrust (EFR

Obstructed — Yes → Go To FBOA CPG / No

Breathing — No → Start CPR, Oxygen therapy → Go To BLS CPG / Yes

Consider Oxygen therapy

Treat life threatening injuries only at this point

Consider Expose and Examine

Assess Pulse, Respiration & AVPU

Formulate RED card information

Maintain care until handover to appropriate Practitioner

RED Card
Information and sequence required by Ambulance
Control when requesting an emergency ambulance
response:
1 Phone number you are calling from
2 Location of incident
3 Chief complaint
4 Number of patients
5 Age (approximate)
6 Gender
7 Conscious?   Yes/no
8 Breathing normally?   Yes/no
If over 35 years – Chest Pain? Yes/no
If trauma – Severe bleeding?   Yes/no

Courtesy of PHECC

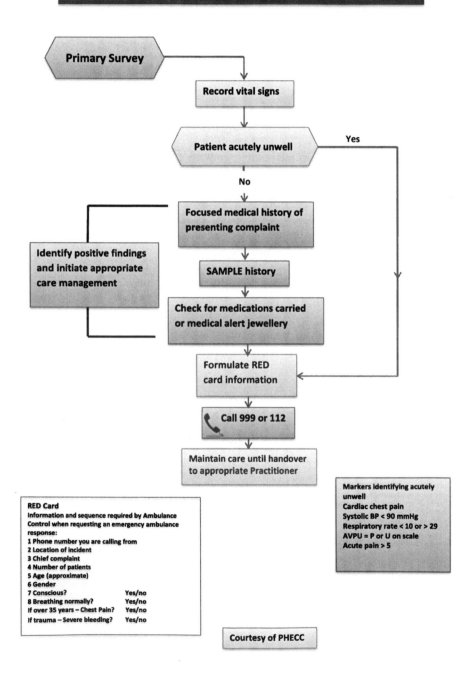

Secondary Survey Medical – Adult   CPG.s for OFA / EFR

Primary Survey

Record vital signs

Patient acutely unwell   Yes

No

Focused medical history of presenting complaint

Identify positive findings and initiate appropriate care management

SAMPLE history

Check for medications carried or medical alert jewellery

Formulate RED card information

Call 999 or 112

Maintain care until handover to appropriate Practitioner

Markers identifying acutely unwell
Cardiac chest pain
Systolic BP < 90 mmHg
Respiratory rate < 10 or > 29
AVPU = P or U on scale
Acute pain > 5

RED Card
Information and sequence required by Ambulance Control when requesting an emergency ambulance response:
1 Phone number you are calling from
2 Location of incident
3 Chief complaint
4 Number of patients
5 Age (approximate)
6 Gender
7 Conscious?   Yes/no
8 Breathing normally?   Yes/no
If over 35 years – Chest Pain?   Yes/no
If trauma – Severe bleeding?   Yes/no

Courtesy of PHECC

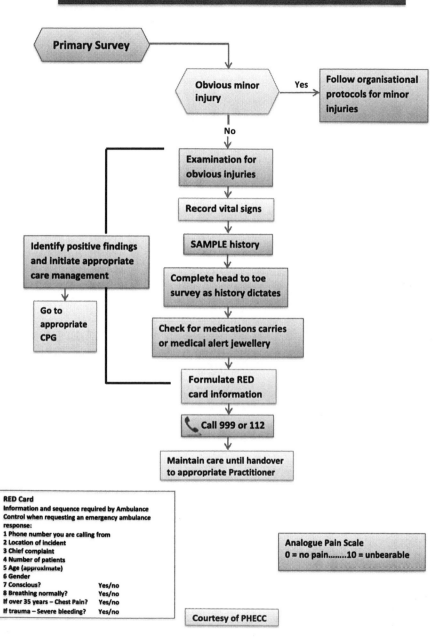

Secondary Survey Trauma – Adult   CPG.s for OFA / EFR

Primary Survey

Obvious minor injury

Yes → Follow organisational protocols for minor injuries

No ↓

Examination for obvious injuries

Record vital signs

SAMPLE history

Complete head to toe survey as history dictates

Check for medications carries or medical alert jewellery

Identify positive findings and initiate appropriate care management

Go to appropriate CPG

Formulate RED card information

Call 999 or 112

Maintain care until handover to appropriate Practitioner

RED Card
Information and sequence required by Ambulance Control when requesting an emergency ambulance response:
1 Phone number you are calling from
2 Location of incident
3 Chief complaint
4 Number of patients
5 Age (approximate)
6 Gender
7 Conscious?   Yes/no
8 Breathing normally?   Yes/no
If over 35 years – Chest Pain? Yes/no
If trauma – Severe bleeding?   Yes/no

Analogue Pain Scale
0 = no pain........10 = unbearable

Courtesy of PHECC

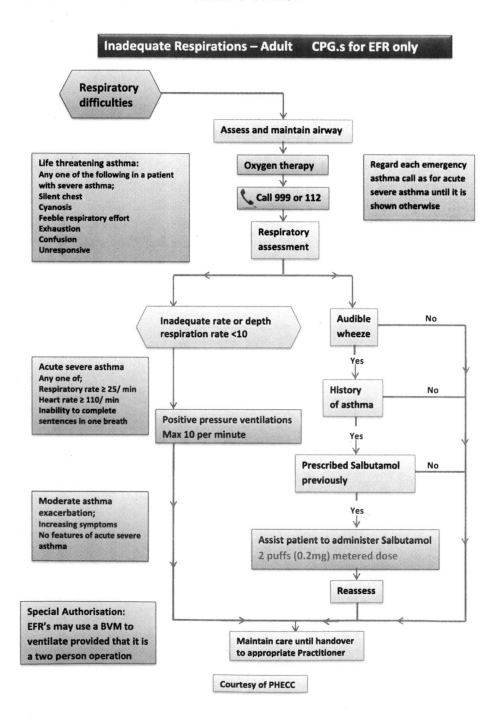

Inadequate Respirations – Adult   CPG.s for EFR only

Respiratory difficulties

Assess and maintain airway

Oxygen therapy

📞 Call 999 or 112

Respiratory assessment

Life threatening asthma:
Any one of the following in a patient with severe asthma;
Silent chest
Cyanosis
Feeble respiratory effort
Exhaustion
Confusion
Unresponsive

Regard each emergency asthma call as for acute severe asthma until it is shown otherwise

Inadequate rate or depth respiration rate <10

Audible wheeze — No

Yes

History of asthma — No

Yes

Acute severe asthma
Any one of;
Respiratory rate ≥ 25/ min
Heart rate ≥ 110/ min
Inability to complete sentences in one breath

Positive pressure ventilations
Max 10 per minute

Prescribed Salbutamol previously — No

Yes

Moderate asthma exacerbation;
Increasing symptoms
No features of acute severe asthma

Assist patient to administer Salbutamol
2 puffs (0.2mg) metered dose

Reassess

Special Authorisation:
EFR's may use a BVM to ventilate provided that it is a two person operation

Maintain care until handover to appropriate Practitioner

Courtesy of PHECC

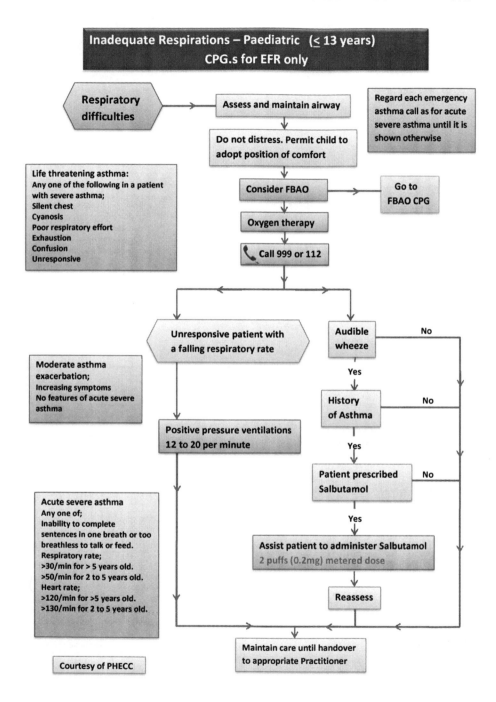

Inadequate Respirations – Paediatric (≤ 13 years)
CPG.s for EFR only

Respiratory difficulties

Assess and maintain airway

Regard each emergency asthma call as for acute severe asthma until it is shown otherwise

Do not distress. Permit child to adopt position of comfort

Consider FBAO → Go to FBAO CPG

Oxygen therapy

Call 999 or 112

Life threatening asthma:
Any one of the following in a patient with severe asthma;
Silent chest
Cyanosis
Poor respiratory effort
Exhaustion
Confusion
Unresponsive

Unresponsive patient with a falling respiratory rate

Audible wheeze — No

Moderate asthma exacerbation;
Increasing symptoms
No features of acute severe asthma

Yes

History of Asthma — No

Positive pressure ventilations 12 to 20 per minute

Yes

Patient prescribed Salbutamol — No

Acute severe asthma
Any one of;
Inability to complete sentences in one breath or too breathless to talk or feed.
Respiratory rate;
>30/min for > 5 years old.
>50/min for 2 to 5 years old.
Heart rate;
>120/min for >5 years old.
>130/min for 2 to 5 years old.

Yes

Assist patient to administer Salbutamol
2 puffs (0.2mg) metered dose

Reassess

Maintain care until handover to appropriate Practitioner

Courtesy of PHECC

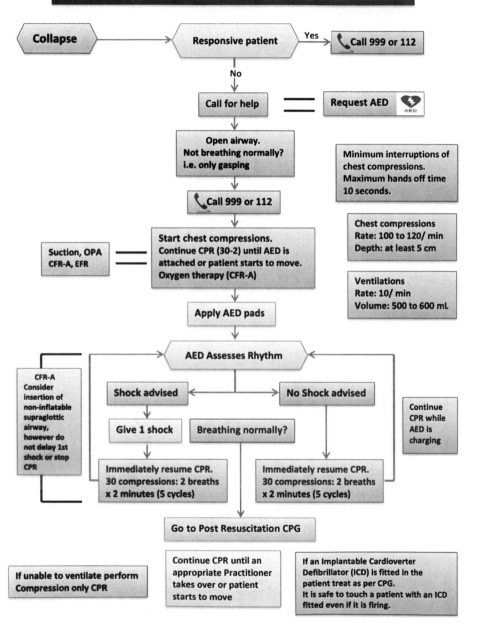

Basic Life Support – Adult   CPG.s for CFR, OFA & EFR

Collapse → **Responsive patient** — Yes → 📞 **Call 999 or 112**

No

Call for help ══ **Request AED** 🔺

**Open airway.
Not breathing normally?
i.e. only gasping**

Minimum interruptions of
chest compressions.
Maximum hands off time
10 seconds.

📞 **Call 999 or 112**

Suction, OPA
CFR-A, EFR ══ **Start chest compressions.
Continue CPR (30-2) until AED is
attached or patient starts to move.
Oxygen therapy (CFR-A)**

Chest compressions
Rate: 100 to 120/ min
Depth: at least 5 cm

Ventilations
Rate: 10/ min
Volume: 500 to 600 mL

Apply AED pads

AED Assesses Rhythm

CFR-A
Consider
insertion of
non-inflatable
supraglottic
airway,
however do
not delay 1st
shock or stop
CPR

Shock advised ← → **No Shock advised**

Continue
CPR while
AED is
charging

Give 1 shock   **Breathing normally?**

**Immediately resume CPR.
30 compressions: 2 breaths
x 2 minutes (5 cycles)**

**Immediately resume CPR.
30 compressions: 2 breaths
x 2 minutes (5 cycles)**

Go to Post Resuscitation CPG

If unable to ventilate perform
Compression only CPR

Continue CPR until an
appropriate Practitioner
takes over or patient
starts to move

If an Implantable Cardioverter
Defibrillator (ICD) is fitted in the
patient treat as per CPG.
It is safe to touch a patient with an ICD
fitted even if it is firing.

Courtesy of PHECC

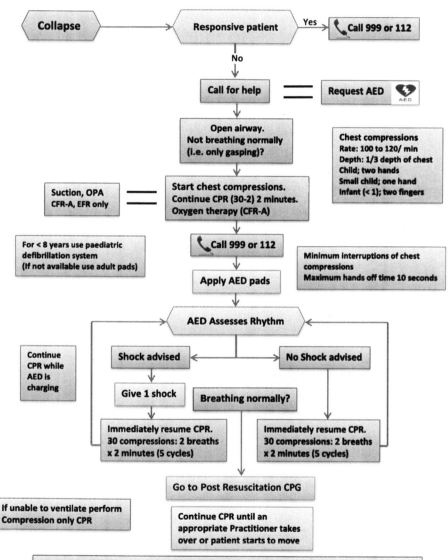

Basic Life Support – Paediatric (≤ 13 Years)   CPG.s for CFR, OFA & EFR

Collapse → **Responsive patient** —Yes→ 📞 **Call 999 or 112**

No ↓

Call for help —— **Request AED** 🔋 AED

↓

Open airway.
Not breathing normally
(i.e. only gasping)?

Chest compressions
Rate: 100 to 120/ min
Depth: 1/3 depth of chest
Child; two hands
Small child; one hand
Infant (< 1); two fingers

Suction, OPA
CFR-A, EFR only —— **Start chest compressions.**
Continue CPR (30-2) 2 minutes.
Oxygen therapy (CFR-A)

↓

For < 8 years use paediatric
defibrillation system
(If not available use adult pads)

📞 **Call 999 or 112**

Minimum interruptions of chest
compressions
Maximum hands off time 10 seconds

Apply AED pads

AED Assesses Rhythm

Continue
CPR while
AED is
charging

Shock advised ← → **No Shock advised**

↓

Give 1 shock   **Breathing normally?**

Immediately resume CPR.
30 compressions: 2 breaths
x 2 minutes (5 cycles)

Immediately resume CPR.
30 compressions: 2 breaths
x 2 minutes (5 cycles)

Go to Post Resuscitation CPG

If unable to ventilate perform
Compression only CPR

Continue CPR until an
appropriate Practitioner takes
over or patient starts to move

Infant AED
It is extremely unlikely to ever have to defibrillate a child less than 1 year old. Nevertheless, if this were to occur the approach would be the same as for a child over the age of 1. The only likely difference being, the need to place the defibrillation pads anterior (front) and posterior (back), because of the infant's small size.

Courtesy of PHECC

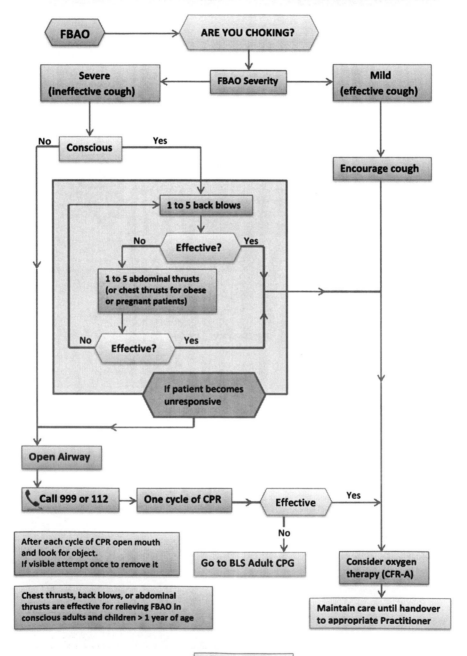

Foreign Body Airway Obstruction – Adult   CPG.s for CFR, OFA & EFR

FBAO → ARE YOU CHOKING?

FBAO Severity

Severe (ineffective cough) ← FBAO Severity → Mild (effective cough)

Severe (ineffective cough) → Conscious

No / Yes — Conscious

Mild (effective cough) → Encourage cough

1 to 5 back blows

Effective? — No / Yes

1 to 5 abdominal thrusts (or chest thrusts for obese or pregnant patients)

Effective? — No / Yes

If patient becomes unresponsive

Open Airway

Call 999 or 112 → One cycle of CPR → Effective — Yes

Effective — No → Go to BLS Adult CPG

After each cycle of CPR open mouth and look for object.
If visible attempt once to remove it

Chest thrusts, back blows, or abdominal thrusts are effective for relieving FBAO in conscious adults and children > 1 year of age

Consider oxygen therapy (CFR-A)

Maintain care until handover to appropriate Practitioner

Courtesy of PHECC

Foreign Body Airway Obstruction – Paediatric (≤ 13 years) CPG.s for CFR, OFA & EFR

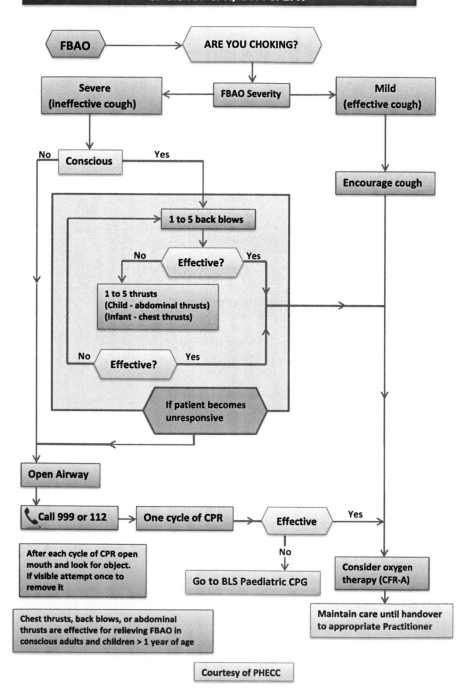

Courtesy of PHECC

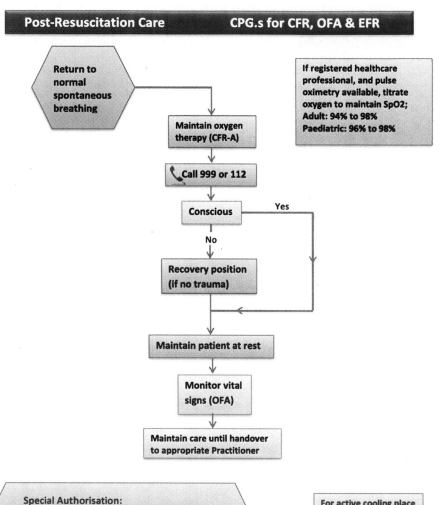

Post-Resuscitation Care   **CPG.s for CFR, OFA & EFR**

Return to normal spontaneous breathing

Maintain oxygen therapy (CFR-A)

If registered healthcare professional, and pulse oximetry available, titrate oxygen to maintain SpO2; Adult: 94% to 98% Paediatric: 96% to 98%

Call 999 or 112

Conscious — Yes

No

Recovery position (if no trauma)

Maintain patient at rest

Monitor vital signs (OFA)

Maintain care until handover to appropriate Practitioner

Special Authorisation: CFR-As, linked to EMS, may be authorised to actively cool unresponsive patients following return of spontaneous circulation (ROSC)

For active cooling place cold packs in arm pits, groin & abdomen

Courtesy of PHECC

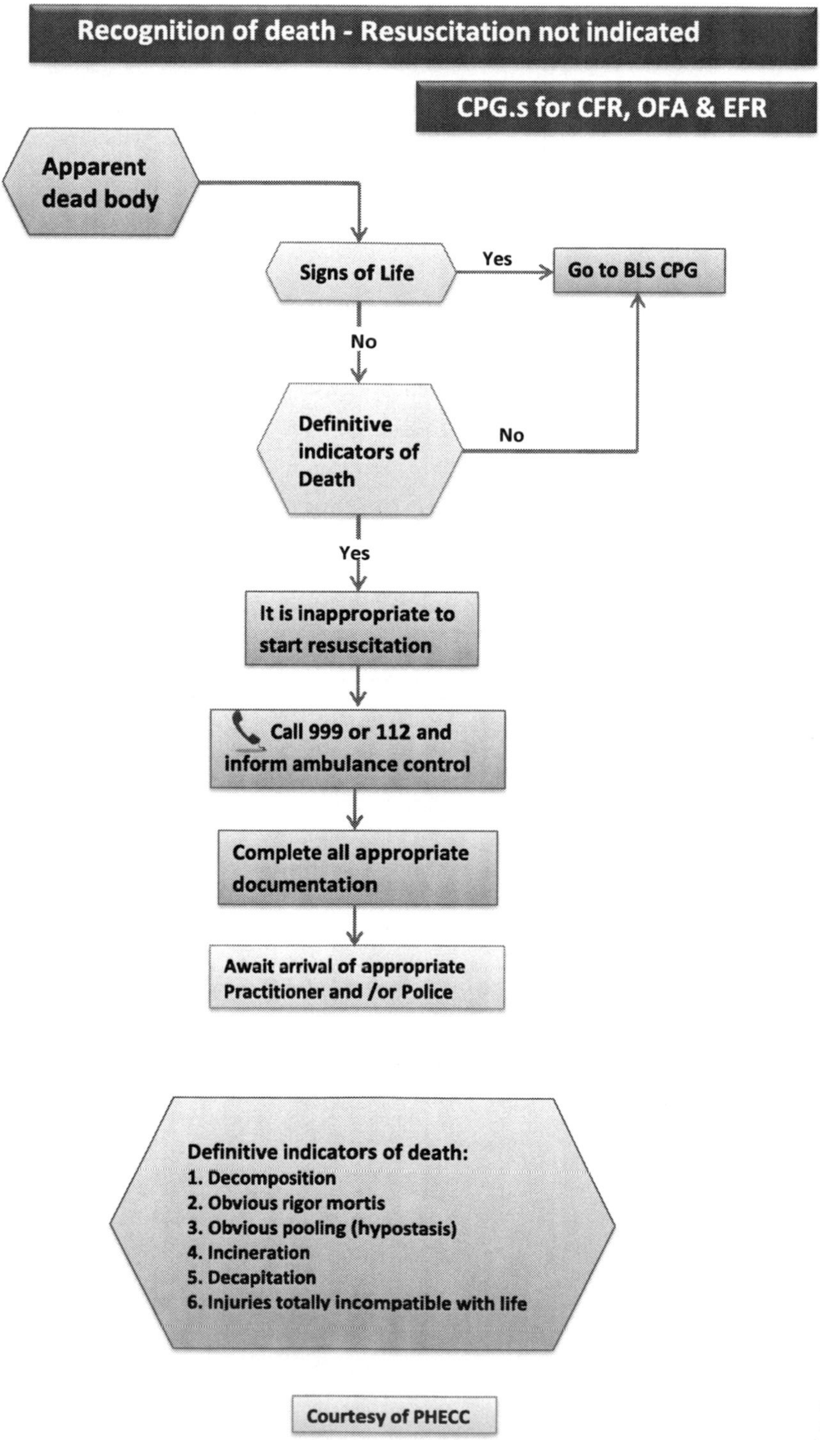

Recognition of death - Resuscitation not indicated

CPG.s for CFR, OFA & EFR

Apparent dead body

↓

Signs of Life —— Yes —→ **Go to BLS CPG**

No ↓

Definitive indicators of Death —— No ——→ (to Go to BLS CPG)

Yes ↓

It is inappropriate to start resuscitation

↓

📞 **Call 999 or 112 and inform ambulance control**

↓

Complete all appropriate documentation

↓

Await arrival of appropriate Practitioner and /or Police

Definitive indicators of death:
1. Decomposition
2. Obvious rigor mortis
3. Obvious pooling (hypostasis)
4. Incineration
5. Decapitation
6. Injuries totally incompatible with life

Courtesy of PHECC

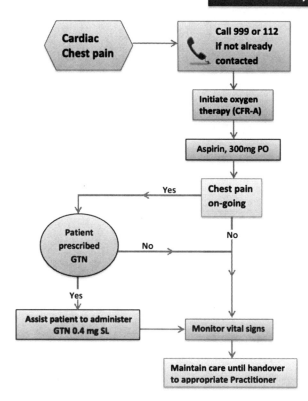

Cardiac Chest Pain – Acute Coronary Syndrome

CPG.s for CFR, OFA & EFR

Cardiac Chest pain → Call 999 or 112 if not already contacted

↓

Initiate oxygen therapy (CFR-A)

↓

Aspirin, 300mg PO

↓

Chest pain on-going

— Yes → Patient prescribed GTN

No ↓

Patient prescribed GTN — No →

Yes ↓

Assist patient to administer GTN 0.4 mg SL → Monitor vital signs

↓

Maintain care until handover to appropriate Practitioner

If registered healthcare professional, and pulse oximetry available, titrate oxygen to maintain SpO2;
Adult: 94% to 98%

Courtesy of PHECC

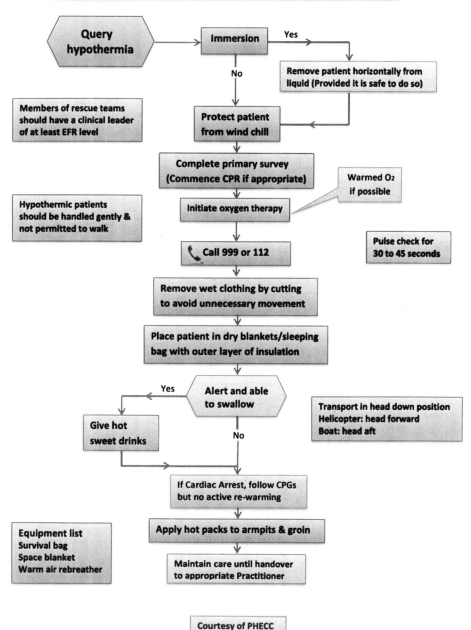

Courtesy of PHECC

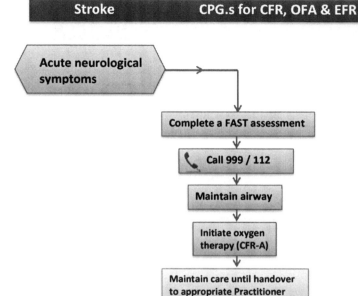

Stroke	CPG.s for CFR, OFA & EFR

Acute neurological symptoms

Complete a FAST assessment

Call 999 / 112

Maintain airway

Initiate oxygen therapy (CFR-A)

Maintain care until handover to appropriate Practitioner

If registered healthcare professional, and pulse oximetry available, titrate oxygen to maintain SpO2; Adult: 94% to 98%

F – Facial weakness
   Can the patient smile? Has their mouth or eye drooped? Which side?
A – Arm weakness
   Can the patient raise both arms and maintain for 5 seconds?
S – Speech problems
   Can the patient speak clearly and understand what you say?
T – Time
   Time to call 999/112 now if positive FAST

Courtesy of PHECC

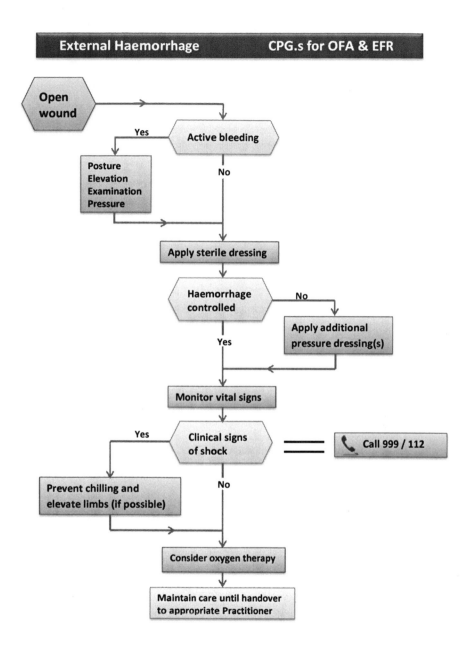

External Haemorrhage   CPG.s for OFA & EFR

Open wound

Active bleeding

Yes

Posture
Elevation
Examination
Pressure

No

Apply sterile dressing

Haemorrhage controlled

No

Apply additional pressure dressing(s)

Yes

Monitor vital signs

Clinical signs of shock

Yes

Call 999 / 112

Prevent chilling and elevate limbs (if possible)

No

Consider oxygen therapy

Maintain care until handover to appropriate Practitioner

Courtesy of PHECC

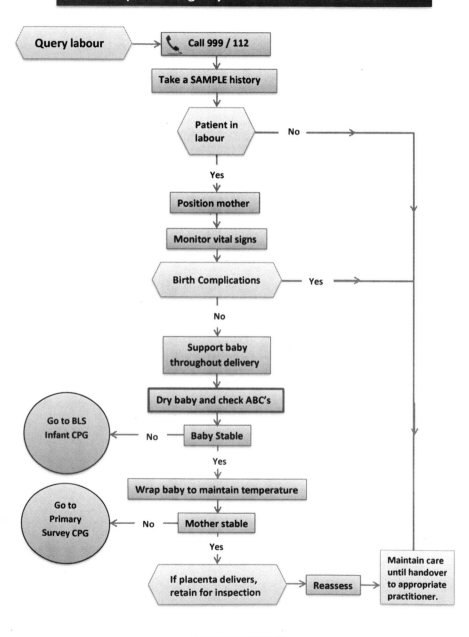

Pre-Hospital Emergency Childbirth   CPG.s for EFR

Query labour → 📞 Call 999 / 112

Take a SAMPLE history

Patient in labour — No →

Yes ↓

Position mother

Monitor vital signs

Birth Complications — Yes →

No ↓

Support baby throughout delivery

Dry baby and check ABC's

Go to BLS Infant CPG ← No — Baby Stable

Yes ↓

Wrap baby to maintain temperature

Go to Primary Survey CPG ← No — Mother stable

Yes ↓

If placenta delivers, retain for inspection → Reassess → Maintain care until handover to appropriate practitioner.

Courtesy of PHECC

Glycaemic Emergency - Adult   CPG.s for OFA & EFR

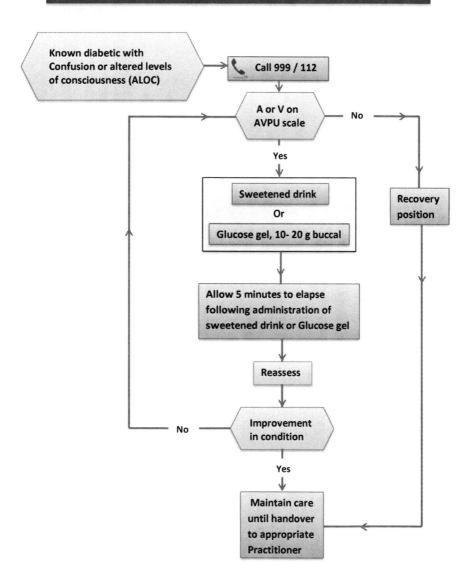

Known diabetic with Confusion or altered levels of consciousness (ALOC)

📞 Call 999 / 112

A or V on AVPU scale

No → Recovery position

Yes

Sweetened drink

Or

Glucose gel, 10- 20 g buccal

Allow 5 minutes to elapse following administration of sweetened drink or Glucose gel

Reassess

Improvement in condition

No

Yes

Maintain care until handover to appropriate Practitioner

Courtesy of PHECC

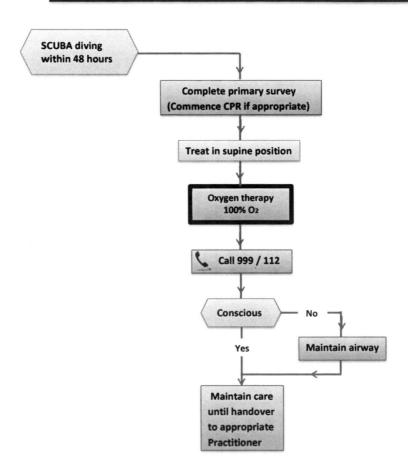

Decompression Illness (DCI)   **CPG.s for EFR**

SCUBA diving within 48 hours

Complete primary survey (Commence CPR if appropriate)

Treat in supine position

Oxygen therapy 100% O₂

Call 999 / 112

Conscious — No — Maintain airway

Yes

Maintain care until handover to appropriate Practitioner

Transport dive computer and diving equipment with patient if possible

Transport is completed at an altitude of < 300 metres above incident site or aircraft pressurised equivalent to sea level

Courtesy of PHECC

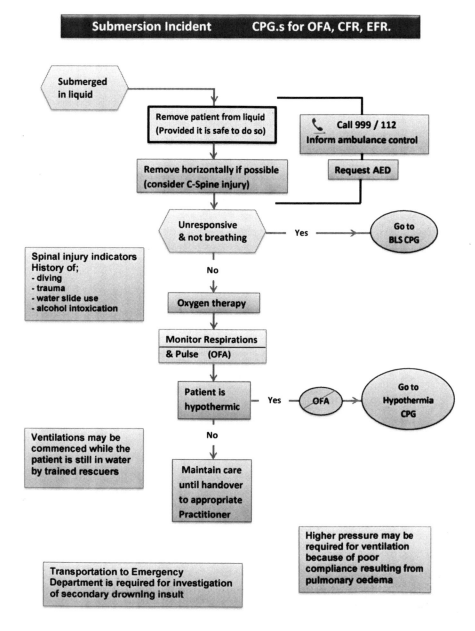

Submersion Incident   CPG.s for OFA, CFR, EFR.

Submerged in liquid

Remove patient from liquid (Provided it is safe to do so)

Call 999 / 112 Inform ambulance control

Remove horizontally if possible (consider C-Spine injury)

Request AED

Unresponsive & not breathing — Yes → Go to BLS CPG

Spinal injury indicators History of;
- diving
- trauma
- water slide use
- alcohol intoxication

No

Oxygen therapy

Monitor Respirations & Pulse (OFA)

Patient is hypothermic — Yes — OFA → Go to Hypothermia CPG

Ventilations may be commenced while the patient is still in water by trained rescuers

No

Maintain care until handover to appropriate Practitioner

Higher pressure may be required for ventilation because of poor compliance resulting from pulmonary oedema

Transportation to Emergency Department is required for investigation of secondary drowning insult

Courtesy of PHECC

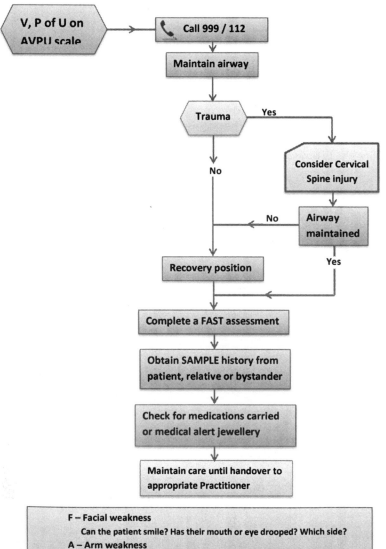

Altered Level of Consciousness - Adult   CPG.s for OFA & EFR

V, P of U on AVPU scale → 📞 Call 999 / 112

Maintain airway

Trauma

→ Yes → Consider Cervical Spine injury

No ↓

Airway maintained

No → (back to main flow)

Yes ↓

Recovery position

Complete a FAST assessment

Obtain SAMPLE history from patient, relative or bystander

Check for medications carried or medical alert jewellery

Maintain care until handover to appropriate Practitioner

F – Facial weakness
    Can the patient smile? Has their mouth or eye drooped? Which side?
A – Arm weakness
    Can the patient raise both arms and maintain for 5 seconds?
S – Speech problems
    Can the patient speak clearly and understand what you say?
T – Time
    Time to call 999/112 now if positive FAST

Courtesy of PHECC

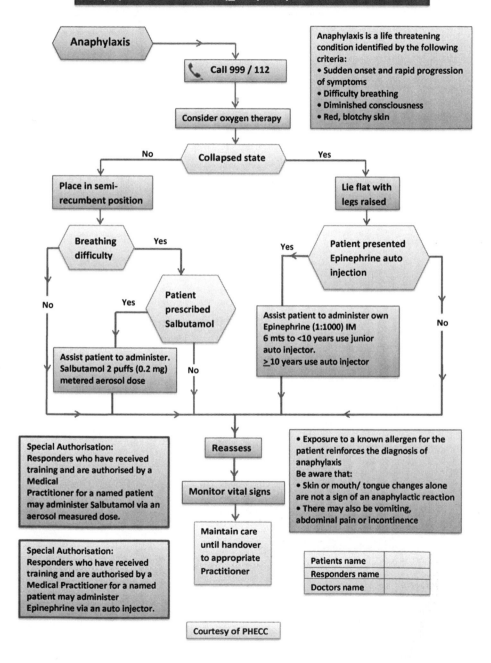

Anaphylaxis – Paediatric (≤ 13 years)   CPG.s for OFA & EFR

Anaphylaxis

Call 999 / 112

Consider oxygen therapy

Anaphylaxis is a life threatening condition identified by the following criteria:
• Sudden onset and rapid progression of symptoms
• Difficulty breathing
• Diminished consciousness
• Red, blotchy skin

Collapsed state   No / Yes

Place in semi-recumbent position

Lie flat with legs raised

Breathing difficulty   Yes / No

Patient presented Epinephrine auto injection   Yes / No

Patient prescribed Salbutamol   Yes / No

Assist patient to administer. Salbutamol 2 puffs (0.2 mg) metered aerosol dose

Assist patient to administer own Epinephrine (1:1000) IM 6 mts to <10 years use junior auto injector.
≥ 10 years use auto injector

Reassess

Monitor vital signs

Maintain care until handover to appropriate Practitioner

Special Authorisation: Responders who have received training and are authorised by a Medical Practitioner for a named patient may administer Salbutamol via an aerosol measured dose.

Special Authorisation: Responders who have received training and are authorised by a Medical Practitioner for a named patient may administer Epinephrine via an auto injector.

• Exposure to a known allergen for the patient reinforces the diagnosis of anaphylaxis
Be aware that:
• Skin or mouth/ tongue changes alone are not a sign of an anaphylactic reaction
• There may also be vomiting, abdominal pain or incontinence

Patients name	
Responders name	
Doctors name	

Courtesy of PHECC

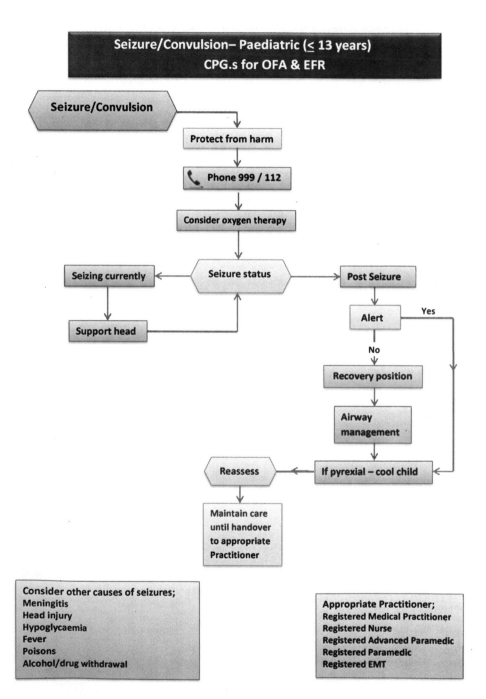

Seizure/Convulsion– Paediatric (≤ 13 years)
CPG.s for OFA & EFR

Seizure/Convulsion

Protect from harm

📞 Phone 999 / 112

Consider oxygen therapy

Seizing currently ← Seizure status → Post Seizure

Support head

Alert — Yes

No

Recovery position

Airway management

Reassess ← If pyrexial – cool child

Maintain care until handover to appropriate Practitioner

Consider other causes of seizures;
Meningitis
Head injury
Hypoglycaemia
Fever
Poisons
Alcohol/drug withdrawal

Appropriate Practitioner;
Registered Medical Practitioner
Registered Nurse
Registered Advanced Paramedic
Registered Paramedic
Registered EMT

Courtesy of PHECC

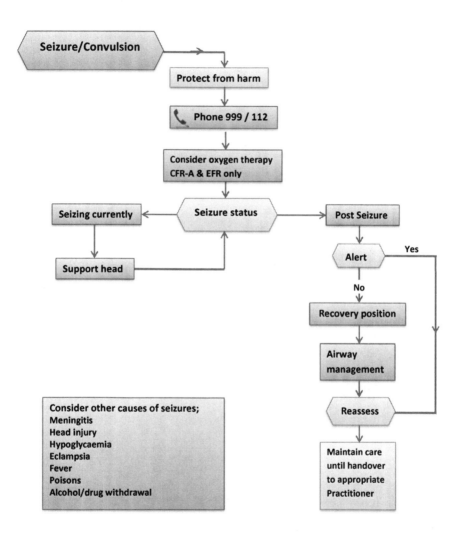

Seizure/Convulsion– Adult   CPG.s for OFA & EFR

Seizure/Convulsion

Protect from harm

Phone 999 / 112

Consider oxygen therapy CFR-A & EFR only

Seizure status

Seizing currently

Support head

Post Seizure

Alert — Yes

No

Recovery position

Airway management

Reassess

Maintain care until handover to appropriate Practitioner

Consider other causes of seizures;
Meningitis
Head injury
Hypoglycaemia
Eclampsia
Fever
Poisons
Alcohol/drug withdrawal

Courtesy of PHECC

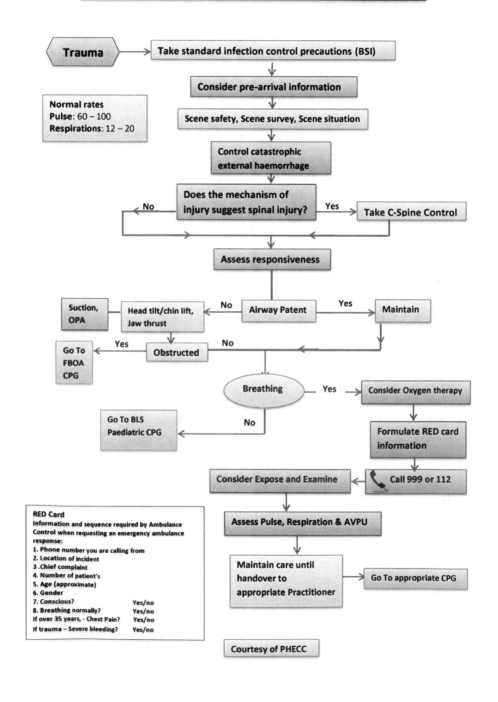

Primary Survey – Paediatric (≤ 13 years)   CPG.s for EFR

Trauma → Take standard infection control precautions (BSI)

↓

Consider pre-arrival information

Normal rates
Pulse: 60 – 100
Respirations: 12 – 20

↓

Scene safety, Scene survey, Scene situation

↓

Control catastrophic external haemorrhage

↓

Does the mechanism of injury suggest spinal injury? — No ← / Yes → Take C-Spine Control

↓

Assess responsiveness

↓

Suction, OPA ← Head tilt/chin lift, Jaw thrust ← No — Airway Patent — Yes → Maintain

Go To FBOA CPG ← Yes — Obstructed — No →

↓

Breathing — Yes → Consider Oxygen therapy

No → Go To BLS Paediatric CPG

↓

Formulate RED card information

↓

Call 999 or 112 → Consider Expose and Examine

↓

Assess Pulse, Respiration & AVPU

↓

Maintain care until handover to appropriate Practitioner → Go To appropriate CPG

RED Card
Information and sequence required by Ambulance Control when requesting an emergency ambulance response:
1. Phone number you are calling from
2. Location of incident
3. Chief complaint
4. Number of patient's
5. Age (approximate)
6. Gender
7. Conscious?   Yes/no
8. Breathing normally?   Yes/no
If over 35 years, - Chest Pain?   Yes/no
If trauma – Severe bleeding?   Yes/no

Courtesy of PHECC

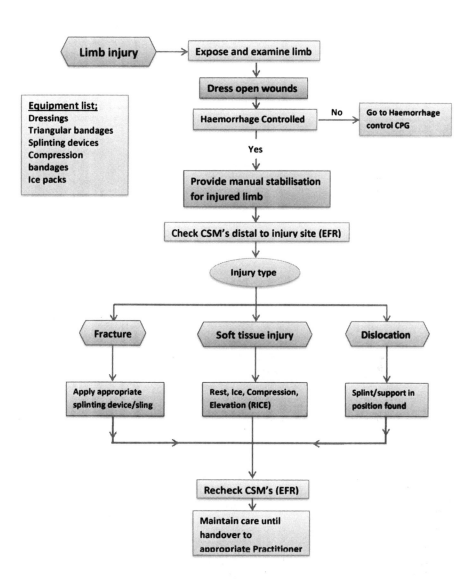

Limb injury   CPG.s for OFA & EFR

Limb injury → Expose and examine limb

Dress open wounds

Equipment list;
Dressings
Triangular bandages
Splinting devices
Compression bandages
Ice packs

Haemorrhage Controlled — No → Go to Haemorrhage control CPG

Yes

Provide manual stabilisation for injured limb

Check CSM's distal to injury site (EFR)

Injury type

Fracture | Soft tissue injury | Dislocation

Apply appropriate splinting device/sling | Rest, Ice, Compression, Elevation (RICE) | Splint/support in position found

Recheck CSM's (EFR)

Maintain care until handover to appropriate Practitioner

Courtesy of PHECC

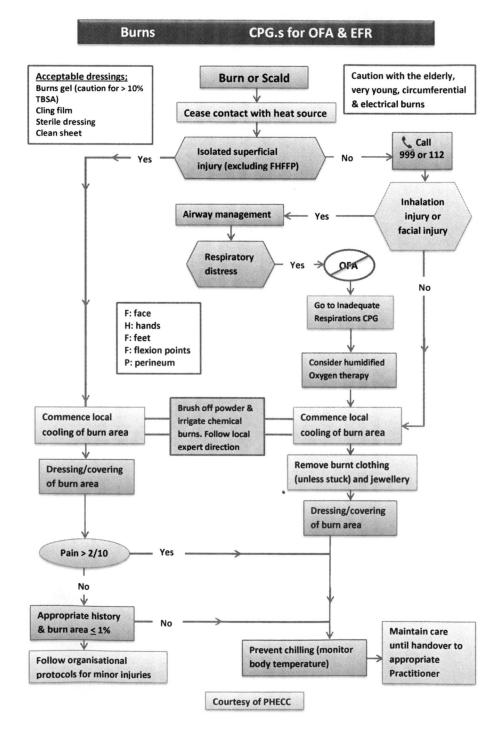

Burns   **CPG.s for OFA & EFR**

Acceptable dressings;
Burns gel (caution for > 10% TBSA)
Cling film
Sterile dressing
Clean sheet

Burn or Scald

Caution with the elderly, very young, circumferential & electrical burns

Cease contact with heat source

Isolated superficial injury (excluding FHFFP) — Yes / No

Call 999 or 112

Inhalation injury or facial injury

Airway management — Yes

Respiratory distress — Yes → OFA

F: face
H: hands
F: feet
F: flexion points
P: perineum

Go to Inadequate Respirations CPG

Consider humidified Oxygen therapy

Commence local cooling of burn area

Brush off powder & irrigate chemical burns. Follow local expert direction

Commence local cooling of burn area

Remove burnt clothing (unless stuck) and jewellery

Dressing/covering of burn area

Dressing/covering of burn area

Pain > 2/10 — Yes

Appropriate history & burn area ≤ 1% — No

Follow organisational protocols for minor injuries

Prevent chilling (monitor body temperature)

Maintain care until handover to appropriate Practitioner

Courtesy of PHECC

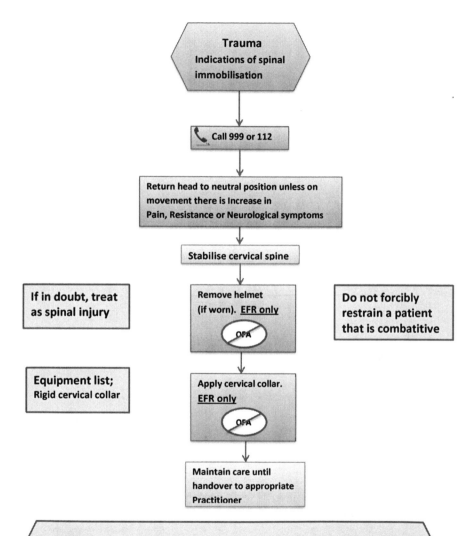

Spinal Immobilisation – Adult   CPG.s for OFA & EFR

Trauma
Indications of spinal immobilisation

Call 999 or 112

Return head to neutral position unless on movement there is Increase in Pain, Resistance or Neurological symptoms

Stabilise cervical spine

If in doubt, treat as spinal injury

Remove helmet (if worn). **EFR only**

OFA

Do not forcibly restrain a patient that is combatitive

Equipment list; Rigid cervical collar

Apply cervical collar. **EFR only**

OFA

Maintain care until handover to appropriate Practitioner

Special Authorisation (EFR):
EFR's may extricate a patient on a long board in the absence of a Practitioner if;
1 an unstable environment prohibits the attendance of a Practitioner, or
2 while awaiting the arrival of a Practitioner the patient requires rapid extrication to initiate emergency care

Courtesy of PHECC

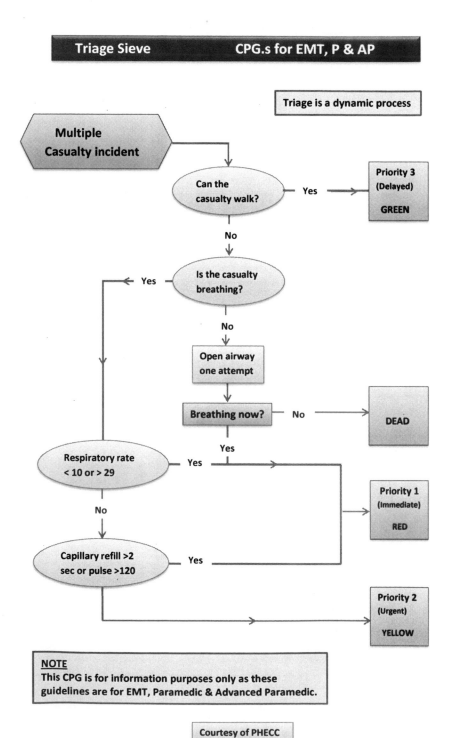

Triage Sieve   CPG.s for EMT, P & AP

Triage is a dynamic process

Multiple Casualty incident

Can the casualty walk? — Yes → Priority 3 (Delayed) GREEN

No

Is the casualty breathing? ← Yes

No

Open airway one attempt

Breathing now? — No → DEAD

Yes

Respiratory rate < 10 or > 29 — Yes →

No

Priority 1 (Immediate) RED

Capillary refill >2 sec or pulse >120 — Yes →

Priority 2 (Urgent) YELLOW

NOTE
This CPG is for information purposes only as these guidelines are for EMT, Paramedic & Advanced Paramedic.

Courtesy of PHECC

15.3. List of Abbreviations and Acronyms

ABC	Airway, breathing, circulation
AcBC	Airway, C-spine breathing, circulation
ABCDE	Airway, breathing, circulation, disability, expose, and examine
AKA	Also known as
ARDS	Adult respiratory distress syndrome
ARF	Acute renal failure
AED	Automated external defibrillator
ALS	Advanced life support
AVPU	Alert, voice, pain, unresponsive
ALOC	Altered level of consciousness
BSI	Body substance isolation
BCLOC	Breathing circulation and level of consciousness
BPM	Breaths per minute
CAB	Compressions, airway breathing
CSM	Circulation sensation and movement
CSF	Cerebrospinal fluid
CPR	Cardio pulmonary resuscitation
CPGs	Clinical practice guidelines
CO2	Carbon dioxide
DOA	Dead on arrival
EMS	Emergency medical services
EFR	Emergency first responder
FAST	Face, arm, speech, time
FBAO	Foreign body airway obstruction
GTN	Glycerol trinitrate
HIV	Human immunodeficiency virus
ICP	Increased intracranial pressure
MCSM	Modified circulation sensation and movement
MI	Myocardial infarction (heart attack)
MSDS	Medical safety data sheet
mg	Milligram
ml	Millilitre
MOI	Mechanism of injury
O2	Oxygen
OPA	Oropharyngeal airway
PAT	Paediatric assessment triangle

PEEP	Posture, elevation, examination, and pad and bandage
PPE	Personal protection equipment
RICE	Rest, ice, compress, elevate
START	Simple triage and rapid treatment
SPLINTS	Swelling, pain, loss of movement, irregularity, numbness, tenderness, shock
SBAR	Situation, background, assessment, recommendation
SOP	Standard operating procedure
SAMPLE	Signs and symptoms, allergies, medication, previous history, last intake, event
TB	Tuberculosis
TBSA	Total body surface area

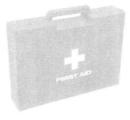

INDEX